Anxiety
Management Training

A Behavior Therapy

THE PLENUM BEHAVIOR THERAPY SERIES
Series Editor: Nathan H. Azrin

ANXIETY MANAGEMENT TRAINING
A Behavior Therapy
By Richard M. Suinn

BEHAVIORAL TREATMENT OF ALCOHOL PROBLEMS
Individualized Therapy and Controlled Drinking
By Mark B. Sobell and Linda C. Sobell

COGNITIVE-BEHAVIOR MODIFICATION
An Integrative Approach
By Donald H. Meichenbaum

PHOBIC AND OBSESSIVE-COMPULSIVE DISORDERS
Theory, Research, and Practice
By Paul M. G. Emmelkamp

THE TOKEN ECONOMY
A Review and Evaluation
By Alan E. Kazdin

Anxiety Management Training

A Behavior Therapy

Richard M. Suinn

Colorado State University
Fort Collins, Colorado

Plenum Press • New York and London

Library of Congress Cataloging-in-Publication Data

Suinn, Richard M.
    Anxiety management training : a behavior therapy / Richard M.
Suinn.
        p.   cm. -- (Plenum behavior therapy series)
    Includes bibliographical references and index.
    ISBN 0-306-43545-4
    1. Anxiety--Treatment. 2. Behavior therapy.   I. Title.
II. Series.
RC531.S85 1990
616.85'223--dc20   90-42069
                                                                   CIP

ISBN 0-306-43545-4

© 1990 Plenum Press, New York
A Division of Plenum Publishing Corporation
233 Spring Street, New York, N.Y. 10013

Printed in the United States of America

1

Anxiety and Stress

- "My life just seems to be one pressure point after another. . . my days are like tightropes, stretched really thin. . . "
- "I'm restless, my head goes a mile a minute, I'm always worrying. . . something I've done, something I should do. . . something I didn't do. . . "
- "Sleeping in the night is hard. . . I lay awake and can't sleep. . . then I toss and turn all night on waves, up and down, in and out of sleep. . . and in the day, I'm constantly fatigued. . . "
- "No, I'm fine. . . just constantly fatigued. . . "
- "I get so uptight about things. . . sometimes it's little things, sometimes it's a booming big one, but I can't let go of being uptight, strung out. . . "
- "My job brings pressure. . . by the very nature. . . it's the due dates for reports, and the environment is demanding, and I'm expecting a lot of myself, and I want to look good all the time. . . I bring my work home. . . seems like my whole life has this one focus. . . "
- "I really want to be a good parent. . . but I don't have any experience. . . and I'm just not confident in myself. . . so I constantly evaluate what I'm doing. . . is it enough, am I not being myself, what does that mean. . . "
- "School's O.K. If my folks would only leave me alone. I feel they're constantly looking over my shoulder, judging me, expecting me to meet their standard. . . it's no wonder I can't concentrate on school work. . . "
- "I'm all right mostly. . . except sometimes I have these attacks. . . my heart beats so fast it feels like it's going to stop. . . can't breathe, I think I'm going to suffocate. . . waves of something dreadful going to come down on me. . . then I can't breathe, and I know I'm going to die. . . and I'm frightened so much you can't know how this feels. . . "
- "I'm frightened of being outside, I just feel safer in my own home where there's just myself. . . I can't even look out the front door, it's indescribable how overwhelming it all is. . . when outside, I wanted to creep along a sturdy wall, but more, to run home. . . "
- "I'm quite normal, calm, in control, organized. . . until I see a dog, and then I'm out of control, I know it's harmless, but I choke in my throat, my knees go weak, I feel helpless and in danger. . . "

The Prevalence of Anxiety and Stress: Epidemiology

The existence of stress and the presence of anxiety appears now to be one of the expected conditions of modern life. Stress and the negative consequences of stress are now recognized by industries and businesses to the degree that stress management programs, especially for executives and managers, have been developed. Although executive fitness programs were mainly associated with the value of physical health and vitality, more and more research is now promoting physical exercise as a means of coping with anxiety and tensions. But we can also note other evidence of the degree to which stress has become an ever-increasing problem. One such confirmation can be found by examining the case load of physicians. Although physicians are the professionals seen by persons in need of help for physical complaints, currently physicians are also the source to whom persons go for mental health complaints (Goldberg, Steele, Johnson, & Smith, 1982; Orleans, George, Houpt, & Brodie, 1985). It is quite revealing therefore that one study of local physicians discovered the most common reasons for a medical visit were for a physical checkup, or for hypertension, pharyngitis, or tonsillitis, or cuts and bruises. However, following quite close behind these reasons was the complaint of "anxiety." And not only was anxiety ranked extremely high, but this complaint as a cause for seeing a physician was more frequent a reason than bad colds or bronchitis (Marsland, Wood, & Mayo, 1976).

Indeed, at one point, the National Institute of Health recognized the need for primary care physicians to receive training in mental health since so many mental health complaints were coming directly to them. Cragan and Deffenbacher (1984) sent out letters to patients in a family practice clinic, offering a program for coping with stress and anxiety. Over 100 persons responded in search of help! These persons ranged in terms of occupations from accountants to secretaries, engineers, factory workers, professors, and construction workers. Interestingly enough, when asked about their major symptoms of stress, these persons listed symptoms that were mainly physical in nature. The most frequent stress symptom was tension in the neck and shoulder region (21.8%), followed by headaches (14.5%), then stomach complaints (13.6%), general tremors and shakiness (10.9%), and, finally, insomnia (6.4%). Epidemiological estimates are that approximately 8.3% of the population, or about 13.1 million people in the United States, suffer from an anxiety disorder (Wilson, 1988). The economic impact is reflected in the annual cost of treating panic and agoraphobic disorders alone, an amount estimated to be between $4.1 and $20 billion.

Another signal of the extreme prevalence of anxiety conditions are

the data on disorders where anxiety is considered a crucial causative factor. Twenty-five million Americans suffer from hypertension; headaches compose the 14th most common symptom in medical general practices (with 80% of these due to tension headaches), and eight million persons have ulcers. At one point, five billion doses of tranquilizers and an equal number of barbiturates have been prescribed each year in the United States (Charlesworth & Nathan, 1981). There are an estimated 12 million who are involved in alcohol abuse. Over $15.5 billion is estimated to be lost by American industries as a result of alcoholism. Of relevance is the fact that alcohol abusers are often using alcohol to attempt to manage their anxieties. Cox, Norton, Dorward, and Fergusson (in press) reported that over 80% of a group of inpatient alcoholic abusers relied upon alcohol as a means of dealing with panic attacks. Chambless, Cherney, Caputo, and Rheinstein (1987) actually found that as many as 40% of another group of inpatient alcohol abusers had also experienced one or more problems which would have been diagnosed as anxiety disorder. Social phobias also seemed common, but studies also discovered the presence of severe agoraphobia among alcohol abusers (Mullaney & Trippett, 1979; Smail, Stockwell, Canter, & Hodgson, 1984). Although previously coronary heart disease had not usually been considered as directly caused by stress, currently stress and arousal have been indirectly implicated through studies of the Type A behavioral pattern. Approximately one-half million Americans die from heart disease annually. About one-fourth of these deaths occur in persons under the age of 65. In effect, cardiovascular disease represents the largest single cause of premature mortality in the United States. As we shall see in a later chapter, cardiovascular disease appears linked not only to heredity, smoking, obesity, diet, lack of exercise, and other risk factors. In addition, showing Type A characteristics seems to be a risk factor (Friedman & Rosenman, 1974; Dembroski, Weiss, Shields, Haynes, & Feinleib, 1978). The Type A pattern includes a "person who is aggressively involved in a chronic, incessant struggle to achieve more and more in less and less time" (Friedman & Rosenman, 1974, p. 67).

If we look at the occurrence of conditions which are directly diagnosed as anxiety disorders, the evidence is even clearer regarding the prevalence of anxiety states. Agras, Sylvester, and Oliveau (1969) surveyed household members living in Burlington, Vermont through direct interviews about their fears. A surprisingly high number, nearly 50% of the sample of 325 persons, acknowledged possessing mild fears, such as of snakes, storms, heights. On the whole, defining phobias as intense fears, the prevalence of phobic disorder in the population was estimated as 7.7%. An additional striking finding was that phobias tended to remain with the affected individual for very long periods. If untreated, an

individual was likely to remain fearful, to at least a mild degree, for a lifetime.

A similar epidemiological interview was conducted by Costello (1982) of 449 women from 10 communities in Calgary, Alberta, Canada. All subjects had been selected at random from five communities representing the "bottom extreme" and from five communities representing the middle level of socioeconomic status (p. 280). All women were interviewed in their homes regarding life events and experiences for the 12 months prior to the interview. Only 16% of the women refused to be interviewed. Results showed that only 26% were completely free of fears, while 23% reported intense levels of fears. In contrast, 19% of the women revealed that the level of intensity was so high as to cause them to resort to avoidance behaviors. The most common phobias for the American sample of men and women included fear of snakes, fear of injury or illness, fear of heights, and fear of either open or closed spaces. For the Canadian women, the most common fears were of animals, heights, closed spaces, and people.

Both studies also traced the prevalence of fears as a function of age. In the American sample, a "mountain peak"-shaped profile appeared— a rising in numbers of phobias from childhood to about middle age, followed by a fairly precipitous decline to age 70 years. The Canadian study covered an older sample, with the range of ages of respondents being from 18 to 65 years. Hence, this research missed those childhood years when fears appear to be at their highest incidence in the Agras *et al.* (1969) report. The Canadian results showed an initial decline between the ages of 18 and 35; but the information for the next ages varied according to whether avoidance behaviors were associated with the fear. For both mild fears without avoidance, and intense fears without avoidance, there was a sharp rise in prevalence during ages 36–45, followed by a decline for the succeeding years. On the other hand, mild and intense fears associated with avoidance behaviors generally followed the early years' trend for a continued decline across the life span.

Among the phobic disorders receiving increasing attention from both researchers and practitioners today is agoraphobia. There is a suggestion that what was once a fairly uncommon disorder is now rapidly on the rise. Agras *et al.* (1969) reported a prevalence rate of about 0.6%. By 1980 the frequency of agoraphobia had dramatically increased. The Epidemiologic Catchment Area (ECA) study of the National Institute of Mental Health covered five geographic study areas, including New Haven, Connecticut, Baltimore, Maryland, and St. Louis, Missouri (Myers, Weissman, Tischler, Holzer III, Orvaschel, Anthony, Boyd, Burke Jr., Kramer, & Stoltzman, 1984). Direct interviews were conducted on up to 5,000 persons within each location, although an overall survey covered approximately 300,000 persons in each geographic target area. In the

initial analysis, the prevalence of agoraphobia was now found to be clearly higher than in the Agras survey, ranging from about 2.7% to as high as 5.8%.

Costello's Canadian study did not directly isolate agoraphobia, but the category of separation fears was interpreted as "subclinical forms of agoraphobia," since it was defined as involving "fears of being alone, traveling, and being in crowds." In this 1982 report, separation fears were found occurring in 13.2% of the women. This points out another interesting and unusual finding, that is, that agoraphobia appears to be epidemiologically gender-related. The ECA research discovered that nearly 75% of the agoraphobic complaints were from women, while Burns and Thorpe (1977) similarly discovered that 88% of their agora-phobic subjects in a national survey were women! The explanation for this is still quite open to speculation. Psychological explanations include the hypothesis that men shift to substance abuse as their means of coping with panic, while women rely upon the avoidance behaviors that is a central criterion for diagnosis of agoraphobia. A psychodynamically ori-ented hypothesis would postulate stronger attachment of female young-sters to the same-sexed primary nurturing parent, and a greater anxiety about separation. A tentative finding did discover that more women agoraphobic outpatients experienced childhood separation anxiety than men agoraphobic patients (Gittelman & Klein, 1985). Furthermore, more women agoraphobic patients fit the category of never being sepa-rated, to go to camp, to socialize outside the immediate family, etc. Such signs of tight attachment bonding occurred in childhood, but espe-cially in adolescence, and may again be reflective of a source of separa-tion fears. A final hypothesis derives from cultural assumptions. Possibly it is more acceptable for women to be honest about and to act upon their fears than it is for men in our society. Similarly, men in the sample may have been those who felt compelled to deny reporting that they were subject to avoidance behaviors, and hence not in control of their lives.

Generalized anxiety disorder, unlike agoraphobia, has long been recognized as a significant psychiatric disorder deserving major atten-tion. Estimates of the occurrence of generalized anxiety disorder range from about 2% to 6.4% of the population in the United States and in Great Britain (Marks & Lader, 1973; Weissman, 1983). A large-scale survey, initially focused on psychotherapeutic drug usage, also collected information on over 3,000 persons regarding anxiety states (Uhlenhuth, Baltzer, Mellinger, Cisin, & Clinthorne, 1983). The researchers con-cluded that generalized anxiety disorder was clearly the most common anxiety disorder, followed by phobias other than agoraphobia, then agoraphobia. This is consistent with a more limited survey of New Haven residents, which also found generalized anxiety disorder to be the most prevalent of the anxiety disorders, more common than phobias

(which were the next most common condition) (Weissman, Myers, & Harding, 1978). Such information has led Cerny, Himadi, and Barlow to consider generalized anxiety disorder to be the "most commonly reported anxiety disorder," and of utmost concern considering that "Anxiety disorders represent the single largest mental health problem in the country, far outstripping depression. . . " (Barlow, p. 22). Although no genetic hypotheses have yet been postulated, it is interesting to note that there is a tendency for relatives of persons with an anxiety disorder to demonstrate similar complaints (Carey & Gottesman, 1981). Thus the rate of anxiety disorder among first degree relatives of anxiety disorders patients has been found in several studies to range in frequency from 14.9 per 100 to 18.4 per 100.

Another anxiety disorder which falls into the category of a serious mental health problem is panic disorder. Until recently, the separate importance of panic disorder was not recognized; instead, it was classified as part of generalized anxiety disorder. A complicating factor is the tendency for panic experiences also to appear in the lives of patients whose primary diagnosis is generalized anxiety disorder or some other psychiatric disorder. Furthermore, persons suffering from panic disorder also seem to be subject to the simultaneous presence of other psychiatric complaints. Barlow, Vermilyea, Vermilyea, and Di Nardo (1984) compared the panic symptoms found in panic disorder patients against panic symptoms reported by patients with other psychiatric diagnoses. There were 74 patients who had met the DSM-III criteria for panic disorder. Among the other diagnostic classifications were obsessive compulsive, generalized anxiety, simple phobic, social phobic, agoraphobic, and major depressive disorder. An amazing 83% of patients with a diagnosis other than panic disorder reported the symptom of at least one panic attack. Six patients who were experiencing symptoms of panic eventually received a consensus diagnosis instead of major depression. Other studies across the world support Barlow *et al.*'s finding that panic attack symptoms can occur with high frequency among patients with psychiatric diagnoses other than panic disorders, such as schizophrenia, antisocial personality, alcohol or substance abuse. For instance panic attacks were found in as many as 62% of schizophrenics, 42% of patients suffering from major depressive disorder, 35% of obsessive–compulsives, 30% of those diagnosed as antisocial personality, 17% of substance or alcohol abuse patients, and 50% of patients diagnosed as manic (Boyd, 1986). Perley and Guze (1962) reported that 64% percent of patients diagnosed as hysterics also experienced panic attacks, and Leckman, Weissman, Merikangas, Pauls, and Prusoff (1983) found that nearly 25% of a group of 133 patients diagnosed as suffering from major depression also met the criteria for panic disorder or agoraphobia with panic. In addition, 40% of cardiology patients examined by Beit-

man, DeRosear, Basha, Flaker, and Corcoran (1987) also were observed to experience severe panic attacks.

All such data suggest that obtaining an accurate estimate of the true prevalence of panic disorder may be difficult. This difficulty is due to the possibility that patients whose primary diagnosis should be panic disorder might actually be misdiagnosed with a different psychiatric classification. Furthermore, patients whose primary diagnosis should be other than panic disorder might actually be misdiagnosed as panic disorder since panic attacks seem to appear among patients other than panic disorder patients. More than likely, the prevalence estimates are low and on the conservative side. The Epidemiologic Catchment Area survey found a range of from 0.3% for males in New Haven to 1.2% of females in Baltimore with panic disorder; the overall rates for both gender ranging from 0.6% to 1.0%. These 1984 data are higher than the 0.4% prevalence rate found by the 1976 New Haven, Connecticut study of Weissman, Myers, and Harding, and again suggest a growing increase of anxiety states among the population.

Although there are very few epidemiological studies of children, a review of seven community surveys led Orvaschel and Weissman (in press) to conclude that anxiety symptoms of all types were quite prevalent for all age children of both sexes. For the category of "fears and worries," the percent of children reporting these symptoms ranged from 4% in Denmark as the lowest to 43% in the United States and Japan as the highest. For separation anxiety, only two reports were cited, with 13.7% of the children in Denmark and 41% of the children surveyed in the United States showing this form of distress. For general tensions or other symptoms of tension, such as nightmares, the Denmark community reported a prevalence rate of 8%, while a U.S. study found a prevalence rate of 18% (Weissman, 1985). Anxiety symptoms appeared to be more commonly reported among girls than among boys, although there was high variation of this gender association, depending upon age and the specific type of anxiety. Anxiety symptoms also seemed more prevalent among black than white children and in lower than higher socioeconomic class children.

Cross-Cultural Prevalence of Anxiety and Fears: Epidemiology

The case of a 32-year-old Chinese man is reported as showing the following clinical history:

> "A 32-year-old single cook from central China sought psychiatric help for complaints of panic attacks and somatic symptoms

including palpitations, breathlessness, dizziness, and numbness of his limbs. For several months he had visited herb doctors who diagnosed his disease as a 'deficiency in vitality' and prescribed the drinking of boys' urine and eating of human placenta to supply energy and blood. . . .

"He had his first attack of somatic syptoms at age 32, consisting of breathlessness, palpitations, dizziness, nausea, etc. . . after intercourse, at which time he often found his penis shrinking into his abdomen. . . he would become very anxious and hold onto his penis in terror, experiencing severe vertigo, palpitations, and fainting spells. . . .

"He made frequent trips to the clinic, in a state of panic, and described his symptoms in an exaggerated manner: 'hands tremble, anguish in the abdomen, penis withdrawing, heart pounds kag-kag, kasu-kasu, I am scared. . . my body trembles at night, it moves, blood does not come up, my body stops moving, my lung gets hot and my head too, my mouth will dry up so that I drink a cup of tea and then I have to urinate. . . I cannot breathe at night, my heart pounds; my head aches if I talk too much, my heart sounds kok, kok-kok, my head sounds zuzu-zuzu.'" (Rubin, 1982, pp. 161–162)

The question of the universality of anxiety states is dramatically illustrated by this case history. Although it has the quality of being a complaint colored by a culturally unique focus of fear (penis loss), certainly the experience of panic, the narrow phobic concern, the physiological reaction, and the insomnia all call attention to the state of anxiety being described. In general, there is a scarcity of information on the prevalence of anxiety around the world that would permit speculating on whether this disorder is simply a product of civilization. It is true that reports on the Aborigines conclude that anxiety is absent. Among the Australians are Aboriginals who are considered to be tied for the rank of being the most primitive and least advanced techological race (along with the Bushmen of Kalahari). These Australian Aborigines have no permanent dwellings, no pottery, no domestic animals or crops. About 10,500 remain in existence, scattered among 11 mission towns and six government towns in northern Australia. A survey under the supervision of the Flying Doctor Service was established in 1971 on a regular basis to provide psychiatric services and to conduct epidemiological study of psychological disorders. Field teams monitored the presence of psychiatric disorders, with these teams being composed of a psychiatrist, a Caucasian nurse from the nearest town, and one or two Aboriginal aides. The conclusion by Eastwell (1982), the psychiatrist in the study, was that free-floating anxiety was almost nonexistent among the true Aborigines. Only 10 patients showed symptoms of anxiety, and five of these were

I

THE NATURE AND
PRESENCE OF ANXIETY
AND STRESSORS

Contents

simultaneously suffering from life threatening disease such as cancer, and hence might be expected to experience anxieties. The remaining five were all considered to have been "acculturated" and therefore now tainted by the influence of civilization. Kidson and Jones (1968) also concluded that anxiety states were absent in their study of a population of over 400 Western Australian Aborigines. Despite a strong statement by Yap of disbelief in such data, other investigations also failed to uncover any major presence of anxiety (Cawte, 1972; Morice, 1978).

One popular interpretation of this low or nonexistent prevalence is that real anxieties are sublimated into a culturally accepted specific target, such as sorcery. According to Eastwell, "The first illness common to the Aboriginals, and the most dramatic, is an anxiety state with paranoid features magnified to psychotic proportions. The patient fears imminent death from sorcery, and the severity of concurrent autonomic signs is a noteworthy feature. Sorcery is part of the psychological reality of the people" (p. 233). In other words, free-floating anxiety becomes displaced to a specific fear stimulus, sorcery. It is also possible that anxiety fails to appear as free-floating because of displacement to other symptoms, such as somatic complaints. Jones and Horne (1973) refer to both the fear of sorcery as well as the somatic expression of anxiety in their comments, ". . . Aborigines are afraid, as they often are of spirits, the dark, witchcraft, strangers and so on. This fear is short-lived and goes when the cause is removed. No intractable symptoms of 'overt anxiety' without a culturally appropriate cause were found. . . hypochondriacal symptoms. . . certainly do exist and may be the Aborigine equivalent of anxiety" (p. 224). Other reasons for the low presence of free-floating anxiety include the general permissiveness and lack of pressure of the people. There is great warmth and extreme permissiveness shown by the mothers, a nearly nonexistent drive for achievement, little sense of penalty for failure, and an acceptance of the realistic limitations to aspirations. Furthermore, there appears a strong social support system provided by kinfolk "who are auxiliary egos. . . who share his conficts" (Eastwell, p. 241).

On the other hand, with the exception of these Aborigines, anxiety disorders do seem to be a shared phenomenon across the world. Good and Kleinman reviewed surveys conducted in urban and in rural environments including villages and small communities. They concluded that anxiety disorders appear at the rate of from 12 to 27 cases per thousand people. For instance, Norwegians showed a rate of 11 cases per thousand for anxiety neurosis; Indians showed rates of 12.0 per thousand; and Iranians had a rate of 71 per thousand in villages for anxiety neurosis (Bash & Bash-Liechti, 1969, 1974; Bremer, 1951; Murphy, 1982). Weissman (1985) summarized the rates from nine community surveys for anxiety states (Table 1.1), finding a range from 5 per thousand in Finland to 54 per thousand in Zurich.

As stated earlier, it is also likely that the way in which anxiety is displayed in other cultures is shaped by the beliefs, taboos, and cultural idioms of that group. Such anxieties of these other societies may well be channeled into culturally relevant forms, instead of appearing as free-floating anxiety. Examples of such forms are readily seen in the various versions of fearfulness:

Koro or *shook yang* in Southeast Asia, involves the fear of disappearance of one's genitals. It seems to be most prevalent among southern Chinese, and is diagnosed through the presence of three elements: delusions that the penis is withdrawing, along with a fear of death; intense panic; and secondary complications resulting from the patient's attempts to physically prevent his penis from disappearing (for instance, by binding the genital organ to a rod). The origins of the term are unknown, but speculation has it that it either came from the Malay term meaning "to shrink" or the Japanese word meaning "tortoise." Associated with these primary symptoms are other characteristics, such as palpitations, sweating, nausea, visual blurring, pain, physical spasms, burning sensation, and loss of breath (Levin & Bilu, 1980). The case cited earlier in this section is an illustration of *koro*. Another illustration is the eight-year-old boy who had been bitten on the penis by an insect. Upon being examined by a friend, it was noticed that the penis seemed to be withdrawing. The friend became alarmed, and tied the boy's penis with a string, bruising it, but to prevent further withdrawal. The apparent shrinking continued, leading to the use of medicinal balm, and the clamping of the

Table 1.1. Community Surveys of Anxiety States: Rates per 1000[a]

Locale (Year) (Author)	Sample size	Prevalence		
		Male	Female	Total
Canada (1952) (Murphy)	1,010	—	—	29
France (1976) (Brunetti)	101	—	—	39
United Kingdom (1977) (Brown et al.)	612	—	15	—
Zurich (1982) (Angst & Dobler-Mikola)	591	40	68	54
Norway (1951) (Bremer)	Entire community	5	12	—
Denmark (1951) (Fremming)	3,467	3	1	—
Sweden (1956) (Essen-Moller et al.)	2,550	13	34	—
Sweden (1966) (Hagnell)	2,658	15	38	—
Finland (1976) (Väisänen)	1,000	—	—	5

[a]From "The epidemiology of anxiety disorders: Rates, risks, and family patterns" by M. Weissman, 1985, in A. Tuma and J. Maser (Eds.), *Anxiety and the anxiety disorders*. Hillsdale, NJ: Erlbaum. Copyright 1985 by Lawrence Erlbaum. Adapted by permission.

penis with chopsticks. This still did not prevent the retraction, and so the child was taken to the hospital. With reassurances from the physician that nothing was wrong, the boy recovered completely (Rubin, 1982).

Latah in Siberia and Malaysia has been attributed to an acute fright which then leads to several symptoms which characterize this disorder. Typical symptoms include high suggestibility, seizures, and acute startle reflexes (Kenny, 1983). When startled, the patient may exhibit an imitating of sounds or behaviors of other persons, or become susceptible to commands. Echolalia and echopraxia appear to be common. In one case, the patient would copy someone who was pretending to drink, by actually drinking to the point of oversatiation and vomiting. This same patient would also imitate a person writing on his skin, but using a cigarette instead of a pen. Another case involved a woman who would croak in imitation of a frog, and who could be induced to disrobe (Aberle, 1952). The most common feature of *latah* is the triggering off of symptoms when the patient is startled by something or someone. This might occur as a result of a sudden loud noise, an unexpected command, or an unanticipated appearance of an animal. The behaviors triggered by the startle includes the imitating, or automatic obedience to even ridiculous commands, or bizarre self-determined actions such as reciting obscene phrases about sexual organs, barking, or attacking pieces of yarn. The religious sect known as the Holy Rollers has been considered by some as involving latah-like actions, for instance the rolling on the ground caused by a sudden sound. In some cases, the etiological event is narrowed to specific experiences. For example, the Ainus of Japan possess a fear of snakes; hence *latah* tends to originate when a person has a frightening experience involving a snake.

Shinkeishitsu in Japan involving a clinical subcategory with anxiety symptoms. *Shinkeishitsu* is roughly translated as neurasthenia, and divided into three subcategories: a neurasthenic condition with hypochondriacal signs; an obsessional-phobic condition involving a fear of being found objectionable because of personal defects; and a condition which involves tension, palpitations, and vomiting similar to a panic attack (Prince, 1987; Reynolds, 1976). An example of this disorder is the patient who restricted himself to his home, was totally withdrawn from company because he believed that he possessed a body odor that would drive others away. He was extremely shy and hypersensitive, would not look others in the eye during conversations, and sat across the room in the most isolated corner. *Shinkeishitsu* is one of the rare cultural disorders for which a specific theory was developed to explain its origins, as well as for which a specific therapy was designed. The disorder is believed to be a neurosis due to a weakness in the nervous system and exhaustion, combined with perfectionistic tendencies and self-consciousness. When an unpleasant event occurs, the patient reacts physiologically (e.g., through blushing), becomes overly sensitive to his or her reaction, obsesses, and becomes more and more withdrawn to avoid embarrassment. The therapy, called Morita Therapy, isolates the patients from social interactions, while assigning activities which focus on nature, such as gardening. The patient is brought to realize that one is not responsible for one's feelings or thoughts, but only for one's actions. Eventually the shame and obsessions are replaced.

Shenjing shuairuo in China and Taiwan involves neurasthenia, anxiety, sleep difficulties, palpitations, stomach complaints, and an "embittered spirit" from feeling oppressed by work or study. Mao Zedong, the past political leader of the People's Republic of China, confessed suffering from neurasthenia at one time (Terrill, 1980). Shenjing shuairuo has been linked to tensional origins, such as high frequency of occupational stress and family conflicts. Consistent with Chinese patterns of mental distress, shinjing shuairuo tends to appear with dominantly somatic complaints, such as dizziness, feeling of swelling in the neck, poor appetite, stomach problems, tingling in the head. There may also be a diminished sense of vital energy, or an excess of hot inner energy, or a fear of excessive loss of semen (Kleinman, 1986). A case illustration is the "Thirty-five-year-old female physician who works in a local factory clinic. . . to heed the Cultural Revolution's call to serve the people. . . Within a year she felt that she had made a mistake and at the same time began to experience headaches, palpitations, insomnia, and agitation. . . she was criticized. . . by her unit leaders for not accepting enough responsibility for her work. . . For the past two months, she has felt a lack of energy. . . poor memory. . . marked restlessness. . . " (Kleinman, 1982, p. 166).

Narahati-e qalb in Iran involves heart palpitations with some patients showing anxiety symptomatology. This "heart distress" is often tied with anger and tensions related to a sense of shame at loss of control over hostility. The physical complaints emphasize concerns over the heart, such as palpitations, pressure in the chest, or a feeling that the heart is being squeezed. When appearing among women, issues might also include conflicts over female sexuality, childbirth and pregnancy, and fertility. Where the focus is loss of control and angry outbursts, the patient may have good insight into the distress which such hostile feelings are causing. An illustration is the male patient who became angry at his spouse and children, shouted at them, and struck his wife. In seeing a physician, he initially complained about feeling pressure on his heart and severe shaking: I was "real nervous. . . (because I) just got angry, when I started shaking (and shouting)" (Good, Good, & Moradi, 1985, p. 400). A factor analysis of narahati-e qalb symptoms among Iranian patients showed a cluster of symptoms which included anxiety, irritability, obsessional ruminations, shortness of breath, numbness, and tingling.

Susto in Latin American cultures involves complaints believed caused by a past trauma or frightening experience. It has been classified as a type of fear reaction, and translated as magical fright or soul loss. When a person is traumatized by an incident, such as witnessing an accident, it is believed that the soul leaves the person's body. The result is that the individual is left anxious, frightened, and weak. Associated symptoms may include anorexia, insomnia, catatonia, painful sensations, and even hallucinations (Comas-Diaz & Griffith, 1988). *Susto* and certain other disorders are considered as sicknesses deriving from a natural response to an event that is a work of God, and is called *males naturales*. On the other hand, a *mal artificial* is a disorder that is willfully caused by another person, rather than being a natural event. In effect, the *mal artificial* is a work of the devil, such as *mal puesto* (sorcery to cause an illness; a hex).

An illustration of *susto* is the seventeen year old Mexican-American woman who had awakened in the middle of the night seeing what she thought was a witch, in the body of a large bird with enormous claws. She started to talk to herself, ignored her friends, and lost interest in her work. Periods of depression alternated with moments of heightened agitation and expressions of fright. She would not talk about her dreamlike experience, but only alluded to having lost her soul to a demon, who "was a jealous neighbor." In seeing a *cuarandera* (a folk therapist), the initial diagnosis was of a *mal puesto* and rituals and herb medicines were prescribed. Later, she was considered to have been visited by a witch from another neighborhood as a result of bad feelings over a boyfriend. The appearance of the witch in a dream was so frightening as to lead to a temporary departure of the woman's soul, which was then hidden away by the witch.

In conclusion, the data appear to confirm the constant and perhaps increasing presence of anxiety states not only in other countries, but especially within the United States. In some cases, such as in the mild fears without avoidance behaviors, the distress may not lead to seeking of psychological help. However, the person's quality of life is definitely impaired. In other cases, such as generalized anxiety disorder and panic disorder, the patient's everyday functioning can be seriously impaired to the degree that psychological treatment, medication, or even hospitalization may be essential.

Contributions to Stress and Anxiety

Major questions involve where does stress and anxiety originate and what contributes to the development of tensional states in individuals? As a broad perspective, at least three major factors can be identified:

cultural, biological, and psychological. These three must always be examined in any attempt to fully understand any single client's circumstances. The next sections will cover these three potential sources of stress and anxiety.

Cultural

In the prior section, the role of cultural beliefs and orientations was pointed out as producing differences in the expression of anxiety, such that each society adds its own distinctive flavor to the characteristic patterns of anxiety (Marsella, 1980). Spiro has offered what is perhaps the best summary of the influence which culture plays on stress and anxiety and the consequences:

> It is my guess. . . that each culture creates stresses and strains—some of them universal, some unique—with which the personality must cope; that the cultural heritage provides, to a greater or lesser degree, institutional techniques for their reduction, if not resolution; that the incidence of psychopathology in any society is a function not merely of the strains produced by its culture but also of the institutional means which its cultural heritage provides for the resolution of strain; that those individuals who, for whatever the reasons, cannot resolve the culturally created strains by means of the culturally provided instruments of resolution resolve them in idiosyncratic ways (neuroses and psychoses); and that to the extent that different cultures create different types of strain, idiosyncratic resolution of strain (neuroses and psychoses) will reveal cultural variability. (1959, p. 142)

Good and Kleinman (1985) have expressed the same ideas through a cross-cultural model for anxiety that includes recognition of biological as well as psychological variables (Figure 1.1). Their model is quite interesting for several reasons. First, it focuses on the ultimate outcome of the interaction between cultural, physiological, and psychological as being the expression of the illness, or the clinical phenomenon of the disorder. Secondly, it emphasizes the interactional nature of the three major variables, for instance, as social and cultural coping resources influence a person's affect; and vice versa, as a person's emotions affect the person's ability to use such resources. Similarly, an individual's cognitions and perceptions color that person's interpretations of the environment as stressors; but in addition, the strains which the society places on the individual influences that person's internal perceptions and thoughts. Thirdly, their model identifies the possible views offered by the society regarding the meaning of stress and stress reactions. Good and Kleinman provide two basic views: a "professional disease model" and "popular illness meanings" (or what I would consider a "folk medicine" viewpoint). In essence this is the filter which interprets the meaning of symptoms to each person, and simultaneously offers a type of resolution congruent with such meanings.

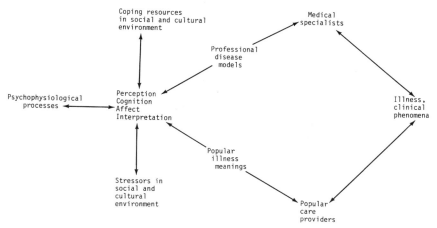

Figure 1.1. A model linking psychophysiological, coping, perceptual, and stress variables to clinical illness. From "Culture and anxiety: Cross-cultural evidence for the patterning of anxiety disorders" by B. Good and A. Kleinman, 1985, in A. Tuma and J. Maser (Eds.), *Anxiety and the anxiety disorders.* Hillsdale, NJ: Erlbaum. Copyright 1985 by Lawrence Erlbaum. Adapted by permission.

Returning to the case of the Chinese cook suffering from heart palpitations, panic, and numbness, the folk medicine herb doctors diagnosed his symptoms as "deficiency in vitality." With this in mind, and consistent with the Asian folk medicine understanding of the proper treatment, the prescription was for intake of boys' urine and human placenta to replenish the lost energy and blood. Other societies offer other meanings. For example, I am familiar with the depression, loss of direction, and listlessness which plagued a Native American following his discharge from military service. A Western psychiatrist might have evaluated the depression as biological and therefore treatable with antidepressants, such as a trycyclic, which might in itself seem incomprehensible and perhaps magical to a non-Westerner. Instead, the tribal witch doctor understood the symptoms to be caused by the presence of a warrior spell which had been cast to permit the boy to successfully go to war, but which had not been lifted and which was inappropriate for adjustment to peaceful living. Removal of this spell provided a straightforward recovery. Naturally, the pattern of thinking which involves the "professional disease model" in Good and Kleinman's conceptual framework for anxiety is the direction that appeals to Western medicine. This direction can be expanded to cover psychiatric as well as psychological professional viewpoints and treatment.

A rather convincing example of what appears to be a culturally formed adjustment problem within the United States involves the sudden increase in eating disorders, with women being the primary victims. In fact, Adler (1982) referred to 1981 in the U.S. as the "year of the binge purge syndrome," while Polivy and Herman (1985) considered "anorexia nervosa the disorder of the 1970's and bulimia the disorder of the 1980's." At least one explanation emphasizes the standard of beauty to which American men appear dedicated, and its impact on those women who internalize such standards, namely of being 'attractively thin.' Garner, Garfinkel, Schwartz, and Thompson (1980) demonstrated convincingly that Miss America contestants and *Playboy* centerfold models actually weighed less than the average American woman. The most startling finding was that the weights of such "ideal beauties" have actually been declining over the last 20 years examined (1959–1978). Most intriguing is the finding that the finalists in Miss America contests have weighed less than the other contestants since 1970. In essence, the argument is that our society's views of what constitutes optimal body weight establishes the goals for some women, leading to the adoption of weight-control behaviors, and leaving such persons vulnerable to eating disorders when such behaviors are carried too far. Striegel-Moore, Silverstein, and Rodin (1986) remind us that women who are now bulimic are the daughters of the first generation of Weight Watchers!

On a more narrow perspective, Spiro also refers to stresses and strains which originate within a society itself. Such intracultural variables have long been recognized in social psychology as including social stratification, neighborhood influences, organization, minority group status, poverty, and environmental factors such as noise pollution and overcrowding. The classic study by Hollingshead and Redlich (1958) is well known for documenting the influence of socioeconomic levels, with families categorized from class I to class V, with I being the highest educational and occupational achievement levels. Anxiety disorders, including phobias and physical conditions affected by psychological factors, were clustered in this study among the class IV persons. In an equally pioneering study by Faris and Dunham of Chicago (1939), the unique stresses of social isolation and community disorganization appeared to create differences in incidence of psychopathology in differing neighborhoods. Regarding urbanization, the data around the world certainly support the contention that urban residents are much more subject to hospitalization for mental disorders than rural residents (Cooper, 1978). This information is quite consistent with the observation cited earlier that the five Australian Aborigines experiencing anxiety states which were not attributable to the presence of a life-threatening disease, were those considered to be "acculturated," that is, integrating into civilized society.

Regarding minority group status, ethnic minority groups are now over 20% of the nation's population, with blacks numbering over 26.4 million, Hispanics 14.6 million, Asians over 3.5 million, and American Indians over 1.3 million (U.S. Department of Commerce, 1986). Unique stresses continue to be part of the consequences of being a member of such a minority population, as a result of conflicts over cultural identity, racism, poverty, status inconsistencies, value conflicts, and social obstacles to aspirations (Albee, 1980). Serious concerns have been raised regarding the unmet needs for services for minority persons.

Environmental factors directly reflect the state of affairs of our society. With increased technology, reliance upon machinery, building construction, affluence leading to multiple car families, air and noise pollution are the modern symbols of city life. Physical health hazards from air pollution and sound pollution have caused the establishment of laws aimed at bringing these problems under control; what is now being recognized are the stresses and mental health issues created by these same factors. At least one study has reported that there are higher admissions rates to the psychiatric hospital for residents living in high noise areas around London, or England's Heathrow Airport than for residents living in low noise neighborhoods (Abey-Wickrama, A'Brook, Gattoni, & Herridge, 1969). Furthermore, when the stress of noise is added to an experiment involving aggression, aggression escalates. Donnerstein and Wilson (1976) gave subjects the opportunity to deliver electric shock to a victim (a confederate of the experimenter). When an angry subject is confronted with unpredictable and uncontrollable noise, the subject would deliver more intense shocks than when noise was absent.

If machinery is one reason for the increase in pollution, the high birth rate, the increase in immigrants, and the attractiveness of city as opposed to rural life, all contribute to overcrowding. Some evidence suggests that being in a crowded area for even a few hours leads to physiological signs of stress, such as increased blood pressure (Aiello, Epstein, & Karlin, 1975). Withdrawal behaviors as a means of coping with such stress have been confirmed as a consequence of not only being faced with a high density social interaction, but also merely expecting to be confronted with such a situation (Baum & Koman, 1976; Joy & Lehmann, 1975). Interestingly enough, and pertinent to our discussion about societal differences, some cultures have evolved their own resolution to such stresses and strains. Faced with high social density and crowded living, the Japanese, for instance, are viewed as having evolved strict rules of behavior and formality, which provide a sense of protection of privacy, even when in the presence of many others.

Biological

The presence of fear was given a reason by Darwin (1872), who viewed this emotion as the consequence of evolution and natural selection. As with his general theory of natural selection, Darwin believed that fear had an adaptive function, this being to arouse and mobilize the organism for coping with danger. In arriving at this conclusion, he took into account the profile of changes that are associated with fear. He observed rapid heart rate, dilation of the pupils of the eyes, dryness of the mouth, rising of the hair, increased rate of breathing, changes in voice quality, and general changes in facial expression. These changes were instinctual and may also have served to signal danger to other animals in the herd. Cannon (1929) suggested that the sympathetic nervous system took over during threat as a means of mobilizing for emergencies and the possible need for intense muscular activity. These sympathetic changes were interpreted as "preparatory for struggle," the fight-or-flight response. Epinephrine is stimulated, which in turn frees stores of glycogen for energy to the muscles and redistributes blood from the viscera to the heart, brain, and extremities. At the same time, blood vessels close to the periphery constrict and blood clotting time shortens, presumably as precaution in the event of wounds. Since saliva and mucus dry up, the size of the air passages to the lungs is increased, thereby providing more air as breathing also increases.

Selye (1956) is often considered the father of modern stress theories, offering one of the first systematic descriptions of the stress response. His was also a biologically oriented approach, covering a sequential description of physiological and tissue changes in response to stressful events. More particularly, these changes are said to occur in his "alarm" phase of his General Adaptation Syndrome. The General Adaptation Syndrome is a pattern of bodily responses resulting from the presence of a stressor. The sequence of events identified by Selye includes several phases starting with an alarm phase as the organism initially reacts. During this phase there is a concentration of energy and a focusing of effort as the organism begins to be alerted. This phase is relatively short and is soon replaced by the resistance stage as the organism attempts to adjust. During this stage, the biological system seeks to adopt the most optimal defense against the stressor. There are attempts to isolate and encapsulate the stress so as to narrow it to the smallest possible site. However, if such defenses are prolonged and the stress is not resolved, then the wear and tear of adapting leads to deterioration. The phase called exhaustion now is said to occur, characterized by tissue damage, disease, and eventually cessation of functioning of the damaged organ or organism. Each organism's unique response to stress is modulated by certain 'conditioning' factors. One such factor involves internal characteristics. This includes hereditary and constitutional factors, as well as 'memory traces' from prior learning and experience. A second factor involves external characteristics. These include climate, time of day, season, and diet.

Lang (1985) has also postulated a theory which hypothesizes certain biological substrates. He proposes that there are phylogenetically inborn survival responses associated with emotions, including those needed to escape from or defend against external threats. He also speculates that these emotional clusters of actions are stored within the organism in a three level hierarchical organization. A "subroutine" serves as the foundation level, and involves specific context-relevant actions, such as attack modes or flight modes. Next are larger "emotional programs," such as fear or anger, which are said to possess some level of response stereotyping, but which can still vary somewhat in the specific actions selected. Finally, there are broad "dimensional propositions" which organize emotions, and which include the dimensions of intensity, direction, and control over the emotional state.

The above conceptualizations are really ways of theoretically lending some organization and meaning to changes which are observed to occur during fear or other emotional states. Are there any experimentally derived evidence that the arousal of such states has a biophysiological base? One line of research extends the evolutionary hypotheses and searched out clinical and laboratory evidence. Seligman and Hager (1972) proposed that phobias have biological significance in that human phobias "are largely restricted to objects that have threatened survival, potential predators, unfamiliar places, and the dark" (p. 465). In further restating the evolutionary hypothesis, they argue that "The great majority of phobias are about objects of natural importance to the survival of the species" (p. 455). Their initial support for their concept of "preparedness" is the observation that there is unequal potentiality for objects to become the target of phobias. If all phobias are a result of learning, then all objects or situations should show the same frequency of becoming part of a phobic disorder. However, as Seligman (1972) points out, fear of heights, animals, and the dark are quite common fears; on the other hand, ". . . only rarely, if ever, do we have pajama phobias, grass phobias, electric outlet phobias, hammer phobias, even though these things are likely to be associated with trauma in our world" (p. 312). This concept of preparedness focuses on the acquisition of phobias, and postulates that we are biologically prepared to acquire phobias to specific stimuli because of evolutionary experiences, while other stimuli are resistant to fear-induction.

Beyond the argument based upon relative frequency of types of phobias, some experimental documentation has also been reported. In an extensive review of the literature, McNally (1987) has summarized the relevant data using the hypothesis that preparedness can be confirmed through studying the easier acquisition, the irrationality, and a greater resistance to extinction of 'prepared' phobias. Overall, there appeared to be experimental support for the hypothesis only in findings that resistance to extinction of electrodermal responses were greater for certain fear stimuli. There are interesting single-case examples, however, that lend some further credence to the speculation of preparedness. Valentine (1978) sought to replicate the classic Watson demonstration whereby fear is precipitated in a young child through conditioning. In an early comment, Valentine interpreted Watson's success as due to the prior innate existence of a fear "as yet unawakened" until the learning experience. Valentine decided on an experiment with his own child, first permitting her to reach for a pair of opera glasses, but then loudly blowing a whistle behind her. Instead of a fear response developing, the child simply quietly turned around to see what the noise was all about. However, when the same procedure was repeated with a caterpillar, the very first sound of the whistle led to the child giving a loud scream, and turning away from the caterpillar. These results led Valentine to propose that some fears can be viewed as "lurking about" until a life situation lets them free.

Although the possibility of innate preparedness appears to be a logical explanation for the discrepant frequencies in types of objects forming phobias, the experimental evidence is still insufficient to make a strong case. On the other hand, the question of biophysiological contributors can be examined in another way. This direction would examine what we know about the neurophysiological basis of emotions, and evidence that anxiety states can be precipitated through the infusion of chemicals. Both anatomical and physiological research have confirmed without doubt that certain brain structures, neural pathways, and endocrine functions are involved in emotions. The limbic system and certain of its structures, such as the hypothalamus, hippocampus, amygdala, septum and cingulate gyrus, are all involved in different emotions (Hornsby, 1987; Nemeroff & Loosen, 1987). In addition, hormones and neurotransmitters are involved in the biochemistry of emotions, such as the corticosteroids in stress, and norepinephrine, gamma-amino butyric acid, and serotonin in anxiety.

The possibility that anxiety states are a result of biological vulnerability receives some support from data that suggest that anxious patients are in a state of hyperarousal physiologically. Barlow (1988) reviewed the literature and concludes that "The one robust finding is that anxious patients are chronically hyperaroused and slow to habitu-ate" (p. 194). This chronic physiological activation can be seen in such patients' increased resting heart rates, higher blood flow in the forearms, more tense electromyographic readings, and higher galvanic skin re-sponse activity (Ehlers, Margraf, Roth, Taylor, Maddock, Sheikh, Kobell, McClenahan, Gossard, Blowers, Agras, & Koppell, 1986; Holden & Bar-low, 1986; Lader, 1980). Not only is there such a hyperarousal under resting conditions, but the anxious patient takes longer to habituate to stimulation, with slower habituation rates being correlated with higher anxiety (Johnstone, Bourne, Crow, Frith, Gamble, Lofthouse, Owens, Owens, Robinson, & Stevens, 1981; Maple, Bradshaw, & Szabadi, 1981). Lader and Wing (1964), for instance, found that it took 20 trials for all of their control subjects to habituate to auditory stimulation, but only six of the anxious patients had been able to return to baseline by the 20th trial.

Is it possible that the chronic hyperarousal of the anxious patient also signifies other basic neurophysiological characteristics? A rather promis-ing direction has been research on an area of the midbrain known as the locus coeruleus. Studies have determined that the infusion of a biochemi-cal substance, yohimbine, creates experiences of panic among subjects, including increases in heart rate, higher blood pressure, dilation of the pupils, and trembling. Patients suffering from agoraphobia with panic or panic disorder reported not only physiological symptoms such as palpita-tions and increased heart rate, but also the subjective experiences they associate with panic or anxiety (Charney, Heninger, & Breier, 1984; Holmberg & Gershon, 1961; Uhde, Boulenger, Vittone, Siever, & Post, 1985). In contrast, normal subjects reported the somatic symptoms but not the psychological symptoms. Yohimbine appears to act by affecting the locus coeruleus. It is interesting to note that the locus coeruleus is associated with parts of the brain traditionally considered associated with the emotions, such as the limbic system. Another piece of information that further implicates the locus coeruleus is the finding that clonidine may be a drug which is capable of blocking panic states (Hoehn-Saric, Merchant, Keyser, & Smith, 1981; Siever & Uhde, 1984). And clonidine appears to derive its effects through being a potent inhibitor of locus coeruleus activity. Among animals, direct electrical stimulation of the locus coeru-leus results in intense fear similar to panic among monkeys (Redmond, 1979); furthermore lesions which block locus coeruleus activity seem to produce results similar to that of antianxiety medication (Gray, 1985). Thus this part of the brain appears suspiciously connected with panic states. However, researchers are still cautious about concluding that the locus coeruleus is the origin of anxiety states (Carr & Sheehan, 1984; Woods, Charney, McPherson, Gradman, & Heninger, 1987).

The search for biophysiological substrates of anxiety has also identified other brain activity. Benzodiazepine is a class of tranquilizer with
successful application to mild anxiety states. Furthermore, a very revealing finding involves the discovery of receptors in the brain with special
affinity for benzodiazepine. These receptors have been found to increase by as much as 20% within as quickly as 15 minutes under conditions of stress (Paul & Skolnick, 1978, 1981). Also, animals which have
been specifically bred for "high emotionality" have been found to possess a lower number of brain benzodiazepine receptor sites (Robertson,
Martin, & Candy, 1978). Of further interest is the information on "anticonflict." In well known studies of experimental neuroses, conflict is
created through pairing mild shock with a reinforcer (Geller & Seifter,
1960). Under such conditions, a state of chronic anxiety becomes established, with hyperarousal and vigilance. However, the introduction of
the benzodiazepines counteracts the conflict situation, that is, acts as
anticonflict agents. Instead of the shock preventing the instrumental
behaviors, the animal now proceeds without fear (Braestrup, Nielsen,
Honore, Jensen, & Petersen, 1983; Haefely, Polc, Pieri, Schaffner, &
Laurent, 1983). Finally, anxiety effects can be returned through the
introduction of agents which are antagonistic to the effects of the benzodiazepines (Insel, Ninan, Aloi, Jimerson, Skolnick, & Paul, 1984).

Given the relationship between the benzodiazepines and their brain
receptors and anxiety, the next question has been to seek the more
specific mechanisms whereby the benzodiazepines have their impact.
One clear association has been to gamma-amino butyric acid (GABA)
activity. GABA appears to have an inhibitory effect, resulting in the
blockage of anxiety. The benzodiazepines have a potentiating effect on
the gamma-amino butyric acid neurotransmitter, facilitating its release at
synapses. This combination of natural GABA activity enhanced by the
introduction of a benzodiazepine has been found to even further reduce
levels of anxieties. Hence a gamma-amino butyric acid model of anxiety
is also under consideration as a possible explanation.

A broader hypothesis is one which examines the entire endocrinological system, the hypothalamic-pituitary-adrenocortical (HYPAC)
system. This system controls a variety of neurohormones which may be
implicated in anxiety. The evidence shows that the HYPAC system is
indeed activated during laboratory-induced stress, such as the viewing of
war battle scenes or being faced with stressful interviews (Bliss, Migeon,
Branch, & Samuels, 1956; Wadeson, Mason, Hamburg, & Handlon,
1963). This same result is also produced during real life stressful experiences, as where a patient is confronted with surgery (Price, Thaler, &
Mason, 1957). Specific hormonal products of hypothalamic-pituitary-
adrenocortical activity which have shown increases under stressful condi-

tions have included cortisol, prolactin, and the thyroid-stimulating growth hormone (Curtis, Nesse, Buxton, & Lippman, 1979; Konincyx, 1978; Rose & Hurst, 1975). One rather major illustration was the study on pilots landing jet fighters on aircraft carriers, an activity which has been associated with extremely high levels of accidents and death to pilots and their crews. This study found a three times higher level of serum cortisol levels among even experienced pilots, despite their rating themselves subjectively as being calm. The increased cortisol secretion was also found during simulated landings (Miller, Rubin, Clark, Poland, & Arthur, 1970). Despite such documentation, the data on levels of hormones under stressful conditions are inconsistent. For instance, Bourne, Rose, and Mason (1967, 1968) found little change in cortisol among helicopter ambulance medics in combat; and Noel, Dimond, Earll, and Frantz (1976) found no increases in prolactin, growth hormone, or thyroid-stimulating hormone before and during the military training jumps.

A different approach to determining whether biophysiological factors are contributors to anxiety states is the study of whether it is possible to induce anxiety through chemical agents. Several different substances have been found capable of producing anxiety responses in human or animal subjects (Charney & Redmond, 1983). These have included yohimbine, isoprenaline (isoproterenal), adrenaline, lactate, caffeine and beta-carboline (Breggin, 1964; Charney et al., 1984; Charney, Heninger, & Jatlow, 1985; Ehlers et al., 1986; Frohlich, Tarazi, & Dustan, 1969; Grant & Redmond, 1981; Ninan, Insel, Cohen, Cook, Skolnick, & Paul, 1982; Pitts & Alley, 1980). Yohimbine, mentioned earlier, and lactate have been among the more closely studied substances in recent years with special regard for their ability to trigger reactions similar to panic disorder attacks (Charney, Heninger, & Redmond, 1983; Ehlers et al., 1986; Liebowitz, Fyer, Gorman, Dillon, Appleby, Levy, Anderson, Levitt, Palij, Davies, & Klein, 1984). In general, the trend has been to discover that the injection of these substances precipitates anxiety among persons with a history of anxiety states, including panic and phobias. For instance, the patients of Frohlich et al. were observed to experience uncontrollable "hysterical outbursts." Interestingly, normal subjects tend to speak of their experiences "as if" they were anxious, noting the presence of physiological symptoms similar to anxiety, but lacking the subjective sense of nervousness or psychological tension.

In contrast, normal subjects have been sometimes found to react with panic-like symptoms where CO_2 has been inhaled, in concentrations sometimes as low as 4–5% (Cohen & White, 1950; Sanderson, Rapee, & Barlow, 1989; Woods, Charney, Goodman, & Heninger, 1987; Waeber, Adler, Schwank, & Galeazzi, 1982). Cohen and White (1950) provided anxious patients and control subjects with oxygen followed by carbon dioxide air. The subjects were 43 patients and 27 controls; the breathing condition involved 12 minutes of inhaling of oxygen followed by 12 minutes of breathing of air containing 4% carbon dioxide. Of the 43 patients, 47% experienced symptoms which they rated as identical to their anxiety attacks, while another 37% developed symptoms which they felt to be similar to their anxiety attacks.

The ability of CO_2 to stimulate panic attacks is rather paradoxical, since CO_2 inhalation has been successfully prescribed as one type of treatment for reduction of anxiety (Wolpe, 1958, 1973). In one study, the panic experience prompted by CO_2 not only reproduced somatic symptoms, but also the cognitive symptoms of a true panic attack, such as a fear of death or loss of control (van den Hout & Griez, 1982). One clinician reports that his patient describes the moments before uncontrollable panic as "if all the air was sucked right out of the room" (Shader, p. 592). However, findings have been inconsistent, with some studies failing to duplicate panic experiences among normal subjects, even though anxiety patients tended to become panicked (Fyer *et al.*, 1986; Woods *et al.*, 1986). In one study, however, an increase in the concentration of CO_2 did seem to bring the panic experience in normals above threshold (Woods, Charney, *et al.*, 1987).

Psychological

Despite the evidence on biophysiological contributors, there still remains room for consideration of psychological factors. In fact, there are clues even among the biophysiological research studies of at least an interactive role of psychological variables. The fact that chemical infusions tend to provoke panic primarily among persons already suffering from anxiety disorders suggests that an important component may be the patients' expectations. As the somatic symptoms are prompted, the ultimate arrival of a panic condition may be because the patients interpret the somatic symptoms as precursors of a complete loss of control. Liebowitz *et al.* (1985) have especially noted that CO_2 inhalation leads to sudden increases in respiration, which may in turn provoke a fear of being "out of control," thereby reintegrating a true panic experience. When panic disorder patients are given prior explanations regarding the expected onset of somatic symptoms from CO_2 inhalations, such instructions reduced the anxiety consequences of the carbon dioxide (Rapee, Mattick, & Murrell, 1986). Of especial interest is the innovative study by Sanderson, Rapee, and Barlow (1988) during which they manipulated the sense of being in control by the subjects. Two groups of 10 panic disorder patients were told that they could regulate the flow of

CO_2 by turning a dial, but that this regulatory function only operated when a panel light was lit. For one group, this light was always on, while for the other the light was never illuminated. Patients who assumed they had control (since their light was on) experienced substantially less anxiety or panic. This is in contrast, however, to results by Bourne, Rose and Mason (1967, 1968) which found that stress *increased* with more responsibility and control. They discovered higher levels of corticosteroids indicative of stress among the experienced officers of a Green Beret combat unit in Vietnam than among the enlisted men. Increased levels occurred in anticipation of and during a Vietcong attack for the officers and the radio operator. On the other hand, the corticosteroid levels for the enlisted men actually fell during the attack, suggesting a lower level of stress with their lower level of responsibility.

Before leaving the hypothesis regarding control or loss of control, there is one other area of study that is pertinent to this psychological variable. The need to retain control or the fear of losing control has been offered as one explanation for the peculiar phenomenon of relaxation-induced anxiety attacks. Borkovec (Heide & Borkovec, 1983, 1984) has observed situations in which increases in anxiety and a fear of losing control occurred among generalized anxiety patients learning relaxation. Fourteen subjects volunteered for brief training for relaxation for tension. Progressive relaxation or focused relaxation was provided; progressive relaxation followed standard instructions for tensing and relaxing muscle groups; focused relaxation involved instructions similar to transcendental meditation. Five individuals experienced clinically observable anxiety symptoms which "required some clinical intervention" (p. 175). One such person experienced such a severe panic attack as to terminate the training immediately: "During the 45-sec practice period. . . she began crying and reported intense anxiety. . . (and) chose to terminate the study because of the reaction" (p. 174). Increased rather than decreased tension was experienced by 30.8% of the group being trained with progressive relaxation, and 53.8% of the group being trained with transcendental meditation. Correlations between measures of fear of losing control and arousal or anxiety showed that high fears of losing control were associated with higher tension following relaxation training (correlations of .22, .25, .34). Therefore there has been much speculation that need for control may be a major factor in anxiety states.

As a final observation on the argument that psychological factors interact with the biophysiological, a conclusion by Stokes (1985) is worth noting. After a comprehensive review of the support for endocrinological influences on anxiety, Stokes still concluded, "Investigations have focused on the HYPAC system and suggest that neuroendocrine responses to anxiety-provoking stimuli are generally excitatory to that system, but the response varies with the individual's *perception* of the stimulus" (p. 75). We will return to this issue of perception or appraisal in a later chapter.

In discussing the psychological theories regarding anxiety, Freud's beliefs deserve recognition. In his early analysis, Freud saw anxiety as the reflection of repressed libidinal energy (1924, 1936). Since this sexual energy was blocked it becomes later transformed into free-floating anxiety. Additionally, Freud accepted the common perspective that anxiety was a signal of threat. However, he added the concept that the threat could be from either external or internal sources. Externally, the source of danger was from the environment, such as from parents. This objective or reality anxiety has motivating features, driving the individual to take steps to protect itself from the danger. The other source of threat is internal, deriving from forbidden and unacceptable impulses. This neurotic anxiety involves a fear that such inner instincts will get out of control, leading to actions which in turn cause punishment. Moral anxiety is also internally generated, amounting to the fear of the super ego functions. This anxiety appears whenever the individual considers doing something that is contrary to the moral training that has been internalized. To the degree that impulses and their consequences have been repressed, then the individual lacks the ability to identify the source of the anxiety, and hence free-floating anxiety is precipitated. If the anxiety cannot be resolved, and the impulses continue, then the ego falls back on unrealistic attempts to deal with the constant pressure. As the anxiety level becomes traumatic, then the person experiences the type of anxiety reminiscent of the early birth trauma.

Cognitive interpretations of anxiety tend to shift the focus away from the physiological condition itself and emphasize cognitive processes instead. As Beck vigorously proclaims, "Anxiety, however, is not *the* pathological process in so-called anxiety disorders any more than pain or fever constitute the pathological process in an infection or injury. We should not allow nature's mechanism for dramatizing the feeling of anxiety to mislead us into believing that this most salient subjective experience plays the central role in the so-called anxiety disorders. Anxiety acts as an attention getter. It draws attention away from the concern or preoccupations and onto this unpleasant subjective experience. . . the main problem in the anxiety disorders is not in the generation of anxiety but in the overactive cognitive patterns (schemas) relevant to danger that are continually structuring external and/or internal experiences as a sign of danger" (p. 15).

According to this view, a person's appraisal and views of reality are the essential sources of anxiety. Hence, Beck proceeds to argue that "The locus of the disorder in the anxiety states is not in the affective system but in the hypervalent cognitive schemas relevant to danger that are continually presenting a view of reality as dangerous and self as vulnerable" (Beck, p. 192). Sarason (1985) defines the cognitive components of anxiety as involving personal beliefs, assumptions, and expectations about how the world works and the person's place in the world. For the cognitive theorist, thought processes seriously color everyday interactions. For instance, two types of cognitive components are said to characterize the anxious person: self-preoccupation and worry. In self-preoccupation, events are reconstrued in personal terms, thereby interfering with objective appraisals or the ability to take the perspective of someone else. There is some evidence that anxious persons may well be characterized by this self-preoccupation (Breznitz, 1971; Doctor & Altman, 1969; Phares, 1968). For instance, test anxious subjects have their test-taking performances impaired because of spending more time in attending to the irrelevant topic of self-criticism (Wine, 1971). Another illustration of the self-preoccupation can be found in the attributions of anxious persons. Weiner, Frieze, Kukla, Reed, Rest, and Rosenbaum (1971) discovered that high-anxiety subjects tended to attribute their failures to internal factors (their ability) and successes to external factors (luck), while low-anxiety subjects attributed success to their own ability and effort. The general negative cognitive activity of worry is also characteristic of anxious individuals. Both test-anxious and socially anxious subjects have been found to share a common tendency to actively worry about events (Leary, 1982; Smith, Ingram, & Brehm, 1983; Wine, 1971). The information processing system of the person suffering from an anxiety disorder is said to be flawed. Returning to Beck, faulty thinking is postulated as characterizing anxious patients in the form of castastrophizing, loss of perspective or objectivity, and dichotomous thinking. Spontaneous thoughts, images, or cognitive sets (bias of selectively enhancing information relating to danger) can all be part of the contributing factors in the onset of anxiety.

Finally, the work of Lazarus should be recognized in its emphasis on appraisal. Anxiety appears when an event is appraised as being a threat, this appraisal being largely a cognitive, symbolic process (Lazarus & Averill, 1972). Lazarus emphasizes that the confusion about understanding stress has been due to the viewing of stress-related emotions as causes of the stress. Instead, he proposes that such emotions are *consequences*, particularly of certain cognitive processes. Instead of simply spending research time examining the emotional states by considering such emotions as effects, he argues for more attention to be paid to understanding the causes of such emotional effects, that is, cognitions and perceptions. Cognitions involve the person's appraisals in two ways: appraisal of an environmental event in terms of its potential to be harmful, and appraisal of one's resources in terms of their adequacy for coping with the threat. Stress is said to exist when the individual both perceives an event as threatening or harmful, as well as perceiving his or her own resources as being inadequate to handle the threat. Stress cannot exist if the individual does not become conscious of an event as harmful, regardless of the actual level of danger of the event. In the same fashion, an event that is in reality of little danger might actually create substantial threat if so appraised by the person (Lazarus & Folkman, 1984). Lazarus' model of threat is one that proposes a dynamic process of events and appraisals, such that perceptions of events may be revised as continuously as self-appraisal of coping abilities may change.

This concept of the role of appraisal as a precursor to affective responding is quite consistent with the comment cited earlier by Stokes, that neuroendocrine stress responses are influenced by the individual's perception of the stimulus. Stokes' conclusion was aimed at explaining the inconsistency of findings regarding the postulated increase in hypothalamic-pituitary-adrenocortical system hormone secretion under stress. As an example, children were expected to show heightened cortisol production upon admission to the hospital for surgery. Instead one group of children showed lower cortisol secretion; but this same group also reported that the hospital experience was less distressing than either being in the clinic or at home before surgery (Knight, Atkins, Eagle, Evans, Finklestein, Fukushimas, Katz, & Weiner, 1979).

Summary

The information in this chapter clearly confirms the need in today's modern world to consider the problem of anxiety and stress. Anxiety states are extremely common and costly, not only in terms of economic consequences, but also in terms of hazards to emotional and physical well-being and one's quality of life. High prevalence has been documented regarding phobic disorders, agoraphobia, generalized anxiety disorder, and panic disorder. And anxiety and stress are not limited to the modern Western world, but represent an issue that has cross-cultural implications. Perhaps only the most primitive Aborigines may be free from stress; there is certainly evidence for the symptoms of stress appearing in other civilized countries and in other cultures. The mode of expression of stress may differ, as each culture appears to put its own stamp on how stress is expressed.

As an overall perspective, this chapter elaborates on various major sources of stress. These include the cultural, biological, and psychological. The meanings that a person attaches to events, as well as the coping resources available, are influenced by one's cultural heritage. New problems can be shaped by one's cultural values and beliefs, as seen in the development of eating disorders in our Western society. Intracultural factors are also important, including ethnic minority status. Biological factors have been cited by Selye in terms of threats to health and physical well-being, by Lang in terms of biological substrates of emotions, Seligman and Hager in terms of preparedness for developing a phobic disorder, and Barlow and others in terms of possible physiological explanations for heightened vulnerability to anxiety states. The research information in support of these hypotheses appears convincing, at least to the degree of convincing us that biological sources cannot be overlooked. Finally, psychological variables must be included among the various sources of stress, even when the primary source stems from a biological event. A sense of control, the nature of cognitive appraisal or meaning attached, the presence of irrational beliefs, the psychodynamics of a person's personality and habit structure—all must be included in a more comprehensive approach to understanding stress.

II

SCIENTIFIC
FOUNDATIONS

EVIDENCE FOR ANXIETY MANAGEMENT TRAINING

Applications to Anxiety States

Case: An engineer unable to maintain employment because she experiences intermittent bouts of generalized anxiety.

Case: A successful mathematician who is prevented from fully enjoying ski outings because his fear of heights is precipitated by being on a chairlift.

Case: An executive who has experienced one heart attack and is at risk for another because of his Type A life-style.

Case: A housewife whose poor health and mild depression can be traced as secondary outcomes from the constant hassles and stresses of everyday affairs.

Case: A member of an Olympic team who feels the intimidation of being in Russia because of a history of harassment by Soviet judges.

Case: A psychiatric patient who is making poor progress in psychotherapy because his anxiety level is so high as to block participation.

Case: A young diabetic whose level of blood sugar appears to fluctuate as a result of uncontrolled frustrations and stresses.

Case: A high school Hispanic student who feels ready to explode in anger in response to the obstacles facing him.

Case: A Vietnam veteran who still experiences through weekly flashbacks the chills and fear of a traumatic evening battle.

The individuals above have all been treated through the behavior therapy technique described in this book, Anxiety Management Training (AMT). Although each case may have differed in content or symptom structure, AMT proved successful, illustrating one of the primary strengths of this therapy - its generalizability. AMT is a coping skills training method, which teaches clients the use of applied relaxation for anxiety control. It is an arousal-induction type of therapy, using imagery to stimulate anxiety, as a means of giving clients first-hand practice in anxiety reduction. Built into the basic five-session training are steps to gradually increase client self-control, with reduced therapist involvement, and steps to increase self-efficacy and generalization to real life events. Anxiety Management Training does not require that clients be conscious of the precipitating cues responsible for their anxiety states, and therefore can be used with generalized anxiety disorder clients. However, one step in AMT involves enabling clients to become more aware of their bodily or cognitive signs of impending anxiety arousal. Where such signs involve thought processes, AMT can break up the cognitions involved in the anxiety state. As we proceed further into this book, more details will be presented on how to conduct AMT sessions and the varied applications.

Need for the Anxiety Management Training Method

Anxiety Management Training was designed in response to the need for a short-term therapy which could help clients suffering from generalized anxiety disorder, or any anxiety state that was free-floating. Desensitization has proven to be a highly effective therapy where the stimulus associated with the anxiety is definable, that is, for phobic disorders. Similarly, modeling appears to be useful in the treatment of phobias and in enhancing self-efficacy. However, neither approach can be applied to generalized anxiety conditions, in which the client is unable to identify even the triggering stress cues. Implosion and flooding could be modified for generalized anxiety, but the process is exhausting for clients, and could exacerbate anxiety if the timing of the exposure is incorrect. Stress Inoculation Training (SIT), with its multimodal orientation, is much more complex and with an emphasis on cognitive or self-talk strategies including some from Rational Emotive Therapy. During the application phase of Stress Inoculation Training, imagery rehearsal is employed, derived from desensitization. Hence, the limitations of desensitization also apply here to Stress Inoculation Training (Meichenbaum, 1985).

My desire to seek a method for the treatment of generalized anxiety disorder (GAD) stemmed from the prevalence and severity of this condition. Furthermore, it made sense that any treatment model which was successful with this syndrome would have major generalizability to other conditions in which anxiety has a major role. Generalized anxiety disorder is the most commonly reported anxiety disorder, with a prevalence of as high as 6.4% of the population (Weissman, 1983). Characteristic of generalized anxiety disorder are autonomic hyperactivity and "apprehensive expectations. . . focused on multiple life circumstances" (Cerny, Himadi, & Barlow, in press). The diagnostic criteria used by the *Diagnostic and Statistical Manual of Mental Disorders* (DSM-IIIR) (Spitzer & Williams, 1987) states that the essential feature ". . . is unrealistic or excessive anxiety and worry (apprehensive expectation) about two or more life circumstances. . . for six months or longer. . . (including) signs of motor tension, autonomic hyperactivity, and vigilance and scanning" (p. 251). Unlike phobic disorder, there is no truly circumscribed stimulus for GAD although there may be circumstances receiving more emphasis. For instance, the person suffering from generalized anxiety disorder may emphasize the circumstances surrounding family members, but the concern itself is an unfocused, generalized apprehensiveness of potential misfortune to one's child (where there is no foundation for such a concern). Among children and adolescents, the circumstances may involve academic, athletic or social performance. Because of such free-floating features and the multiplicity of circumstances, generalized anxiety disorder has been particularly resistant to behavioral theories regarding ways of treating it (Suinn & Deffenbacher, 1985).

Beyond the importance of generalized anxiety disorder as a disorder deserving treatment, there is heuristic value from any therapy which can successfully impact on this disorder. Specifically, any treatment which can control the anxiety levels inherent in generalized anxiety disorder should prove useful for other disorders or conditions in which anxiety is a core causative factor. The various cases cited at the beginning of this chapter all have anxiety in common. Thus, the therapeutic approach for generalized anxiety disorder should have beneficial applications for phobic disorders or situation specific anxieties (such as social, test or speech anxiety); physical or health problems with an anxiety component (such as hypertension, ulcers, dysmenorrhea, tension headaches, or Type A behavior patterns); psychological conditions which appear secondary to anxiety (such as certain depressive states); conditions associated with trauma (such as post-traumatic stress disorder); or settings in which anxiety is an obstacle to psychological gains (such as effective use of psychotherapy or vocational counseling). Finally, a treatment model applicable to generalized anxiety disorder would also have relevance for adjusted persons where stressors inhibit their performance levels, such as athletes, musicians, and theatre arts performers.

As we commented earlier, the primary motivation leading to the development of the AMT technique was the search for a treatment for generalized anxiety disorder. Given that desensitization, a behavior therapy, was having such great success with phobias, the principles forming the foundation for AMT also came from behavioral psychology. A major hope was that the short-term treatment program characterizing desensitization would also be feasible with AMT; hence, the basic AMT training is designed to involve about 6–8 sessions. In fact, the first published research study involved therapy completed in $2\frac{1}{2}$ weeks (Suinn & Richardson, 1971). In addition, the reliance upon imagery as a possible method for anxiety induction, rather than the use of *in vivo* stimuli, also derived from the success of imagery in desensitization. Furthermore, using imagery appeared to be a safer approach since it can be readily discontinued, whereas *in vivo* exposures might be more subject to precipitating high levels of anxiety that is uncontrolled. Finally, the history of AMT reflected some of the emphases in behavioral therapy regarding the importance of actual practice of desired behaviors, the relevance of homework for generalization beyond the therapy office, and the desirability of self-control orientations.

Overview of Research

From its earliest inception in 1971, the efficacy of Anxiety Management Training has been tested through research. The history of such research has proven to be quite exciting as new discoveries and applications have occurred. Of interest to clinical practitioners is the fact that many reports have tested the long-term effects of AMT, such that AMT has been shown to be a therapy with a convincing accumulation of evidence on its stable effects.

The first series of studies on AMT were conservative in the choice of client problems. Phobic conditions were selected rather than the potentially more difficult generalized anxiety disorder. University students were selected rather than psychiatric patients in order to have a less complex client sample. Our hope was that AMT could be validated, and that we could learn about whether the technique needed to be revised in content, approach, or length. The content involved anxiety induction followed by some type of coping control to eliminate the anxiety. The approach for anxiety *induction* in the first study included arousal by imagery rehearsal of a prior anxiety experience as well as the use of audio recordings (actually 78 rpm phonograph disks!) of fear-arousing material, specifically a segment of the narrative of Edgar Allan Poe's *Tell-Tale Heart* horror tale (Suinn & Richardson, 1971). The approach to anxiety *control* was twofold: the use of applied relaxation and relaxation imagery, and the use of competency imagery.

Subjects were university students suffering from mathematics anxiety, as measured by the Mathematics Anxiety Rating Scale (Suinn, Edie, Nicoletti, & Spinelli, 1972). As a behavioral index of performance on mathematics tasks, the numerical section of the Differential Aptitude Tests was administered. We assumed that the presence of mathematics anxiety would hinder performance; similarly that performance would improve upon the removal of mathematics anxiety. There were 24 students included in behavior therapy treatment, and 119 control students who agreed to a test-retest format. The controls would provide baseline data on the changes occurring in test results due to the experience of being retested and not due to any interventions.

The results were more than satisfying; not only were there substantive decreases in the level of anxiety from this short treatment program, but there were also some improvements in performance on the mathematics skills test. Specifically, mathematics anxiety levels for the treated subjects decreased from a mean of 242 to a mean of 180. Norms for the mathematics anxiety scale used indicate that a score above 225 places the person above the 75th percentile (Richardson & Suinn, 1973). On the other hand, the mean for a normal, nonanxious subject who has retaken this mathematics anxiety test would be 180. In other words, the subjects treated with AMT showed a significant reduction of their anxiety level, dropping from being in an abnormally high level to the level of normal subjects. The subjects treated with AMT also showed an increase in their performance on the numerical section of the Differential Aptitude Test. Although the increase on the Differential Aptitudes Test was only three points, this was in contrast with a control group which showed a mean increase of only 0.61 points.

An interesting side note is the fact that subjects were also given the Suinn Test Anxiety Behavioral Scale (Suinn, 1969), a measure of test anxiety. As it turned out, although these students were not seeking treatment for test anxiety, their initial mean scores placed them in the 80th percentile on test anxiety. Following AMT, which the subjects understood was a treatment to help their mathematics anxiety, scores on test anxiety also showed a reduction. This reduction did not reach the level of normal subjects, but did drop from the initial 80th percentile to the 60th percentile, and was only 15 points from being at the 50th percentile. In other words, even in this initial study, there was evidence of the generalization of treatment effects from AMT.

Furthermore, we discovered that imagery alone was sufficient to produce the necessary anxiety induction and so, with great relief, we quickly discarded the phonograph materials (I had always harbored the concern that hearing Basil Rathbone acting out Edgar Allan Poe would strike some modern young student as hilarious, rather than frightful. . . leading to outbursts of giggling, which would then utterly destroy the serious clinical atmosphere we were trying to create). We also concluded that relaxation seemed to be as useful as competency imagery in providing the clients with a means of controlling their anxiety. Since psychiatric patients or outpatients with long histories would not be expected to recall many recent examples of being competent in life, the use of competency imagery was also discarded. Eliminating the identification of competency scenes removed the possibility of a lengthy debate with a client who might insist that the request was an impossible one.

Initial Studies on Situation-Specific Anxieties: The Surprising Superiority of AMT over Desensitization

Since this first article in 1971, a series of early studies were conducted at Colorado State University on the revised AMT technique (without audio recordings or competency imagery). The target problem continued to be situation specific anxieties, such as mathematics, test, and public-speaking anxieties. Nicoletti (1971) found AMT effective in the reduction of public-speaking anxiety. His clients were volunteers from the counseling centers of two universities in Colorado, as well as a control group of students in an Introductory Psychology course. The clients were those whose primary complaint was public-speaking anxiety; 25 such clients comprised this group. Of the 25 clients, half were randomly assigned to a wait-list control group, with the remaining half receiving AMT immediately. For a second control group, a random sample of test scores of 20 students from a larger pool of 92 students was used. These were students who were not complaining about anxiety experiences, and hence formed a no-problem control group. As measures of anxiety, the IPAT Anxiety Scale was used to assess general anxiety, while the Public Speaking Anxiety Inventory was devised to measure public speaking anxiety for this study (Cattell & Scheier, 1963; Nicoletti, Edie, & Spinelli, 1971). The Public Speaking Anxiety Inventory required clients to rate their levels of anxiety associated with each of 50 situations involving speaking, for example, "Giving an impromptu speech before a small group," and "Being asked to express your opinion by a group that does not share your views." AMT treatment involved five sessions of two hours each, spread over three weeks, with two sessions each week. Clients were seen in group sessions.

Results involving analysis of covariances showed that the AMT treated clients were significantly different from the wait-list clients on both the public speaking and general anxiety measures. On the Public Speaking Anxiety Inventory, the treated clients dropped in scores from 176 to 136, compared to a reduction from 159 to 148 for the wait-list group. Furthermore, although the client groups were significantly higher than the no-problem control group on pretesting, the AMT-treated group reached a level at posttesting that was comparable to that of the no-problem subjects (AMT post = 135, No-problem post = 138). In terms of the IPAT, all of the groups scored at similar levels on pretesting; however, at posttesting, the AMT-treated group were significantly lower than the wait-list group. The treated clients showed a reduction of IPAT scores from 47 to 40, while the wait-list group dropped only two points (from 50 to 48), and the no-problem subjects showed no change (35 at pretest, 35 at posttest). Nicoletti concluded that AMT was an effective treatment, not only for public speaking anxiety, but possibly for general anxiety. As a way of further understanding how the clients perceived the treatment, he also reported on some of the comments made by clients. Among those he received were comments such as, "I don't feel as help-less about controlling my anxiety," "The technique has really helped me to become aware of when I am nervous," "I had a chance to use it this last weekend and I could shut off the anxiety," and "I don't feel the same about the anxiety when it occurs, I feel like I can control it before it gets out of hand" (p. 108). From such observations, Nicoletti concluded " . . . there seem to be two main benefits gained from the treatment: 1. The awareness of the physiological symptoms associated with anxiety and thus providing a means for identifying anxiety early; (and) 2. Providing a nonspecific technique for controlling anxiety regardless of the specific stimulus conditions" (p. 108).

Mathematics anxiety was targeted by Richardson and Suinn (1973a). The subjects were again volunteers from a counseling center, this time from a university in Missouri. This study sought to compare the results of AMT therapy with desensitization, with the Mathematics Anxiety Rating Scale and the Differential Aptitude Test. The Differential Aptitude Test, numerical section was given with a 10-minute time limit to add time pressure. Twenty students were in the desensitization group, 13 in the AMT group, and 18 in a no-treatment control group of students from an education course who were not seeking treatment. The desensitization clients were seen in nine treatment sessions, meeting three times each week for three weeks. The AMT group format was as described previously in the Suinn and Richardson study. The results showed that both treatment approaches reduced the levels of anxiety from above the 80th percentile to the 50th percentile on a measure of mathematics anxiety. Although the Differential Aptitude Test results were close to but still failed to reach statistical significance, the treatment groups did show greater improvements in comparison with the control group (desensitization gained 4 points, AMT gained 3 points, control group gained 1.6 points).

Richardson and Suinn (1973b) not only examined the effectiveness of AMT on another situation-specific anxiety, test anxiety, but also attempted an even briefer version of AMT. In this study, AMT was provided in only three hours of total treatment time. Forty student volunteers had responded to a newspaper advertisement announcing a behavior therapy program for test anxiety, sponsored by the university's counseling service. Test anxiety was determined by a clinical interview and substantiated by scores on the Suinn Test Anxiety Behavioral Scale (Suinn, 1969). Three behavioral treatment approaches were used. Standard desensitization was provided through six one-hour sessions, meeting three times weekly for two weeks. An accelerated form of desensitization, called accelerated massed desensitization, offered treatment through two sessions one week apart (Suinn, Edie, & Spinelli, 1970). Session one involved relaxation training for one hour. Session two involved two hours, during which the top one-third of a standard test anxiety hierarchy was used. For AMT, treatment was through two sessions, a week apart. Session one focused on relaxation training, while session two involved two hours of anxiety-arousal and relaxation control. All treatment was through audiotape recordings, although the therapist-experimenter was present at all times during the treatment sessions. In comparison with a wait-list control group, all treatment groups showed significantly lower test anxiety scores following treatment. Furthermore, all treated clients' posttreatment test anxiety scores were either at or below the mean of a normal group of university students. The reductions from pretest to posttesting were highest for the standard desensitization clients (57 points), next for the accelerated massed desensitization clients (43 points), and next for the AMT clients (25). The wait-list subjects showed a slight increase over the same time period (of 1.8 points). The most interesting aspect of this study is the extremely brief treatment exposures. It raises the possibility that AMT and desensitization can both achieve effects without a protracted treatment schedule, at least for a simple condition such as test anxiety.

Other researchers such as Deffenbacher and Shelton (1978) continued to confirm the initial findings on the efficacy of AMT with test and mathematics anxiety. However, these two psychologists also added some exciting new information. Their sample involved 43 clients volunteering for behavior therapy from the university's counseling service for test anxiety. These clients were randomly assigned to either standard desensitization or anxiety management training. Treatments consisted of five total weeks of treatment, meeting for about one hour once each week. Both desensitization and AMT were conducted in group sessions involving 6–10 members per group. Results on test anxiety confirmed the type of findings we just reported on situation-specific anxieties. Specifically, both desensitization and AMT led to significant reductions in test anxiety following treatment, with the level of gains from the two therapies being quite similar. On the other hand, Deffenbacher and Shelton also uncovered some dramatic new findings as they proceeded to determine if AMT was able to contribute in ways different from desensitization. In addition to evaluating gains at immediate termination of treatment, they also collected follow-up data six weeks after treatment. Furthermore, in addition to measuring test anxiety—the concern for which the clients sought help—they also obtained measures of trait anxiety. The Spielberger Trait Anxiety Inventory (Spielberger, Gorsuch, & Lushene, 1970) was used as a measure of trait anxiety.

Their first new discovery was that AMT clients continued to show reductions in test anxiety during the follow-up. In comparison, the desensitization clients actually showed some minor increases: the mean for the AMT clients on the Test Anxiety Scale was 29 pre-therapy, 23 post-therapy, and 22 at follow-up; the mean for the desensitization clients was 30 pre-therapy, 23 post-therapy, and 25 at follow-up. On the Suinn Test Anxiety Behavior Scale, the findings were in the same direction: mean for AMT clients on pretest was 160, on posttreatment 132, and 129 on follow-up; mean for desensitization clients on pretest was 165, 114 on posttreatment, and 132 on follow-up. In essence, the AMT clients' reductions in test anxiety were maintained, with a trend toward continued improvement. Further, these gains were such that the AMT clients showed a significantly lower level of test anxiety at follow-up when compared against the desensitization clients.

A second major discovery by Deffenbacher and Shelton involved the results when the trait anxiety scores were examined. The AMT clients showed decreases in trait anxiety from pretest to termination of therapy, with these gains continuing through follow-up (means of 48, 42, and 38). In contrast, the desensitization group showed essentially no changes over the three measurement periods (means of 46, 45, and 45). Not only was the level of trait anxiety for the AMT group at follow-up significantly lower than the level for the desensitization group, but the actual mean value was now at the mean for normal subjects on the Spielberger scale. Deffenbacher and Shelton compared the results of AMT against other anxiety reduction behavioral therapies, such as self-control desensitization and found that ". . . the results of anxiety management training appear as robust, if not more so, than other self-control interventions" (p.

281). Further, in their opinion, when compared with standard desensitization, AMT was viewed as "superior" and as possessing the advantages of both "remedial and preventive counseling functions" (p. 277).

Not satisfied with the six-week follow-up, Deffenbacher conducted another treatment study, but with follow-up one year after therapy (Deffenbacher & Michaels, 1981a) (see Figure 2.1). In this study AMT was provided to test-anxious and to speech-anxious subjects, over six weeks, meeting once per week. Test anxiety was measured by the Achievement Anxiety Test (Alpert & Haber, 1960), while speech anxiety was assessed by the Personal Report of Confidence as a Speaker (Paul, 1966), and general anxiety was measured by Fear Inventory (Wolpe, 1969) and the Spielberger Trait Anxiety Inventory. A no-treatment control group also received the same tests. The findings confirmed the continued improvement on debilitating test anxiety by the AMT group, including retaining a level of test anxiety significantly lower than that of a control group at posttesting. Similar findings were also reported for the speech-anxious clients. Finally, although no changes were found on the trait anxiety measure, the AMT group did show continuous reduction in general anxiety scores across time, and their posttest scores were significantly lower than those of the control group. During the various testing periods, the control group showed essentially no improvements in their levels of anxiety on any scales.

Deffenbacher and Michaels (1981b) also obtained a 15-month follow-up on another of Deffenbacher's treatment studies (Deffenbacher et al., 1980). In the initial study, AMT was compared against self-control desensitization with clients suffering from test anxiety. Levels of test anxiety were measured through the Achievement Anxiety Test, general anxiety levels were measured through the Fear Inventory, and trait anxiety through the Spielberger Trait Anxiety Inventory. Both AMT and self-control desensitization groups achieved levels of debilitating, general, and trait anxiety lower than that of a control group at the 15-month follow-up. The trends for AMT and self-control desensitization clients were similar in that both types of clients tended to show lower anxiety test scores at each testing period. However, the AMT clients were slightly lower than the self-control desensitization clients on test anxiety and general anxiety scales at 15-month retesting: AMT test anxiety = 25.4, desensitization = 27.9; AMT general anxiety = 175.1; desensitization = 181.8. Furthermore, on trait anxiety, the two groups achieved comparable levels at follow-up, but the AMT clients had started at a slightly higher level on pretest: AMT pretest—50, follow-up—40; desensitization pretest—47, follow-up—40.

In summary, research appears to support the contention that anxiety management training is effective in the reduction of situation-

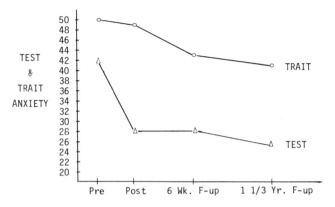

Figure 2.1. Continuing benefits of AMT. (From Deffenbacher & Michaels, 1981.)

specific anxieties, such as test and mathematics anxieties. In addition, there is some documentation which suggests that anxiety management training enables clients to maintain and perhaps even improve on their coping, such that decreases in levels of anxieties continue across long periods of follow-up.

Generalized Anxiety, Trait Anxiety, Generalized Anxiety Disorder: The Confirmation of AMT for General Anxiety Patients

Although the prior studies supported the conclusion that AMT was useful for situation-specific anxiety, and the superiority of AMT in generalization and on follow-up, the fact still remained that AMT was designed for general anxiety problems. Edie (1972) produced the earliest attempt to measure reductions on general anxiety. Clients were solicited from university counseling centers for general anxiety, as well as test and public speaking anxiety. These students were from a state university and a state college in Colorado, all of whom were referred to the behavior therapy program from the counseling centers. Their year in school covered a full range from freshmen to advanced graduate students. Two types of control groups were constituted: a wait list control, and a no-problem control. The no-problem control group were 20 students participating in this research study for research credit for an introductory psychology course. This no-problem group was randomly drawn from an initial sample of 92 participants. The participants from the counseling centers involved 40 total students: 30 were assigned to AMT treatment groups, with the remaining 10 being the wait-list control sample.

   This study really had two unique objectives. The first was to determine whether general anxiety test scores would show improvements; in
effect this was therefore the first attempt to validate the role of AMT in
treating general anxiety. A second objective was a type of component
analysis. Specifically, the question was whether changing the content of
the anxiety part of AMT session made a difference. The usual format
for AMT is to have the client achieve anxiety arousal by first visualizing
themselves in detail in an anxiety-provoking experience. Then, the client
is to use the details of this experience to trigger physical/physiological
anxiety reactions.[1] In Edie's research, he separated the clients into three
treatment groups: AMT I subjects were instructed to emphasize attending to the physical/physiological cues, with the details of the anxiety
scene being minimally described; AMT II subjects were provided the
usual AMT instructions, that is, with equal attention to carefully visualizing the details of the anxiety setting, followed by attending to the resulting physical/physiological reactions; AMT III subjects were given instructions to precipitate noting details of the anxiety setting in order to
relive the anxiety situation, but the consequent physical/physiological
reactions were not emphasized. It should be noted that subjects were not
prevented from elaborating on either the scene details or the consequent
physical/physiological reactions; the study merely reduced the level to
which the therapist directed the client to spend time in focusing on such
details.
   Although some of the clients had been referred for a situation-
specific anxiety, the data confirmed that all clients were significantly
higher on general anxiety scales (IPAT Anxiety Scale and Taylor Manifest Anxiety Scale) as compared with the no-problem normative sample.
As can be readily seen from Table 2.1, the no-problem patients' mean on
the Manifest Anxiety Scale was 20.9 as compared with 31.4 for the wait-
list group, 32.2 for AMT I, 31.0 for AMT II, and 30.5 for AMT III.
Scores on the IPAT scale for the AMT groups and the wait-list group
were also higher than the scores for the no-problem group on pretesting. Results supported the validity of AMT in reducing clients' levels of
manifest anxiety to that of the normal sample. By posttesting, the AMT-
treated groups evidenced a decrease, but the means were still higher
than that of the no-problem control group. If we inspect the results
directly, however, it can be noted that the actual differences between the
no-problem group's mean and each of the AMT groups was no more
than six points. Furthermore, the wait-listed group remained over 13
points higher than the no-problem group at posttesting.

―――――――――――――――――――――

[1]The AMT procedures have been revised such that the standard format now includes
  recognizing cognitive as well as physical or physiological cues.

Table 2.1. Three Variations of AMT for General Anxiety, Wating-List Control Group, and No-Problem Group[a]

Group	Scales	Pre Mean	S.D.	Post Mean	S.D.	Absolute differences between means
Treatment I	IPAT	47.20	9.58	40.00	10.01	− 7.20
Physiological cues	MAS	32.20	7.39	23.30	7.78	− 8.90
($N = 10$)	PSI	160.10	33.34	135.50	36.89	−24.60
	ASCL	291.00	68.84	250.50	62.65	−40.50
Treatment II	IPAT	39.70	10.31	36.30	9.56	− 3.40
Physiological cues	MAS	31.00	6.25	23.70	10.25	− 7.30
plus scenes	PSI	149.00	27.30	124.20	24.36	−24.80
($N = 10$)	ASCL	285.20	65.84	225.10	46.48	−60.10
Treatment III	IPAT	49.30	5.91	41.30	4.81	− 8.00
Scenes only	MAS	30.50	7.18	23.30	5.91	− 7.20
($N = 10$)	PSI	150.60	32.22	128.50	28.08	−22.10
	ASCL	273.40	56.91	231.60	59.90	−41.80
Waiting-list	IPAT	50.60	11.50	48.70	13.60	− 1.90
control	MAS	31.40	10.30	33.20	9.73	+ 1.80
($N = 10$)	PSI	168.50	44.13	164.00	45.12	− 4.50
	ASCL	296.00	88.89	291.60	98.04	− 4.40
No-problem	IPAT	35.70	10.26	35.35	9.70	− .35
no-treatment	MAS	20.95	7.67	18.90	7.01	− 2.05
control	PSI	149.35	18.93	138.55	24.90	−10.80
($N = 20$)	ASCL	201.15	32.88	192.10	35.13	− 9.05

[a]From Edie, 1971.

Regarding the question of whether the different emphases in the instructions for AMT I, II, or III made any differences in outcomes, Figure 2.2 best illustrates the findings. In effect, all three approaches achieved highly similar results in general anxiety reduction.

Edie reported an interesting observation as a result of his interviews with the clients following each AMT session. He comments, "During brief interviews with treatment *Ss* there was an indication that some clients tend to repress or deny the existence of physical aspects of anxiety verbally while appearing (behaviorally) tense and hypermanic. (But). . . many clients (later) comment that the AMT procedures which make use of physiological cues have enabled them to become more aware of how they express anxiety physically, recognize it earlier, and consequently do something about it before it gets out of control" (p. 140).

This experience represents one of the earliest observations during a research study which confirms our later beliefs about the value of the AMT method which includes instructions for the clients to notice their

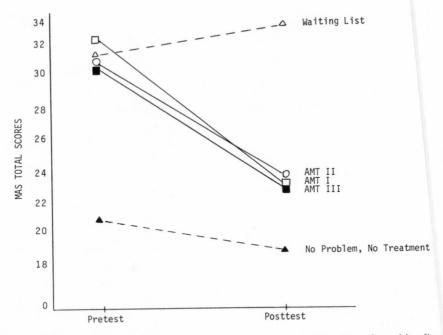

Figure 2.2. Mean pretest and posttest MAS scores for three AMT groups, the waiting-list control group, and the no-problem, no-treatment control group. (From Edie, 1972.)

physical and physiological reactions. Although many generalized anxiety disorder patients may be initially unable to identify the conditions associated with their anxiety, and are often vague about how they experience anxiety, AMT sessions frequently lead to greater insights. Our clinical experiences have been that AMT enables clients to begin not only to become more conscious of their anxiety responses (whether these show up as physiological changes, or catastrophic thoughts or worries, or as behavioral symptoms), but also more aware of some of the core events which precipitate anxiety reactions.

As follow-up to the study, Edie conducted brief 10–15 minute interviews of clients two weeks following termination of the study. Some of the reports were clinically interesting. Clients reported that continued success in using AMT in their daily lives improved the more they used AMT. In other words, continued practice strengthened the efficacy of AMT. For about 50% of the clients interviewed, they reported that their control was automatic, that is, they were able to prevent anxiety from developing without doing anything consciously when they were faced with a new source of tension. Four subjects mentioned that "they felt more socially secure and attributed the feeling to the loss of their previous fear that they might lose control of their anxiety at any moment. It would appear that the experience of control over a previously uncontrollable response was one of the most reinforcing events that the. . . AMT *Ss* had experienced since the completion of treatment" (p. 142). Finally, Edie commented that he observed "that some *Ss*, after anxiety reduction, were less inhibited about expressing other emotions and revealing more of a personal nature about themselves." He concludes that AMT might therefore be an adjunct to other forms of psychotherapy: "It seems plausible that the reduction of anxiety by AMT as an adjunct to insight-oriented therapy could lead to more relevant expression and self-understanding more quickly than the approach of letting the client become comfortable with the situation by himself before he is expected to get down to the work of therapy" (pp. 142–143). As we will see later, this early insight by Edie was examined and proven accurate in a research study on schizophrenics undergoing psychotherapy.

Soon after, Suinn (1976) reported on a case of a 37-year-old woman who was quite successful in many ways. She was a partner in a growing business in which she only served part-time. Nevertheless she had gained a regional reputation, but most important a sense of personal gratification at her ability to achieve. In spite of this positive side, she also had bouts with a general tensional state. This condition exhibited itself in "diffuse emotionality," which often swept her out of control. She saw herself as an intense person who seemed to have only strong emotions, ranging from anger to the point of 'bursting' with joyful excitement, with happiness 'welling up inside.' Among examples of her inability to control her emotional states were:[2]

- When appearing in court over a minor car accident, she became upset at losing, and followed the attorney down the hallway, yelling at him.
- She became so involved in a school issue that she cried and experienced a stomachache after reading a newspaper article referring to the topic.
- When anxious, she would compulsively engage in self-disclosing statements, revealing her personal feelings and anxieties. The sheer volume and intensity of these statements often became aversive to her listeners, leading to their discomfort and withdrawal.
- As she became aware of her emotionality, she began to spend entire mornings fretting and being on edge before a meeting on any topic which had personal relevance to her.

[2]Some details of these real cases have been altered in order to protect the anonymity of the clients.

The basic high levels of daily tension and anxiety appeared to be the basis for her quick irritability, explosive anger, and steep slides into depression. Because of the nonspecific and more general nature of her tensions, Anxiety Management Training was considered as a potentially useful approach. My own prior observation was that, "In a way, she was acting as does the tense executive under work pressure who suddenly blows up angrily over a trifling matter that she would not have reacted to under calmer conditions" (p. 322). AMT was also considered in the hope that the self-control training would generalize to emotional reactions in addition to the anxiety. Anxiety management training was provided over 12 sessions with excellent results that were maintained two years later. She learned to introduce the relaxation as a method to keep herself from becoming overemotional and out of control. She also learned to identify her overtalkativeness as a sure index of anxiety, and was now able to substitute greater calm for the intense need to talk. The number of settings which could prompt tension and emotionality were now much reduced. Finally her view of herself changed from a perception of being a person at the mercy of her emotions to a person who was confident about dealing with a variety of life stresses.

The work of Deffenbacher (Deffenbacher & Shelton, 1978; Deffenbacher & Michaels, 1980, 1981; Deffenbacher *et al.*, 1980) mentioned previously added to the belief that AMT has value with trait anxiety as measured by scales such as the IPAT Anxiety, the Taylor Manifest Anxiety, and the Spielberger State-Trait scales. Daley, Bloom, Deffenbacher, and Stewart (1983) provided even more support using trait anxiety measures over a seven week follow-up. The clients were volunteers with complaints of general anxiety who scored in the upper 15th percentile on the Spielberger Trait Anxiety Inventory, that is, with scores greater than 44 on this scale. The study also had the objective of determining whether a small group treatment format, with no more than 11 clients per group, or a large group format, involving 22 students in a single group, had differential treatment outcomes. There were a total of 22 students in the small group intervention format, and 20 students assigned to a wait-list control group. The AMT treatment was conducted once a week, for 60 minutes per session, over seven weeks. In addition to the Spielberger Trait Anxiety Scale, the Psychological Screening Inventory, a measure of neuroticism, was also administered (Lanyon, 1973). This measure included scores on discomfort/ distress.

Results on the Trait Anxiety Inventory demonstrated that significant reductions occurred for the small group format AMT clients, such that their posttest scores were lower than that of the wait-list clients (39.1 versus 46.7). At seven week follow-up these gains were maintained, with the mean for the small group format being 38.9 compared to 45.1 for the wait-list clients. This finding led the authors to conclude that post-treatment "consolidation" of treatment outcomes is a positive consequence of AMT. Although the large group format clients showed some evidence of reductions in trait anxiety, the levels were not substantial enough to distinguish them from the reductions over time observed in the untreated wait-list group (posttest mean = 43.6; follow-up = 42.2). In addition, formal feedback from the clients in the large group format indicated that these clients were less pleased at the size of their group than the small group clients. Furthermore, more large group format clients missed sessions (an average of one session). Regarding the value of a large group format as a more efficient treatment approach, Daley, Bloom, Deffenbacher, and Stewart (1983) concluded that "increasing group size was. . . a failure" (p. 107). Nevertheless, we should not lose sight of the fact that the "small" group size was still reasonably efficient in that up to 11 clients were, in fact, treated simultaneously. Finally, they also reported reduction on the discomfort subscale of the neuroticism measure.

Hutchings, Denney, Basgall, and Houston (1980) also treated students with high general anxiety. However, they added a placebo control group as well as measures of maladaptive cognitions. The clients were volunteer university students who scored during prescreening in the upper 15th percentile on both the Taylor Manifest Anxiety Scale and the Neuroticism Scale from the Eysenck Personality Inventory (Eysenck & Eysenck, 1968). Prior to assignment to treatment, these students were again screened with the two scales, and only those retained who again scored within the upper 15th percentile. In addition to these scales, other outcome measures included the Anxiety Symptom Checklist which assesses the frequency, intensity, and level of interference of 40 physical and psychological symptoms of anxiety (Nicoletti, 1972), and the Digits Backward subscale of the Wechler Adult Intelligence Scale given under stress instructions. During the Digits Backward, pulse rate, blood volume, skin resistance, and blood pressure readings were obtained. Another performance measure of stress was the Anxiety Performance Test, which consisted of 24 anagram, analogy, and multiple-choice items, also administered under stressful instructions. Hence, the numbers of digits backward recalled, the physiological data during digit span recall, and the score on the Anxiety Performance Test were all considered as performance measures of stress or anxiety. Self-report measures of anxiety involved both Spielberger's Trait and State Anxiety Inventories. Finally, the Cognitive Coping Questionnaire was designed to assess negative cognitions during the various tasks. Follow-up testing was conducted 12 months later with the Taylor Manifest Anxiety Scale, the Neuroticism Scale, and the Anxiety Symptom Checklist.

The final sample was composed of 70 students. Treatment was conducted in groups of five-seven students apiece, meeting once a week for 75 minutes per meeting, across six weeks. The placebo control group was "fashioned after T-scope therapy (Marcia, Rubin, & Efram, 1969). Subjects were shown six one-hour videotaped programs dealing with topics relating to psychology (e.g., depression, sex roles, aggression). Vaguely distinguishable images of people's faces, blurred movement, fire, etc., were superimposed on the tapes for random intervals of 1–1.5 seconds. . . Subjects were told that subliminal frames containing a variety of anxiety-provoking stimuli had been implanted in the tapes. . . to 'unconsciously extinguish' the subjects' anxiety" (p. 184). A relaxation-only treatment group was also included, involving only relaxation instructions, and homework practice in relaxing, but no instructions on the active use of relaxation for coping with anxiety. Finally, a no treatment control group was used to obtain pretest, posttest, and follow-up data only.

A number of results were significant in confirming the efficacy of AMT. First, the AMT group of clients scored significantly lower on posttest than clients in the relaxation-only, placebo or untreated groups on the Trait Anxiety Inventory, and the Neuroticism Scale (see Table 2.2). The AMT group continued to have the lowest scores on these two scales during the one year follow-up. Although not statistically significant, the AMT group's Manifest Anxiety Scale posttest scores were still lower than the levels of any of the other groups, a finding which continued through follow-up. Second, the AMT clients also received significantly lower posttest scores than the untreated controls on the frequency, and intensity subscales of the Anxiety Symptom Questionnaire, and lower scores on the interference subscale than the untreated controls and the placebo groups. These scores for the AMT group continued to be the lowest for all groups at one year follow-up. Third, although no significant differences were found across groups on the Anxiety Performance Test, the AMT group showed lower state anxiety than the untreated control subjects while taking this performance measure of stress. Fourth, although the physiological results did not reach significance, the AMT group reported lower anxiety during the digits span stress task, and achieved higher recall than the control groups. Finally, the AMT group exhibited the least amount of ineffective cognitions during the stress tasks than the control groups (AMT = 14%; relaxation-only = 60%; placebo = 57%; untreated control = 33%).

In other words, using a stringent screening method, Hutchings, Denney, Basgall, and Houston (1980) confirmed that AMT helped in reducing general anxiety, state anxiety during a laboratory stressor condition, and in improving performance on a task under stress. In addi-

Table 2.2. Means[a,b] from AMT for General Anxiety versus Relaxation, Placebo, and Control Group

Measure		Anxiety Management Training ($N = 14$)	Relaxation only ($N = 10$)	Placebo ($N = 14$)	Untreated control ($N = 10$)
Manifest Anxiety	Posttest	10.6	14.4	12.6	13.4
Scale	Follow-up	6.8	10.6	9.1	14.7
State/Trait-trait score	Posttest	57.9	63.2	63.9	67.4
State/Trait-state score	Posttest	38.7	45.4	46.6	53.7
Anxiety Symptom Scale:					
Frequency	Posttest	89.8	96.0	100.8	109.8
	Follow-up	70.9	90.4	81.3	99.9
Intensity	Posttest	86.2	86.3	94.2	99.6
	Follow-up	70.5	81.4	73.4	101.7
Interference	Posttest	68.4	74.3	81.6	89.6
	Follow-up	62.0	69.4	66.1	88.0
Anxiety Performance Test	Posttest	15.4	15.2	13.5	14.9
Neuroticism Scale	Posttest	12.7	16.1	16.5	17.3
	Follow-up	8.6	14.4	11.8	14.8

[a]Reprinted with permission from *Behaviour Research and Therapy, 18,* D. Hutchings, D. Denney, J. Basgall, and B. Houston, "Anxiety management and applied relaxation in reducing general anxiety." Copyright 1980 by Pergamon Press. Adapted by permission.
[b]Lower scores indicate lower anxiety or neuroticism.

tion, the AMT group showed continued reductions in neuroticism measures over time. Interestingly, although physiological measures did not differentiate across groups, the measure of disturbing cognitions and maladaptive preoccupations showed a greater reduction for the AMT group than the placebo group over a one-year follow-up period. This finding raised the possibility that AMT might have effects on cognitive activities, even though AMT had been initially theorized to be solely a physiologically oriented or behaviorally oriented form of therapy. On the other hand, it is historically interesting that both Michael Mahoney and Donald Meichenbaum, just prior to this period (around 1974), suggested to me that AMT was really classifiable as a form of cognitive behavioral therapy. I confess not being ready to share their perspective, since the AMT procedure emphasized situational cues, and physical or physiological signs of anxiety, but had not yet incorporated any instructions involving cognitions. As we shall see in our chapter describing the current AMT method, AMT now does involve cognitive components as a result of Mahoney's and Meichenbaum's viewpoints and Hutchings *et al.*'s types of findings.

Another study from Deffenbacher *et al.* (1980) deserves being cited for its unusual approach to AMT as a treatment providing general anxiety control, or as a "nonspecific" behavior therapy for anxiety control (the initial title of my first AMT publication). He selected persons who were either suffering from test anxiety or speech anxiety. Test anxious clients were those defined as scoring in the upper 10th percentile on the Debilitating scale of the Achievement Anxiety Scale (Alpert & Haber, 1960). Speech-anxious clients were those defined as scoring in the upper 14th percentile on the Personal Report of Confidence as a Speaker (Paul, 1966). Included in the outcome measures were measures of trait anxiety, state anxiety, worry, emotionality, and for the test-anxious subjects, semester grades in a Psychology course and performance on a digit symbol test. The innovation involved combining the test-anxious with the speech anxious clients in the same AMT group, labeled the "heterogeneous AMT group" for this research report. If AMT was indeed nonspecific in format, then clients suffering from different types of anxiety conditions should be equally treatable under a single group format. As comparison groups, Deffenbacher *et al.* also provided a no-treatment control group, and "homogeneous AMT groups," that is, AMT treatment groups with either only test-anxious clients or public-speaking-anxious clients. The AMT treatment was conducted once a week, for 50-minute sessions, over six weeks. Follow-up testing was also obtained seven weeks after termination of treatment.

Results involved analysis of covariance, with pretreatment scores covaried against posttreatment and follow-up scores. For clients suffering from test anxiety, both heterogeneous and homogeneous AMT groups were similar in leading to significantly lower debilitating anxiety, state anxiety, and emotionality than observed in the control group. There were no significant differences between the AMT groups and the controls on grades, the performance task, or worry scores; however, the AMT clients tended to achieve a higher semester grade than the controls (grades of B for both AMT groups, compared with C+ for the control group). By follow-up, again both AMT groups showed significantly lower Spielberger Trait Anxiety scores than the control group. On the Fear Inventory, the homogeneous AMT clients reported lower scores at follow-up than the heterogeneous AMT clients. For clients suffering from speech anxiety, both AMT groups exhibited greater reduction in speech anxiety as compared with the control group. In addition, the heterogeneous group were significantly less speech anxious than the homogeneous AMT clients.

Deffenbacher *et al.* adopted a conservative attitude in interpreting their findings. Thus, they recommended heterogeneous AMT, even though homogeneous AMT also seemed effective with speech anxiety. Nevertheless, they preferred the heterogeneous approach "since heterogeneous AMT was effective and has the potential for rapid, flexible service delivery to large numbers of clients" (p. 633). With the forming of heterogeneous groups, these results added another piece of documentation that AMT was really a nonspecific approach to anxiety reduction, and hence had general applications, in contrast to the narrow focus of desensitization. It might be noted that the study failed to find significant differences in worry and negative distractions; although the AMT groups did show lower worry scores on follow-up than the control group (heterogeneous AMT = 9.1; homogeneous AMT = 9.5; control = 10.9).

At this point, all of the studies involved treating persons who, although showing elevated general anxiety, were still not considered as representative of psychiatric patients. The critical test of the efficacy of AMT with general anxiety still needed research with psychiatric patients. Berghausen (1977) extended the research sample from university students to a highly anxious adult sample, although these were still only volunteers responding to a research project and not diagnosed patients. The subjects were individuals from the San Francisco Bay area responding to newspaper, radio, and other announcements of the availability of a research program for controlling general anxiety. Potential clients were interviewed and considered appropriate if they reported both cognitive and physiological symptoms of anxiety, such as catastrophic ideation and gastrointestinal disturbances, sufficiently severe to impair day-to-day functioning, for instance, causing the person to miss work. Excluded were volunteers reporting a history of psychiatric hospitalization, use of major tranquilizers, or symptoms suggestive of psychosis. Among the instruments used were the IPAT Anxiety Scale, the Spielberger Trait Anxiety Inventory, the Spielberger State Anxiety Inventory, and a revised version of the Profile of Mood States (McNair, Lorr, & Droppleman, 1971). The clients were seen for six 45-minute sessions over a 3-week period. A placebo control group was also conducted involving lectures on sources of anxiety (irritation, hopelessness, expectancies, restraint, and obligations), and encouragement to seek behaviors to reduce feeling overburdened and to improve relationships. AMT treatment and placebo treatment were presented through audiotapes, played with the therapist present.

Berghausen's data found that the AMT volunteers showed a statistically significant reduction from pretest to posttest on all four scales: the IPAT, trait and state measures, and the mood scale. However, the level of improvement turned out to be similar to that achieved by the placebo group, except on the state anxiety measure, on which the AMT group scored lower than the placebo subjects. One possible interpretation is that AMT was not effective, if one also assumes that the placebo treatment was truly an inert method. However, Berghausen compared his results on the IPAT with the report by Edie, which had also used the same scale. In Edie's sample, pretest IPAT scores for the three AMT groups were similar to the pretest score of Berghausen's: Edie AMT I = 47.2; AMT II = 39.7; AMT III = 49.3; Berghausen = 46.2. On posttesting, the Berghausen results were nearly identical with those achieved in Edie's study: Berghausen = 41.1; Edie AMT I = 40.0; AMT II = 36.3; AMT III = 41.3. In comparison, whereas the pretest to posttest changes in IPAT scores for Edie's wait-list control group was 1.90 points, the reduction from pretest to posttest for Berghausen's placebo group was found to be 3.43. All of which led Berghausen to maintain that AMT did show active treatment results in reducing general anxiety, but that the placebo procedure appeared also to have active treatment outcomes. Berghausen also examined his data in terms of the percentage of his clients showing anxiety reduction benefits from AMT versus placebo, and reports the following: IPAT = 79% of AMT, 64% of placebo; trait anxiety = 93% versus 86%; state anxiety = 86% versus 64%; mood = 64% versus 64%. Finally, Berghausen added a comment on an especially beneficial clinical outcome in one case of a person who "experienced a virtual cessation of debilitating headaches by the end of AMT treatment" (p. 154). In essence, if we accept Berghausen's interpretation of the placebo data, then his study could be viewed in perspective as an early success of AMT with subjects other than university students. However, it was Shoemaker who eventually studied the efficacy of AMT on an actual client population.

    Shoemaker's (1976) sample consisted of 60 community mental health clients diagnosed as anxiety neurotics (the prior nomenclature for generalized anxiety disorder) and who also scored above the 75th percentile on the IPAT test. Excluded were any patients who were already receiving either psychotherapy or medication. As part of the study, patients were randomly assigned to AMT training, implosive therapy, placebo, or wait list groups. The placebo treatment method was the same procedure described previously in our discussion of the Berghausen study but involving five meetings. The implosive therapy procedure was based upon the method used by Prochaska (1971), which relied upon three 23-minute-long general anxiety situations. Such scenes were revised to be less geographically specific than Prochaska's original procedure, and evaluated by personal communication by Prochaska (1975) and Sipprelle (1975) as being suitable for implosion. In order to standardize the treatment instructions, all sessions involved audiotaped presentations with the therapist also present. All sessions were conducted as individual sessions, for a total of five sessions over a two-week period. In the event that a patient was observed to become acutely anxious or agitated during the taped sessions, the therapist was ready to intervene with supportive help. However, such intervention never proved necessary. Instruments that were used involved the IPAT Anxiety Scale and the Spielberger Trait Anxiety Inventory and the Spielberger State Anxiety Inventory. Follow-up data were also obtained 30 days after the study ended.

Results confirmed that the AMT clients showed significant reductions on the IPAT, trait anxiety, and state anxiety in comparison with the implosive therapy, placebo, and wait-list groups. Specifically, pretest to posttest changes on the IPAT, trait, and state anxiety scales dropped no more than two points on any of these scales for the implosion, placebo, or wait-list clients. In contrast, the AMT clients reduced their IPAT scores from 47.2 to 40.5, their trait anxiety scores from 52.6 to 43.8 (see Figure 2.3), and their state anxiety scores from 52.0 to 41.9. The most dramatic reduction clinically appears to be represented by the trait and state anxiety scores. The trait anxiety showed reduction from a mean which initially was at the 67th percentile on psychiatric norms to the 41st percentile; while the state anxiety fell from the 63rd percentile to the 34th percentile. The IPAT values decrease of 6.7 points proved to be statistically significant, and compared favorably with Edie's wait-list control group which showed only a 1.9 point decrease. The gains made by the AMT group also appeared to be maintained during the one-month follow-up period.

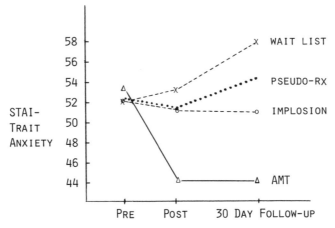

Figure 2.3. AMT and anxiety neurosis. (Adapted from Shoemaker, 1976.)

In his clinical interviews following the completion of the study, Shoemaker uncovered some fascinating clinical observations during his interviews of patients. A number were now seeking therapy, not for general anxiety attacks, but instead for more specifically identified problems, such as deficits in interpersonal skills. In fact, after additional diagnostic interviews six patients were rediagnosed with the following classifications: two were now considered suffering from "social maladjustment," one considered "adjustment reaction of adult life," a fourth as "marital maladjustment," a fifth as "nonspecific condition," and the sixth as "no mental disorder." Of course, all of these had initially been diagnosed at the beginning of the study as suffering from "anxiety neurosis."

Shoemaker's first conclusion was of course that AMT appeared to be successful to the degree that the anxiety symptoms were no longer the major presenting features of these clients, as reflected by the change in their diagnoses. However, the interesting additional finding was the uncovering of more specific complaints. Shoemaker speculated that the AMT success enabled the clients to reduce the extreme anxiety that had blocked efforts to develop adaptive behaviors. Once this anxiety was controlled, the clients were either able to develop insights and identify other, lesser problems, or finally to be able to confront problems that had originally contributed to the prior anxiety. Without the threat of uncontrollable anxiety recurring, the clients could more directly deal with deficiencies. This finding is quite similar to the observations by Edie, in which he noticed a greater openness, self-disclosure, and willingness to go into depth on personal conflicts following AMT treatment. Nicoletti had comparable experiences with his clients when he noticed that: "An interesting indirect result of treating generalized anxiety with AMT is the expression of other feelings. . . after the treatment sessions [such as]. . . anger, sex and insecurity. One possible explanation for the expression of other feelings could center around the fact that anxiety was reduced which made possible the expression of some of the less acceptable feelings" (p. 109). Nicoletti also added the same speculation that was also stated by Edie: "If having Ss express other emotions is a common result of AMT treatment, then the technique itself would have some potential value as an adjunct to psychotherapy. AMT could contribute to the therapeutic process by decreasing inhibitions caused by anxiety" (p. 109). This foresight will later prove to be accurate as our history of interesting research findings unfolds, with actual confirmation for Nicoletti's and Edie's suggestions coming in a report by Van Hassel, which we will describe later.

Continuing our review of the studies on psychiatric outpatients, Jannoun, Oppenheimer, and Gelder (1982) also worked with patients from a psychiatric hospital, whose major complaints involved generalized anxiety. Clinical researchers were apparently developing confidence in AMT and willing to test its efficacy with real patients in real settings. The reputation of AMT was also spreading internationally. In fact, the Jannoun *et al.* study was supported from a research grant from the Medical Research Council of the United Kingdom, and was conducted at the Warneford Hospital in England. The patients studied represented a group with complex symptoms, including agoraphobia, panic, depression, and substance abuse. However, the primary symptoms of the 26 patients were those of severe generalized anxiety and panic attacks. Patients were all eventually placed in an AMT treatment group, but varying in the length of time they waited for treatment to start. During the waiting period, which was at least one month, a baseline was obtained on several measures. The data from these periods were then used to form data for essentially a wait-list group. Assessments involved the Leeds Self-Assessment for Anxiety and Depression scales (Snaith, Bridge, & Hamilton, 1976), the Spielberger Trait Anxiety Inventory, and psychiatric assessments of anxiety and depression by an independent psychiatric observer. Follow-up data were obtained four weeks and 10 weeks after treatment. AMT treatment involved five treatment sessions over a six-week period, followed by one "booster" session six weeks after the termination of treatment.

Results on the Leeds subscale on anxiety, the trait anxiety scale, and the judge's rating of anxiety all showed significant reductions from pretreatment to posttreatment. These reductions were also maintained at the two follow-up periods, with a slight trend for the anxiety levels to fall to an even lower level by the 10-week follow-up period. In contrast, no reductions at all were found for the wait-list group over the four-week period. Although depression was not the focus of treatment, the various depression scores (Leeds, judge-ratings) also showed significant reductions following treatment. Again these were maintained at follow-up and seemed to be further reduced between the four- and 10-week follow-up periods (see Figure 2.4). A rather impressive finding was the substantial reduction of reliance upon anxiety medication by the patients. Prior to AMT treatment, 22 of the 26 patients were regularly taking anxiolytic drugs. Just prior to AMT, five stopped their medications and three decreased, leaving 14 who were still taking drugs. By the end of AMT treatment, 15 patients had now stopped taking medications, six were now showing a decrease, and only five remained the same on medication levels. Overall, there was a 60% decrease in medication usage following treatment and throughout follow-up.

Of related interest is the work of Brown (1980) with community mental health patients who had previously been hospitalized for psychiatric reasons. Brown does not identify the specific diagnoses connected

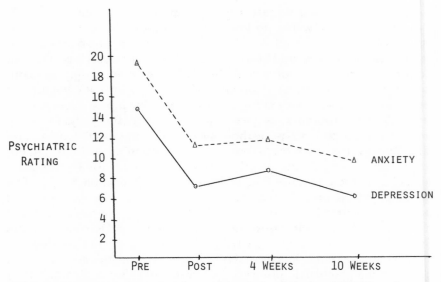

Figure 2.4. Observer ratings of anxiety and depression following AMT. (From Jannoun, Oppenheimer, & Gelder, 1982.)

with such hospitalization, but did report that the AMT group's mean number of hospitalizations was 2.9 for a mean time in the hospital of 11.5 months. A total group of 40 patients were involved in the treatment study, as well as 20 county employees who represented a no problem control group. Although the patients were not specifically selected for a diagnosis of generalized anxiety disorder, it is clear from the test data that the patients were clinically anxious, scoring on the IPAT Anxiety Scale higher than the mean of diagnosed anxiety neurotics (Krug, Scheier, & Cattell, 1976). Other instruments used in assessment included the Fear Survey Schedule (Wolpe & Lang, 1964), the Rathus Assertiveness Schedule (Rathus, 1973), and the Tennessee Self-Concept Scale (Fitts, 1964). Records on rehospitalization were also examined as part of outcome analyses. These hospital records were searched one year after posttesting to determine the number of patients who had been rehospitalized. Posttesting was also accomplished three months after termination of treatment.

The interventions involved two types. A 'coping skills training' intervention was made up of AMT, social skills and assertive training, and discussions of self-reinforcement principles. This coping skills group of 10 clients per group met twice a week for ninety minutes and covered 10 weeks. The AMT component of the intervention actually comprised one-third of the treatment, being conducted over sessions one through seven. Social and assertive skill training was conducted in sessions eight through fifteen, and self-reinforcement was covered in sessions 16 through 20. In addition to the no problem control group, an intervention control group was also formed. This was a "group therapy control group" which involved discussions by clients regarding their problems with anxiety, interpersonal relationships, feelings of self-confidence, and lack of personal control. Although this group was considered a control group, its characterisics were actually similar to traditional group therapy, including the stated goal of achieving insights.

Results showed that gains in anxiety reduction by the behavioral coping skills group were significantly greater than for the verbal psychotherapy group at posttesting on the IPAT, the Fear Survey Schedule, and the Rathus Assertiveness Schedule. Although scores on the Tennessee Self-Concept Scale also improved for the coping skills group, the level of improvement was equivalent to that of the group therapy clients. On three month follow-up, the coping skills group's gains continued to be maintained, with their levels of anxiety and assertiveness again significantly better than that of the group therapy clients.

Brown was also interested in determining whether the level of improvement of the coping skills group reached a clinically significant level. He pointed out that statistical significance need not mean that the patients were clinically recovered. In order to determine this, he compared the test scores of the treated clients against the scores of the no problem control group. He first discovered that the IPAT scores of the coping skills group decreased to a mean which was equivalent to that of a normal group (the coping group decreased from 50.9 on pretest to 29.8 on posttest). Brown then calculated the percentage of coping skills group and group therapy group clients who scored within one standard deviation of the means of the normal control subjects on each test. Chi square analyses confirmed that a greater percentage of coping skills clients improved to a "normal" level as compared with the group therapy clients, on the IPAT and Rathus Assertiveness Scale.

Specifically, 80% of the coping skills clients showed normal scores on the IPAT compared with 20% of the group therapy clients at posttesting. Similarly, 70% of the coping skills group achieved normal scores on the Fear Survey Schedule, as contrasted with 50% of the group therapy clients. These differences were also maintained at follow-up. For example, 78% of the coping group maintained a normal IPAT score three months later, compared with 36% of the group therapy persons; 72% of the coping group maintained normal Fear Survey Schedule scores at follow-up versus 52% of the group therapy clients.

Finally, hospitalization records showed that the behaviorally treated patients showed a much lower rate of rehospitalization for psychiatric reasons than the psychotherapy patients, one year after treatment. Only one (5%) of the coping skills clients was rehospitalized for psychiatric reasons as compared to seven (35%) of the group therapy clients. Although Brown's work was not solely a test of AMT, his general findings must be viewed as adding further support to the value of AMT found by studies on AMT alone. Furthermore, his data on one year follow-up are also quite consistent with other research we have cited that demonstrated the ability of AMT-treated clients to maintain their gains from therapy.

One dramatic final study is deserving of mention even though the patients were not suffering from generalized anxiety disorder. Van Hassel, Bloom, and Gonzales (1982) were interested in the application of AMT with a psychiatric patient population that was severely disturbed, but with anxiety as a major complicating factor. They selected chronic schizophrenic patients whose test results indicated high levels of anxiety. The patients were 39 outpatients at a Veterans Administration hospital in Colorado, all of whom had been diagnosed as suffering from a schizophrenic disorder. Of these, 62% had been diagnosed as of the chronic undifferentiated type, 28% as paranoid, and the remaining 10% as representing other forms of schizophrenic disorders. Given the seriousness of the disorder, most of the patients (that is, 72%) were either on antipsychotic or tranquilizing medications. All patients were also being continued in traditional psychotherapy; hence this study examined the role of AMT as an adjunct to psychotherapy. Assessments included the Spielberger Trait Anxiety Inventory, and ratings by the patient's therapist on variables such as level of anxiety, ability to work effectively in psychotherapy, ability to manage anger, ability to achieve personal goals, ability to manage emotions, and psychiatric status. Anxiety levels were rated based both on reported anxiety as well as anxiety symptoms observed by the therapist. The therapists providing the ratings were blind for the conditions of the research.

Patients were assigned to one of three groups: an AMT group, an applied relaxation group, and a wait-list control group. The AMT group of three to eight patients convened for 45 minutes once a week for six weeks. The applied relaxation group was similar to AMT in training the patients in the application of relaxation to controlling anxiety, once aroused. Its main difference from AMT, however, was that AMT used stressful scenes for practicing anxiety control, whereas the applied relaxation group relied upon naturally occurring *in vivo* conditions during homework assignments.

A major initial concern was that the anxiety arousal step of AMT might precipitate further symptoms, or that the reliance on imagery would precipitate fantasy symptoms. However, Van Hassel *et al.* were quickly reassured: they observed ". . . no exacerbation of psychotic symptomatology. . . by any patient in the program. Additionally, problems of poor attention and inability to utilize imaginal stimuli, reported by other researchers (Cowden & Ford, 1962; Serber & Nelson, 1971), were not noted in this study" (p. 13). Instead, ". . . most patients reported that they felt the program was of benefit to them and that they were applying anxiety management techniques to everyday stresses. Many reported a feeling of greater control over their lives as a result of the program."

In order to adjust for possible differences in pretest scores, analysis of covariance was used. Results indicated that the AMT patients' posttest adjusted treatment means were significantly lower than that of the wait-list group on the trait anxiety measure, on ratings of subjective anxiety level, overt anxiety level, and overall psychiatric status. The applied relaxation group did as well, although the AMT patients' results were typically in the direction of greater improvement. For instance, 86% of the AMT group improved on ratings of observed anxiety, compared with 50% of the applied relaxation group; 71% of the AMT group improved on the trait anxiety scale compared with 57%; and 64% of the AMT group improved on anger control verus 43% of the applied relaxation group. Regarding emotions and anger, the results on the ratings on ability to manage emotions were not significant, but both treated groups showed significant improvement on ratings regarding the ability to manage anger. The treatment groups also showed significant improvements in the ability to reach personal goals.

Given the prior speculations of Edie and Nicoletti regarding the use of AMT as an adjunct to psychotherapy, the therapists' ratings on their patients' ability to work effectively in psychotherapy was of great interest. The findings showed that the AMT group and the applied relaxation group were both rated as having improved in psychotherapy as compared to the wait list group of patients. In other words, the earlier predictions by Edie and Nicoletti regarding the value of AMT as a means of helping patients become more open in psychotherapy appears to have been substantiated by Van Hassel et al.'s findings. In addition, following the initial study, the wait-list patients were provided with AMT treatment. Results on subjective anxiety and overt anxiety confirmed the findings of the initial group. In addition, the treated wait-list group also showed positive gains on their ability to achieve personal goals, an activity again pertinent to progress in psychotherapy.

The Van Hassel et al. study was considered an important landmark because it appears to remove a doubt about how severe a patient population can be and still show positive response to AMT. Taking all the studies on psychiatric patients into account, it now seemed that AMT helps rather than exacerbates generalized anxiety disorder patients, that schizophrenic patients can learn AMT skills and complete training without developing side reactions, and that AMT has not only direct benefits in anxiety reduction for patients, but also added benefits such as being a useful adjunct to psychotherapy, and relieving depression and neuroticism. Unlike many other research studies, Van Hassel *et al.* also obtained brief reports from patients on their reactions to the AMT experience. In addition to the expected comments on the relevance of AMT for anxiety control, some of the more interesting patient quotations were as follows: "It has lessened my fear of losing control"; "This skill (I've learned) appears like the ability of some others to be relaxed and unflappable no matter what. I always thought you were born with it"; ". . . I can think better (now) and problems that seemed overwhelming are not so overwhelming to me anymore"; "(AMT generated) self-confidence in creating a clear mind and subdued body pain" (Van Hassel, 1979, p. 24).

Summary

This chapter reviews the prior and current history of AMT. It was initially designed in response to the need for a treatment appropriate for generalized anxiety disorder. The earliest study to test the efficacy of AMT involved a conservative design with mathematics anxiety as the problem area being treated. With the success of this initial study, the AMT procedure was immediately revised to utilize only imagery to achieve anxiety arousal, and only relaxation to achieve anxiety reduction. The use of external, artificial aids for anxiety arousal, such as phonograph records and the use of competency imagery for anxiety reduction were eliminated from the AMT steps.

The research that followed tended to have the same pattern: focus on situational anxieties such as test anxiety, public speaking anxiety, or general anxiety in university students or clients in a university counseling center. Results continued to confirm the viability of AMT, not only when conducted over a reasonable time span, but also when offered as a briefer two-session program. Further investigations into the characteristics of AMT provided information that AMT was as effective as desensitization at post-therapy, but that AMT positive improvements seemed to continue over follow-up periods of over one year. In other words, compared to desensitization effects which stabilize, AMT led to continued reductions in anxiety over time. In addition, AMT provided gains in the reduction of general anxiety, even though clients had been under treatment for a situational anxiety.

The application of AMT for general anxiety was again initially studied with university counseling center referrals, where general anxiety was now a primary presenting problem. The first study by Edie discovered that a number of AMT clients had acquired the AMT skills so well that their application of the relaxation for coping was an automatic process. Later research actually selected subjects who were extremely high on general anxiety scales, with AMT continuing to prove itself as helpful. Hutchings *et al.* added a placebo control group and a relaxation only group, and found AMT to be superior in the reduction of trait anxiety, neuroticism and negative cognitions. Perhaps the most important findings on actual patients were those by Shoemaker, with anxiety neurotic community mental health center patients. AMT again proved superior in the reduction of both trait and state anxiety, in comparison to results from a placebo and a wait list group. Gains were of such a level that the diagnoses for these patients, initially classified as anxiety neurotics, now changed to other psychiatric categories. Additional clinical results involved the greater openness of the patients to uncovering other problems, which had been suppressed or repressed prior to the anxiety reduction. Shoemaker, Edie, and Nicoletti's views all converged on their feeling that AMT might well be having some additional side benefits beyond simple reduction of anxiety. They were observing and commenting on the value of AMT in promoting self-disclosure, more ability to confront emotional problem areas, and the release and expression of feelings.

The work of Van Hassel with anxious schizophrenics undergoing psychotherapy confirmed the speculations of Shoemaker, Edie, and Nicoletti that AMT could be a very useful adjunct to psychotherapy, through the release of feelings and the enhancing of self-insight and personal self-confrontation. Van Hassel not only demonstrated that seriously ill schizophrenics could be treated with AMT, but that the anxiety reduction was associated with improvements in the use of psychotherapy.

Overall, starting with the conservative early research with mild situation anxiety among student subjects, the history of scientific study on AMT confirms the validity of AMT. AMT appears useful not simply with situational anxieties, but also with general anxiety, including the intense level of general anxiety among mental health patients. The next chapter will review the additional findings as AMT's application is extended from situational and general anxiety cases to other anxiety conditions.

3

EVIDENCE FOR ANXIETY
MANAGEMENT TRAINING

Other Clinical
Applications of the
AMT Method

The previous chapter has reviewed the early studies on AMT and the research relevant to generalized anxiety disorder since these tested the basic validity of AMT and its premises. A number of these studies also added interesting documentation of the added strengths of AMT, such as in superior gains on follow-up to other treatment approaches, and its impact on secondary symptoms such as depression, anger, maladaptive cognitions, and general neuroticism. Additional studies have now accumulated over time which provide the evidence for the extension of AMT to other applications. Essentially, such applications all have the common foundation in viewing AMT as a valuable means for treating anxiety where anxiety is the foundation of the client's problem. This chapter will offer a discussion of results whereby AMT has been applied to such other anxiety conditions. Table 3.1 summarizes the various applications of AMT, while Table 3.2 highlights some of the results of outcome studies.

Behavioral Medicine

In these applications, the assumption is that anxiety and stress form the origins of the physical symptoms. Illustrations include hypertension, ulcers, dysmenorrhea, diabetes, and the Type A behavioral pattern associated with heart disease.

Table 3.1. Applications of AMT

General anxiety:	Generalized Anxiety Disorder—psychiatric outpatients
	General anxiety or trait anxiety-nonhospitalized clients
Situational anxiety:	Test anxiety
	Mathematics anxiety
	Public speaking
	Stuttering
	Social anxiety
Performance anxiety:	Music performance
	Theater or dance
	Athletic performance
Behavioral medicine:	Essential hypertension
	Diabetes mellitus
	Duodenal ulcers
	Dysmenorrhea
	Type A behavioral pattern
Maladaptive cognitions:	Depressive beliefs
	Negative self-evaluation
	Maladaptive cognitions or coping
	Vocational indecision
Unique patient groups:	Anxious schizophrenics
	Anxious delinquents
	High anger clients
	Minority adolescents

Hypertension

Jorgensen, Houston, and Zurawski (1981) demonstrated significant reductions in systolic and diastolic pressure under a stressful task for AMT patients when compared to a control group. Following the initial case report by Suinn and Bloom (1978), which we will describe shortly, this was the first controlled research study on AMT and hypertension. The subjects were patients in the hypertension clinic of a Veterans Administration center in Kansas. Clients had been diagnosed as suffering from essential hypertension before age 55, and were free of any psychiatric diagnosis. The age criterion was to rule out any hypertension that might have been a function of aging. Twenty-one patients were randomly assigned to either an AMT group or a wait-list group. The AMT group was made up of from three to five patients, lasted 75 minutes per session, convened once a week for six weeks. Except for one patient, all were still taking medications for hypertension.

Blood pressure was measured under resting and under a stress condition. The measurements were obtained with a Narco Bio-Systems Automatic Cycling Cuff, recorded on a Narco Bio-Systems Physiograph. The mild stress condition involved verbally identifying the color of ink

Table 3.2. Outcome Studies Involving Anxiety Management Training

Study	Sample	Outcome[a,b]
Situation-specific Test anxiety:		
Deffenbacher & Shelton (1978)	Test anxiety (college)	AMT = SD, test anxiety AMT = SD, general fearfulness AMT > SD, trait anxiety
Deffenbacher & Michaels (1981a)	Test and speech anxiety (college)	1-year follow-up of Deffenbacher, Michaels, Daley, & Michaels (1980), (MAMT = HMAT) > C test and speech anxiety AMT > C general anxiety on one of two measures HAMT = MAMT = C grade point average
Deffenbacher & Michaels (1981b)	Test anxiety (college)	15-month follow-up of Deffenbacher, Michaels, Michaels, & Daley (1980), (AMT = SCSD) > C test anxiety and general anxiety
Deffenbacher, Michaels, Daley, & Michaels (1980)	Test and speech anxiety (college)	For test-anxious subjects, (HMAT = MAMT) > C, test anxiety, general anxiety, and state test anxiety in performance analog HAMT = MAMT = C, performance analog and introductory psychology grades For speech-anxious subjects, MAMT > HAMT > C, speech anxiety MAMT > C, general anxiety MAMT = HAMT = C, introductory psychology grades
Richardson & Suinn (1973b)	Test anxiety (university)	SD > accelerated AMT = accelerated SD > C, test anxiety SD = AMT accelerated = accelerated SD, general fearfulness
Speech anxiety: Nicoletti (1971)	Public speaking (university counseling center)	AMT > C, public speaking anxiety, AMT = No problem control, public speaking anxiety
Resick, Wendig- gensen, Ames, & Meyer (1978)	Chronic stutterers	No control, multiple baseline Post > pretest, conversation, reading, telephone conversation 6-month follow-up > pretest, conversation, reading
Mathematics anxiety: Richardson & Suinn (1973a)	Math anxiety (counseling center)	AMT = accelerated SD = SD > C, math anxiety AMT > accelerated SD = SD = C, math performance test
Smith, Ingram, & Brehm (1983)	Math anxiety (university)	AMT = SD > C, math anxiety AMT > SD = C, math performance

(continued)

Table 3.2. (*Continued*)

Study	Sample	Outcome[a,b]
Suinn & Richardson (1971)	Math anxiety (college)	AMT = SD, math and test anxiety; SD improved math performance with AMT producing similar nonsignificant gain
Social anxiety: Hill (1977)	Social anxiety (students)	AMT = Beh Prac > C, self-esteem, social anxiety
Pipes (1982)	Social anxiety	AMT + Prac > Pr = C, self-esteem, social anxiety AMT = Prac = C, social activity AMT + Prac > C = Pr 4-week follow-up, social anxiety AMT = P = C, esteem
Generalized anxiety Brown (1980)	Community mental health (patients prior psychiatric hospitalization)	AMT + Assertiveness + Self > verbal group therapy, general anxiety, assertiveness AMT + Assertiveness + Self = verbal group, self-concept 3-month follow-up: AMT + > verbal group, general anxiety, assertiveness 1-year follow-up: AMT + > verbal group in rehospitalization
Daley, Bloom, Deffenbacher, & Stewart (1983)	Generally anxious (college)	SAMT > C, general anxiety and neuroticism SAMT = LAMT = C, personality factors and grades
Edie (1972)	General anxiety, public speaking anxiety (univ. counseling center)	AMT = no problem control > C, general anxiety, public speaking anxiety, physiological anxiety (frequency, intensity) AMT = C physiological anxiety (interference)
Hutchings, Denney, Basgall, & Houston (1980)	Generally anxious (college)	AMT > (PR = P = C), general anxiety and neuroticism AMT > C, reported physiological anxiety symptoms (AMT = RC) > C state anxiety in stress analog AMT = RC = PR = P = C, physiological arousal in analog AMT > C, general anxiety and anxiety symptoms at 1-year follow-up
Jannoun, Oppenheimer, & Gelder (1982)	Generalized anxiety and panic disorder (psychiatric outpatients)	AMT > C, general anxiety, external ratings of anxiety, and anxiety medication AMT = C, depression

Table 3.2. (*Continued*)

Study	Sample	Outcome[a,b]
Shoemaker (1976)	Anxiety neurotic patients	AMT > C,P, general anxiety, state anxiety PR = IT = C,P, general anxiety IT > PR = C,P, state anxiety IT = C,P, state anxiety
VanHassel, Bloom, & Gonzalez (1982)	Schizophrenic outpatients	(AMT = RC) > C, trait anxiety and therapist ratings of anxiety, anger, ability to work, profitability in therapy, and overall psychiatric status

Behavioral medicine
Type A behaviors:

Study	Sample	Outcome[a,b]
Baskin (1980)	Type A persons	AMT > C Type A, learned helplessness
Hart (1984)	Type A persons	AMT > C, total JAS, speed/impatience, hard-driving
Suinn, Brock, & Edie (1975)	Type A persons	AMT > C, Type A behaviors, cholesterol
Southern & Smith (1982)	Type A persons	AMT > C, trait anxiety, AMT post > pre Type A improvements
Jenni & Wollersheim (1979)	Type A persons	(AMT = CC) > C, state anxiety CC > (AMT = C), Type A behavior AMT = CC = C, general anxiety, cholesterol, and blood pressure
Kelly & Stone (1987)	Type A persons	AMT = AMT + SIT = AMT + VC, Type A behavior and cognitions AMT + SIT > AMT, anxiety reduction
Suinn & Bloom (1978)	Type A persons	AMT > C, Type A behavior, state and trait anxiety AMT = C, blood pressure, cholesterol, and triglyceride levels
Lobitz & Brammell (1982)	Type A stressed adults	Exercise > AMT = C, Type A behaviors AMT > Exercise = C, trait anxiety AMT = Exercise > C, state anxiety, systolic blood pressure AMT > Exercise = C, diastolic blood pressure

Hypertension:

Study	Sample	Outcome[a,b]
Bloom & Cantrell (1978)	Hypertension	Single case study, blood pressure decreased from hypertensive to normal level with AMT
Drazen, Nevid, Pace, & O'Brien (1982)	Borderline hypertensives	Assertiveness + RET = AMT = Info only, diastolic pressure RET = AMT > Info only, systolic pressure
Jorgensen, Houston, & Zurawski (1981)	Hypertensive (medical male outpatients)	AMT > C, resting systolic blood pressure and systolic and diastolic blood pressure recovery following a mild stressor

(continued)

Table 3.2.   *(Continued)*

Study	Sample	Outcome[a,b]
		AMT = C, resting diastolic blood pressure though difference approached significance ($p < .06$)
Miscellaneous:		
Brooks & Richardson (1980)	Duodenal ulcer (patients)	AMT + Assertiveness > P, symptom-free days, antacid medication $3\frac{1}{2}$ year follow-up AMT > P, relapse
Deffenbacher & Craun (1985)	Anxious/stressed (gynecological patients)	Multiple case study, AMT lowered general anxiety, stress reactions, physiological arousal, and gynecological symptoms, posttreatment and at 2-year follow-up
Quillen & Denney (1982)	Dysmenorrhea (patients)	AMT > C, menstrual pain, autonomic symptoms, time loss due to and interference from dysmenorrhea, and general discomfort both posttreatment and at 2-year follow-up
Rose, Firestone, Heick, & Faught (1983)	Diabetes	Multiple case study, AMT led to lower glucose levels and improved diabetic control even though no anxiety reduction reported
Emotionality and anger		
Deffenbacher, Demm, & Brandon (1986)	High general anger (college)	AMT > C, general anger, personal-situational anger, and in an analog provocation, state anger, verbal antagonism, physical antagonism and constructive coping AMT = C, daily anger level and general anxiety AMT > C, general anger and general anxiety 1-year follow-up
Hazaleus & Deffenbacher (1986)	High general anger (college)	(AMT = CC) > C, general anger, anger-related physiological arousal, daily anger levels, and in analog provocation, state anger and verbal antagonism CC > C, constructive coping in the analog and general anxiety AMT = CC = C, personal-situational anger, coping via physical antagonism and physiological arousal in the analog, and depression (AMT = CC) > C, general anger at 1-year follow-up CC > C, general anxiety at 1-year follow-up
Deffenbacher, Story, Brandon, Hogg, & Hazaleus (1988)	High anger (college)	(AMT + CC) > C, general anger, personal-situational anger, physiological arousal, and in analog, dysfunctional coping

Table 3.2. (*Continued*)

Study	Sample	Outcome[a,b]
		AMT + CC = CC = C, state anger in analog, daily anger, and outward expression of anger
		(AMT + CC = CC) > C, general anxiety
		15-month follow-up: gains maintained in general anger, personal-situational anger, physiological arousal, general anxiety
Deffenbacher & Stark (1990)	High anger (college)	(AMT = AMT + CC) > C, general anger, personal-situational anger, daily anger levels, intensity, physiological arousal, and in analog, state anger and dysfunctional coping
		(AMT + CC) > C, general anxiety
		AMT = AMT + CC = C, self-esteem
Deffenbacher, Story, Stark, Hogg, & Brandon (1987)	High general anger (college)	(AMT + CC = SS) > C, general anger, suppression of anger, outward expression of anger, and in analog, state anger and constructive coping
		(AMT + CC) > C, personal-situational anger
		AMT + CC = SS = C, physiological arousal, daily anger intensity, and general anxiety
Deffenbacher (1988)	High general anger (college)	(AMT + CC = SS) > C, general anger, personal-situational anger, arousal at 1-year follow-up
		(AMT + CC = SS) > C, general anxiety
Deffenbacher, McNamara, Stark, & Sabadell (in press a)	High anger (college)	(AMT + CC + SS) > C, general anger, outward expression of anger, physiological arousal, intensity, and in analog, verbal antagonism and constructive coping
		(AMT + CC + SS) > C, general anxiety
		(AMT + CC + SS) > C, physiological arousal and trait anxiety at 1-year follow-up
Deffenbacher, McNamara, Stark, & Sabadell (in press b)	High anger (college)	(AMT + CC = PGT) > C, general anger, anger suppression, personal-situational anger, arousal, and in analog, state anger and dysfunctional coping
		(AMT + CC = PGT) > C, general anxiety
		15-month follow-up: gains maintained in general anger, personal-situational anger, physiological arousal, and general anxiety
Problems secondary to anxiety		
Nally (1975)	Adjudicated delinquents	AMT > C, general anxiety, state anxiety, self-concept, prosocial behavior

(*continued*)

Table 3.2. *(Continued)*

Study	Sample	Outcome[a,b]
Cragan & Deffenbacher (1984)	Generally anxious/stressed (medical outpatients)	(AMT = RC) > C, general anxiety, stressful situations, physiological anxiety, depression, and hostility

Cognitive/intellective performance

Mendonca & Siess (1976)	Vocationally anxious and indecisive (college)	AMT + PS > (PS = P = C), vocational exploration AMT + PS > (AMT = PS = P) > C, problem-solving (AMT + PS = PS) > (P = C) and PS > AMT > C, information gathering AMT = PS > C, generating alternatives AMT + PS = AMT = PS = P = C, decisional and general anxiety
Thompson, Griebstein, & Kuhlenschmidt (1980)	Academic underachievement (college)	AMT = RC > C, state anxiety, somatic/cognitive anxiety (intensity) RC = AMT = C, trait anxiety, somatic/cognitive anxiety (frequency) 3-month follow-up AMT = RC > C, state anxiety, somatic/cognitive (intensity); AMT = RC = C, trait, somatic/cognitive (frequency) Fall AMT = RC > C, biofeedback-augmented AMT, RC, on GPA Spring AMT + biofeedback > C = all other therapies, on GPA

Performance enhancement

Mathis (1978)	Music students (university)	AMT > C, general anxiety, performance anxiety, performance behaviors AMT = C, audio ratings, performance behaviors
Ziegler, Klinzing, & Williamson (1982)	Athletes	AMT > C, oxygen consumption

[a]The > sign indicates significant between-group differences in the logical direction of improvement, e.g., lowering anxiety and improving performance. The = sign indicates that groups are not statistically different.

[b]AMT = anxiety management training; C = control; CC = cognitive coping skills; HAMT = homogeneous AMT (all clients in group have same presenting problem); LAMT = large group AMT ($n = 27$); MAMT = mixed AMT (clients in group have different presenting problem); P = placebo; PGT = process group therapy; PR = passive relaxation; PS = problem-solving; RC = relaxation coping skills; SAMT = small group AMT ($n = 6-7$); SCSD = self-control desensitization; SD = systematic desensitization; SS = social skills; VC = values clarification.

used to print color words displayed on colored backgrounds, the Stroop task. Follow-up measurements were also obtained six weeks after treatment.

Blood pressure results showed a significant reduction from pretest to posttest in both systolic and diastolic blood pressure for the AMT patients compared to the wait-list group. The usual definition of hypertension involves systolic over diastolic readings of 140/90. On pretest, the AMT group had readings of 139/88, which were reduced on posttest to readings of 120/77. These gains were maintained during the six-week follow-up, with systolic readings of 111 and diastolic readings of 70. No differences between groups were obtained on diastolic blood pressure under the mild stressor, although the AMT group showed higher increases on systolic pressure; on the other hand, the AMT group demonstrated the predicted greater recovery rate following the stressor on both systolic and diastolic blood pressure. In other words, AMT appeared to be helpful in reducing resting levels of blood pressure, and in increasing recovery rates during a stressor. Moreover, the improvements in level of resting blood pressure appeared to continue across time, with further reductions after six weeks.

The authors reported on some spontaneous comments made by clients during the study that indicated gains. "Four subjects reported that family members and/or coworkers had found them to be more relaxed or easier to get along with. Another subject reported that Anxiety Management Training seemed to help decrease his stuttering because the use of relaxation improved his ability to organize thoughts before speaking" (p. 473). Once again, the research data appear to lend support to our earlier conclusions that AMT can have not only long term gains, but can also generalize for coping with problems other than those identified in the original treatment plan.

Bloom and Cantrell (1978) reported on a single case study, relying upon AMT for a hypertensive, pregnant woman, for whom hypertensive medication was considered dangerous. They reported fetal mortality rates to be as high as 50% with evidence of severe hypertension; however, because of possible side effects of medication, AMT was sought as an alternative. The AMT program involved 50-minute sessions once a week over six weeks. Anxiety scenes used for anxiety arousal included receiving word of a lower than expected salary raise, and waiting in her physician's office. The client's blood pressure was taken using a standard mercury sphygmomanometer, obtained once per week for seven weeks before treatment, once per week during the six weeks of treatment, and once per week for eight weeks after treatment.

Prior to treatment, the baseline readings were 133/88; this was followed by a mean of 125/79 following treatment, and 123/81 during the follow-up. As a context, Bloom and Cantrell shared the information that a typical progression of blood pressure changes associated with pregnancy is for blood pressure to rise during the last trimester of the pregnancy to levels above that of the first trimester. The AMT program was such that the third trimester corresponded to the last four weeks of AMT treatment and posttreatment period. Hence, although the reductions in blood pressure following AMT were by themselves worthy of notice, the fact that such reductions occurred during the trimester in which blood pressure increases normally occur gave added meaning to the efficacy of AMT. As a rather nice follow-up commentary, Bloom and Cantrell report that "the client gave birth to a healthy 8 pound, 12-ounce boy. The size and health of the child were further indications that the hyptertension had been effectively controlled" (p. 381).

Suinn and Bloom (1978) did not find significant reductions in blood pressure among Type A subjects treated with AMT. However, systolic pressure did decrease by 14 mm Hg and diastolic pressure by 2.4 mm Hg for the AMT group, compared with 6.1 mm Hg systolic decrease, and 1.3 mm Hg diastolic increase for the control group. The subjects were Type A persons volunteering for a stress management program in the community. AMT was conducted in six sessions, meeting twice weekly for an hour per session. The group of 14 subjects were treated in two groups of seven per group. In addition to the reductions in blood pressure, the AMT group also showed significantly lower Spielberger Trait Anxiety Inventory and State Anxiety Inventory scores as compared with a wait-list control group. For both scales, the AMT subjects anxiety scores were reduced to a level equivalent to that for normal subjects (pretest trait = 47.5, posttest = 37.5; pretest state = 51.3, posttest 37.1).

Drazen, Nevid, Pace, and O'Brien (1982) compared AMT with a program combining rationale emotive therapy with assertive training (RET/AT). A third group was conducted as a control group, involving group discussions on blood pressure monitoring, nutrition, the value of reducing smoking and making life style changes. The groups met for 40 minutes weekly for 10 consecutive weeks. The subjects were 22 workers employed at the General Motors Building in New York City, recruited through a blood pressure screening program, as persons who were hypertensive. Blood pressures were measured prior to treatment, at the end of treatment, and at two-month follow-up. The RET/AT group showed significant reductions in both systolic and diastolic blood pressure from pre- to post- and to follow-up (systolic means = 162.5 mm Hg, 141.20, 146.2; diastolic means = 96.5 mm Hg., 85.0, 88.2). The AMT group showed reductions in blood pressure, but only the diastolic reached significance levels from pre- to post- and pre- to follow-up (systolic means = 150.3, 139.5, 137.4; diastolic means = 93.3, 86.7, 81.7). Some reductions occurred for the control subjects, but these did not reach significance (systolic means = 140.8, 128.3, 133.7; diastolic means = 90.2, 82.3, 79.3.

Ulcers

Brooks and Richardson (1980) compared a combined program of AMT and assertiveness against a placebo group for ulcer patients. The patients were 22 persons who had duodenal ulcers confirmed by X rays, and who were in treatment at a Veterans Center in Texas. Patients were using antacid medication, and their consumption was used as one outcome measure. Other measures included the Spielberger Trait Anxiety Inventory, the Constriction Scale 2 as a measure of inhibition (Bates & Zimmerman, 1971), and the Lazarus Assertiveness Questionnaire (Lazarus, 1971). In addition to the amount of use of antacids, pain ratings were also obtained as well as posttreatment X rays. The treatment program involved a combination of AMT and assertiveness training; four sessions focused on AMT, with the remaining four being involved with assertiveness training. The anxiety control segment also identified anxiety-provoking thoughts.

For instance, one patient felt that the "red tape" of his work environment frequently prevented him from doing his job properly, a situation he interpreted as a personal affront. His anxiety-producing self-verbalization were described as: "This is unfair to the patients and to me; I shouldn't be expected to tolerate this; this is tearing me apart" (p. 202). The treatment program was conducted over a two-week period, meeting in eight 60–90 minute sessions. Follow-up data were collected 60 days later, and hospital records were examined 42 months later. Half the patients were assigned to the active intervention, with the remaining half being in an "attention placebo" group. This placebo group "encouraged patients to talk about their anxieties as they related to ulcer problems but offered mainly support and a little common sense advice" (pp. 202–203).

Results on posttesting indicated that the AMT group was significantly lower than the control group on the constriction and assertiveness measures. Although the trait anxiety scores were also reduced for the AMT/assertiveness group, and these scores increased for the control group on posttesting, the differences did not reach statistical significance. Further analysis of the regression slopes suggested the conclusion that "treatment patients low on self-reported anxiety at pretesting differed little from control patients at post- and follow-up testing . . . (but) treatment patients high on anxiety at pretesting show a relatively much greater difference from the control group at post- and follow-up testing" (p. 204).

Table 3.3. AMT and Assertiveness for Ulcers

	Therapy	Pseudotherapy
Symptom-free days	36	21
Over 60 days		
Antacid consumption (oz.)	63	196
Relapse after 3½ years	1 of 9	5 of 8

On other types of data, the results demonstrated that the AMT/assertiveness group of patients experienced fewer symptomatic days, consumed less antacid medication over a 60-day period for their ulcers, and exhibited less severe pain symptoms when their symptoms did act up. In actual figures, the AMT/assertiveness group had 23.7 days during which symptoms occurred compared with 38.5 days of symptoms experienced by the control patients. In antacid consumption, the AMT/assertiveness group consumed 63.2 ounces of antacid over a 60-day period, in contrast to the 195.7 ounces used by the control patients. Only one of the AMT/assertiveness patients had to return for surgery as a result of the later seriousness of the ulcer, while five of eight control patients needed to have surgery. Of the AMT/assertiveness patients, 67% were able to reduce future hospital visits over the next 42 months to one visit or less; in contrast, 83% of the control patients became ill enough that they returned for treatment.

In other words, the various data confirmed that the AMT/assertiveness program resulted in lower levels of anxiety, increase in assertiveness, decrease in reliance upon medication, and decrease in ulcer symptoms. Furthermore, the study also confirmed the long-term value of the treatment through a three-and-half year follow-up, with only an 11% relapse rate for the therapy group but a 62% relapse for the placebo group (Table 3.3).

Dysmenorrhea

Quillen and Denney (1982) adopted AMT for training primary dysmenorrhea subjects in pain management. They hypothesized that an anxiety management program could be helpful in reducing the pain and bodily discomfort of women suffering from menstrual discomfort. Their subjects were 24 college women volunteers. Measures were the Menstrual Symptoms Questionnaire (Chesney & Tasto, 1975a) and a daily log rating pain, general discomfort, and overall interference of daily activities, as well as recording the amount of time loss from school, work, recreational/social activities. The AMT procedure was modified, with a scene of menstrual discomfort substituting for the usual anxiety

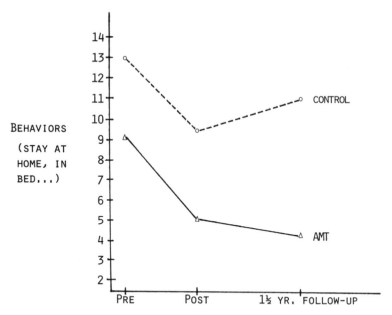

Figure 3.1. AMT effects on behavior from dysmenorrhea. (From Quillen & Denney, 1982.)

scene. An example of such a modification can be found in Chapter 10, with a case history illustrated in Chapter 5. For Quillen and Denney's study, the AMT menstrual discomfort scenes were varied, and included being in class during a lecture, on a dinner date with a boyfriend, awakening at home at night, etc. The intervention covered four two-hour individually administered treatment sessions, one week apart. Follow-up was obtained 18 months later. The women were also categorized either as spasmodic dysmenorrhea or congestive dysmenorrhea. Spasmodic dysmenorrhea involves acute pain usually confined to the pelvic region; while congestive dysmenorrhea involves more diffusely distributed, dull pains. Since Chesney and Tasto (1975b) had discovered that these two types of dysmenorrhea were differentially responsive to therapy, the classification was used for the AMT study.

Results on posttesting found that the AMT-treated women scored significantly lower than the control subjects on four outcome measures from the daily log: level of pain, overall general discomfort, intensity of interference, and amount of time loss from activities. These significant differences were maintained at 18-month follow-up on pain, discomfort, and amount of time loss, but not on interference. Similar results were obtained on the Menstrual Symptoms Questionnaire with significantly less pain and autonomic distress reported by the AMT group as compared with the control group. By 18-month follow-up, the AMT group also showed significantly lower concentration problems or behavioral changes (e.g., taking naps, staying in bed) than the control group (Figure 3.1). Improvements were equivalent for both the acute type of spasmodic dysmenorrhea and the more diffuse congestive dysmenorrhea.

Diabetes

Rose, Firestone, Heick, and Faught (1983) used AMT with juvenile diabetics on the premise that control over emotional stress would reduce metabolic dysfunction and hence stabilize glucose levels. Patients were five adolescent diabetic patients from the Diabetic Clinic of a Canadian children's hospital. All subjects had been diabetic for at least three years, with the mean age of onset of the diabetes being nine years.

The study covered a total of 150 days in order to obtain multiple baselines for each subject, inasmuch as the baselines themselves varied for each adolescent, ranging from 21 days to 54 days. In addition to the baseline condition, measures were also obtained during an attentional control condition, followed by an AMT treatment condition. During the attentional control, which ranged from 14 to 29 days, psychological testing was involved, including the Minnesota Multiphasic Personality Inventory (Hathaway & McKinley, 1967) and the Wechsler Intelligence Scale for Children-Revised (Wechsler, 1967) or the Wechsler Adult Intelligence Scale (Wechsler, 1955). The AMT condition covered seven hours of AMT over a two-week period.

The major interest was in the physiological measures of diabetes. Urine testing was conducted three times daily, with an average recorded for the day. Urine glucose was assessed with both the Diastix method and 24-hour fractional quantitative glucose method (Forman, Goldstein, & Genel, 1974). On all five patients, after AMT treatment Diastix-measured improvements in metabolic regulation shown in daily urine glucose levels were clearly significant in comparison with baseline and control condition measurements. Similar evidence of improvements were found in four of the five patients on the weekly 24-hour fractionated urine glucose analyses, ranging as high as a 69% decrease in glucose. Although the authors did attribute the improved functioning to reductions in stress, they also had an unexplained finding in that subjective reductions in anxiety were not found. Therefore their findings can be considered as promising but must still be interpreted with caution.

Type A Behaviors

The convincing material on the role of Type A behaviors in increasing risk of cardiovascular disease led Suinn, Brock, and Edie (1975) to seek a method for intervention. They hypothesized that change would only occur when stress reduction was learned by the Type A patients. A program combining AMT with behavior rehearsal was provided to patients in rehabilitation following myocardial infarctions. All patients were undergoing the same rigorously controlled exercise, dietary, and medical rehabilitation regime and were identified by the medical director as meeting Type A characteristics. Twenty patients formed the study, with 10 assigned to the behavioral training group, and 10 being a wait-list control. Lipid laboratory data provided information on cholesterol levels, and a program evaluation questionnaire was obtained at the end of treatment. Since prior research had suggested that stress was associated with increases in cholesterol levels, and since the behavioral program emphasizes AMT for control of stress, the lipid data were viewed as important outcome measures. The intervention program involved five total hours, over five weeks, meeting for about one hour per session. The behavioral rehearsal component used imagery to enable patients to rehearse alternative behaviors to their Type A behaviors, including relaxing while waiting in line to cope with impatience, and moving more deliberately, instead of rushing.

The questionnaire involved a simple evaluation of the overall program. One hundred percent indicated that the training helped them to control their tensions; 83% indicated that the program was significant in helping them change their life styles. Examples of such changes included, "I've learned. . . to delegate more authority and responsibility to my employees. . . ," "I feel that I could accomplish as much or more without the previous stress that I put on myself," "It's easier for me to cope with matters than it was. . . I don't fly off the handle at every little thing" (Suinn, 1974, p. 16).

On the lipid analyses, the treated patients showed significant reductions in cholesterol levels, while the control group showed no changes. Since both groups were in a rehabilitation center, and under strict exercise and nutrition control, the changes were interpreted as related to stress reduction. Not only was the degree of change significant for the treated group, but the level was reduced from a clinically abnormal one to a level considered within a normal range. Eight of the treated patients showed reductions in their cholesterol levels compared to five of 10 controls. Because of the success of the program, a second group of 17 patients were provided with the training. Again, results indicated substantial and statistically significant reductions in cholesterol levels, although the posttesting levels were still within the abnormal range (pretest = 262.5; posttest = 243.4).

Since the Suinn, Brock, and Edie study did not measure Type A characteristics with a standardized scale, Suinn and Bloom (1978) designed a study measuring changes in Type A behaviors through the commonly used Jenkins Activity Survey (JAS) (Jenkins, 1972). This is the same study we described previously under the section on blood pressure, inasmuch as systolic and diastolic blood pressure was also measured. Subjects represented a broad range of occupations, including municipal official, dentist, mathematician, executive secretary, farmer, and regional sales representative. Results confirmed reduction in trait anxiety, and showed reductions in blood pressure; however, the blood pressure changes did not reach statistical significance, nor did the cholesterol data (possibly due to the initially low cholesterol levels of the subjects). On the Type A scale, however, the AMT-treated subjects showed a significant reduction in the Jenkins Speed/Impatience subscale as well as on the Hard Driving/Competitive subscale score, compared to the control subjects. While the overall Type A score did not reach statistically significant levels, inspection of the data showed that the AMT-treated subjects had a reduction in their A/B total score from 11.1 to 6.8, compared to a reduction of 9.9 to 9.8 for the control sample.

Kelly and Stone (1987) screened an initial sample first with the JAS, and then with the Structured Interview, the two most reliable Type A diagnostic procedures. As an indication of the severity of these subjects' Type A behaviors, the authors reported that the median Jenkins Activity Survey Type A score was at the 97th percentile. The subjects were volunteers and involved 31 persons from a variety of occupational backgrounds, including executives, professors, sales managers, office workers, lawyers, and interior decorators. In addition to the Type A measures, subjects also were given the Spielberger Trait Anxiety Inventory, the Spielberger State Anxiety Inventory, and a thought listing task to assess cognitive coping.

Viewing AMT as "among the most popular of the behavioral approaches" (p. 47) for Type A treatment, the authors conducted three groups of treatment: AMT alone, AMT plus cognitive behavior therapy, and AMT plus values clarification. The basic AMT group involved one hour per week for six weeks. The AMT plus cognitive therapy group was exposed to three weeks of AMT, followed by six weeks of cognitive therapy training, each session being 90 minutes. The AMT plus values clarification group also started with three sessions of AMT, followed by six weeks of values training, in 90-minute sessions. The cognitive therapy approach emphasized cognitive coping strategies to Type A circumstances. The values clarification emphasized reevaluation of personal values and self-imposed standards.

Results indicated that AMT treatment alone achieved levels of reduction in Type A behaviors which were not improved upon by combining AMT with either cognitive therapy or values clarification. Specifically, all three groups achieved significant reductions in Type A scores, with none of the groups reaching a posttest level that distinguished them from another treatment group's results. Similar results were obtained for the cognitive coping measure. Regarding the anxiety measures, the AMT plus cognitive therapy treatment produced significant reductions compared to the AMT only and the AMT plus values clarification groups. The authors recognized the greater impact of the AMT plus cognitive combination if anxiety reduction was the sole issue. Nevertheless, in their discussion, they pointed out that the major goal was change in Type A behaviors of these very extreme Type A subjects. Therefore, from the standpoint of achieving Type A changes, they noted that "impressive gains were effected in 6 weeks" by AMT alone, and concluded AMT alone "to be the short-term treatment of choice" (p. 52).

An interesting extra finding of this study came from information on self-monitoring. Subjects were separated into a high self-monitoring and a low self-monitoring group. High self-monitoring involves a tendency to attend to situational cues in order to guide one's behaviors. Low self-monitoring involves lowered sensitivity and lowered responsiveness to situational cues which might indicate which behaviors are appropriate. The results indicated an interaction between self-monitoring and the effects of treatment on anxiety. High self-monitoring seemed to be facilitative in enabling the treatments to reduce anxiety levels. To my knowledge, such a finding has never been followed up by other studies. It suggests an intriguing implication which is deserving of further study. As the AMT method has been conceived, there is a major self-monitoring component built in. Clients are trained to pay attention to "how you experience anxiety." Further, through the use of anxiety imagery representing situations which prompt anxiety, clients are also trained to attend to environmental situations (leading some of them eventually to identify the specific cues that trigger their general anxiety reactions). Finally, homework is assigned which also involves monitoring. Perhaps Kelly and Stone were identifying subjects who were already sensitive monitors prior to treatment, and who hence found the tasks of treatment to be readily developed.

Hart (1984) approached the topic of Type A change indirectly. Instead of using AMT for stress management, he adopted it for anger control, on the premise that anger represented a key component in Type A behaviors. The really fascinating background for his study was that he designed it while he was still a beginning graduate student, as part of a clinical course assignment. We had conversed over the long-distance telephone about his ideas, and his results were so interesting that I encouraged him to submit it for publication in Wolpe's journal.

The subjects were volunteers who had shown high scores on the Jenkins Activity Survey scale. Five persons were in the AMT treatment group and another five were in a no-treatment control group selected with the same scale. AMT was introduced as a way of mastering stress for the benefit of protecting their physical energy reserves, since stress drained energies. The actual AMT training focused on anger, hostility, and impatience, and was conducted in 10 sessions over three and one-half weeks, each session lasting two hours.

Hart found that AMT for anger did have consequent results on Type A measures. His results confirmed the earlier results of Suinn and Bloom in reductions on the Hard Driving/Competitive and Speed/Impatience subscales of the JAS for the treated as compared to the control group. In addition, he found significantly lower total Type A/B scores for the treated as compared to the untreated group. In many ways Hart's work was a precursor of what have become current beliefs in the core role which anger/hostility plays in a Type A person's risk for heart disease. Furthermore, his is the first study to demonstrate the validity of revising AMT to provide control over anger.

The usefulness of AMT for Type A persons has also been reported by Southern and Smith (1982) who combined AMT with cognitive behavior therapy and problem solving. The subjects were 30 volunteers who were classified as Type A on the Jenkins Activity Survey. Half were assigned to a treatment group, and the other half to a no-treatment control group. The treatment was conducted weekly in 90-minute sessions, which covered five elements. The first element was information on Type A behaviors and cardiovascular disease; the second element/session involved AMT treatment; the third session introduced subjects to applied behavioral analysis for designing changes in their behaviors; the fourth element covered self-statements for coping; and the fifth covered problem-solving techniques. Measures included daily logs regarding aggressive behaviors, speed and impatience, and hard driving/competitive behaviors, and the Spielberger Trait Anxiety Inventory and the Spielberger State Anxiety Inventory. A four-week follow-up was obtained as well.

The results indicated a significant reduction in total Type A characteristics, aggressive behaviors, speed and impatience, and hard driving/competitive behaviors. These gains were maintained through the follow-up. On the trait anxiety measure, the treated subjects showed significant reductions from pretest to follow-up when compared to the control group. Although the state anxiety scores did not reach statistical significance, the treated group did show some small reductions, while the control subjects showed some small increases.

Lobitz and Brammell (1981) obtained 18 volunteers who reported themselves to be under high levels of stress. Using the Jenkins Activity Survey, subjects were stratified by Jenkins' scores, then randomly assigned to an AMT group, an exercise group, or a no-treatment control group. Other measures included the Spielberger Trait Anxiety Inventory, the Spielberger State Anxiety Inventory, blood pressure measures, and lipid laboratory measures. The AMT program involved one-hour sessions, meeting twice a week for seven weeks. The exercise program involved one hour aerobic conditioning for three times a week over seven weeks. None of the subjects showed a medical history of cardiovascular disease, hypertension, or other significant medical problems. Unlike other reports, the AMT group showed no changes in Jenkins total scores; subscale scores were not reported. However, the exercise group did show significant decreases in total A/B scores. Both AMT and excercise subjects did show significant decreases in state anxiety; however, only the AMT group showed significant decrease in trait anxiety scores. The exercise group showed a significant decrease in heart rate, while the AMT group exhibited no such changes. Both the AMT and the exercise subjects showed significant decreases in systolic blood pressure, and the AMT group showed a reduction in diastolic blood pressure which approached significance. None of the groups exhibited significant reductions in cholesterol. In their discussion, Lobitz and Brammell indicate that their findings partially supported the Suinn and Bloom research. However, Lobitz and Brammell also add the caution that their study did not have subjects who would be considered as pathological either on the Type A measure or on the anxiety measures.

Finally, Jenni and Wollersheim (1979) selected 42 volunteers screened as being Type A with the Structured Interview. Seven of the subjects had previously experienced at least one heart attack. AMT was offered one evening per week for 90-minute sessions over six consecutive weeks. Cognitive therapy was based upon cognitive restructuring, involving identifying irrational thoughts, challenging these, and substituting more reasonable ones. A wait-list control group was also formed. Several measures were used, including Bortner's Type A questionnaire, the Spielberger Trait Anxiety Inventory, the Spielberger State Anxiety Inventory, cholesterol data, and blood pressure data. A six-week follow-up was also obtained.

On the Bortner scale, only the cognitive therapy group showed a significant reduction. Both the AMT and the cognitive therapy groups showed significant reductions on trait anxiety, which were maintained during the six-week follow-up. The AMT group appeared to continue to show trait anxiety reductions across time, while the cognitive therapy group appeared to stabilize at post-testing. On state anxiety, both treatment groups showed significant reductions in state anxiety, although this was not maintained in follow-up. On cholesterol levels, the AMT group showed a significant increase, while neither the cognitive therapy nor the control group showed significant changes. Jenni and Wollesheim also reported that nine of the 10 subjects in the AMT group showed increases in their cholesterol levels. No changes were noted in blood pressure measures across time for any of the groups. The authors conclude that AMT did effect reductions in anxiety of the Type A subjects in partial support of the Suinn and Bloom study, but failed to demonstrate any effects on the Bortner measure of Type A behaviors, nor on physiological measures.

Situation-Specific Anxieties

As we discussed earlier, AMT would be expected to work favorably with phobic conditions if this treatment in fact trains persons to cope with anxiety states as a generalized treatment procedure. And certainly the initial studies with test anxiety and mathematics anxiety support this expectation. Other examples of the application of AMT have also been reported for public speaking, social anxiety, and, possibly, anxiety experienced by agoraphobics.

Speech Anxiety

Deffenbacher (Deffenbacher, Michaels, Daley, & Michaels, 1980; Deffenbacher & Michaels, 1981a,b) has been responsible for a superb series of studies which often had more than one hypothesis being tested. In these three reports, the first primary objective was to validate the applicability of AMT to speech anxiety. Since we described these studies earlier, you will recall that the Deffenbacher *et al.* (1980) project used homogeneous AMT groups in which only speech-anxious or test-anxious subjects were clustered together for treatment, and heterogeneous AMT groups, which were composed of a mixture of speech and of test-anxious subjects. The subjects were selected on the basis of having extreme scores on either a measure of debilitating test anxiety or a measure of speech anxiety. A no-treatment control group was also formed. Follow-up testing was conducted six weeks after posttesting.

Regarding speech-anxiety results, AMT clients in both homogeneous and heterogeneous groups showed significant reductions in their anxieties, compared to a control group. A second objective of the research was to continue to test the efficacy of AMT over an extended time following the end of therapy. In this case, the follow-ups were at six weeks and again after over one year (Deffenbacher & Michaels, 1981a). As with earlier studies, the AMT clients not only maintained their initial gains, but also tended to show further reductions in their anxiety levels. A third and extremely important objective was to test the usefulness of the heterogeneous treatment format, which mixed clients with different presenting problems together in one treatment group. Results on this variable demonstrated that clients in heterogeneous groups experienced recovery significantly lower than control group subjects. Furthermore, on speech anxiety the heterogenous group achieved significantly lower anxiety levels than the homogeneous group. Thus, the mean scores on the speech-anxiety measure turned out to be as follows: heterogeneous AMT—pretest = 25.2, posttest = 12.8, follow-up (six months) = 12.6, follow-up (one year) = 10.8; homogeneous AMT—pretest = 23.3, posttest = 17.0, follow-up (six months) = 14.7, follow-up (one year) = 13.6.

Resick, Wendiggensen, Ames, and Meyer (1978) combined two weeks of AMT with practice involving speaking slowly. Clients were six adults who had been stutterers since childhood and had received speech therapy at some time during their lives. The behavioral program covered 10 sessions, meeting one hour per day over two weeks. Each client was seen individually. During the first half hour of each session for the first week, AMT was practiced. In addition to the usual AMT relaxation instructions, a biofeedback apparatus measuring galvanic skin response changes was also used. This unit emitted a tone that decreased or increased in pitch as a reflection of skin-conductance changes. The biofeedback equipment was considered an optional part of actual training, although most therapists used it as a way of determining how well the clients were doing in controlling their level of relaxation. The anxiety-producing imagery used by the clients involved any experience associated with anxiety, not necessarily connected with speech situations. During the second half-hour of the first week and for the entire second week, the clients were taught systematic slow speaking. This procedure involved reading aloud from a book which had been marked off into 50-word segments. The clients were initially instructed to slow their rate of speech until it took one minute to read a passage. They were then asked to speak to the therapist at this same rate. Later, the clients were instructed to speak at a slightly higher rate until they reached the pace of 90 words per minute.

The assessment involved tape recordings of each client reading, talking to a stranger on the telephone, and having a conversation with a stranger. Dysfluencies were counted if there was a repetition of all or part of a phrase, or if there was a silent or vocal block prior to the onset of a word or syllable. Follow-up was obtained after one month, three months, and six months. The results confirmed a substantial significant reduction of dysfluent stuttering on all three tasks at the termination of therapy with the stuttering remaining low through follow-up. For instance, on the task of conversing with a stranger, the pretest showed that 23.3% of the words were stuttered; this dropped to 6.3% at posttest, and was 7.5% at one month, 4.3% at three months, and 8.7% at six months. For reading, stuttering started at 12% of the words stuttered, declined to 0.7% at posttest, was 1.5% at one month, 0.2% at three months, and 0.5% at six months follow-up. Only the telephone task failed to reflect a retention of the improvements. On this task there were initial improvements but a relapse at six months: pretest = 23.8%; posttest = 7%; one month = 11.8%, three months = 7.3%, six months = 17.2%.

Social Anxiety

Pipes (1982) combined AMT with another training, practice in social skills. AMT plus practice proved superior in anxiety reduction and increase of self-esteem. The practice in social skills, called Friendship Interaction, involved clients having to make two contacts with another member of the group whose names they were given each week. This practice went on for four weeks. The AMT plus Friendship Interaction group added one AMT group meeting each week, involving one and one-half hours of AMT training for a total of five sessions. A wait-list control group was also formed. The subjects were 73 volunteer clients who had indicated experiencing "anxieties about friendships," that is, social anxiety. The measurements used included three measures of social anxiety: the Fear of Negative Evaluation and the Social Avoidance Distress Scale (Watson & Friend, 1969), and the Social Anxiety Inventory (Richardson & Tasto, 1976). In addition, a measure of self-esteem was used, the Texas Social Behavior Inventory (Helmreich & Stapp, 1971). Follow-up was obtained after four weeks' posttreatment.

The results indicated that the AMT/Friendship Interaction group showed signficantly lower scores on the Fear of Negative Evaluation and Social Avoidance scales, and the Texas Social Behavior Inventory when compared against the Friendship Interaction group's results. In addition, the combined AMT/Friendship Interaction group was also superior in improvements on the Social Avoidance Distress scale and the Texas self-esteem scale in comparison to the control group. On follow-up, the combined AMT/Friendship Interaction group continued to be superior to the Friendship Interaction-only group on social anxiety as measured on the Fear of Negative Evaluation scale, and superior to the control group on the Fear of Negative Evaluation scale and the Social Anxiety Inventory. No significant changes occurred, however, on the behavioral logs. Hence it would appear that AMT adds an important impact in reducing social anxiety and increasing self-esteem, even though behavioral changes did not seem to occur.

Hill (1977) compared AMT alone with behavioral practice, and found that both treatments decreased social anxiety and increased levels of self-esteem when compared with a control group. However, there was a trend for AMT clients to show greater increases in dating frequency than the behavioral practice clients.

Finally, in one of my private cases, I found AMT to be helpful in eliminating a performance anxiety for a musician. He had difficulty in playing the organ when faced with audiotape recording and hence was unable to accept contracts to record movie sound tracks. As part of my procedure to determine his progress, I asked him to identify an *in vivo* experience that might be a relevant test. Since we were not in his home area, he could not access an organ that duplicated his own special instrument. Instead, he proposed to attend a concert to see how he felt about seeing someone else perform. Although this was not a very good test, it was all that was available at the moment. However, when he reported back, he announced that he had substituted a different task. He admitted that he was homophobic but tested his anxiety level by approaching a strange person at the concert and arranging a date. The success of this rather unexpected circumstance therefore lends some case history support for AMT's ability to generalize to social anxiety.

Agoraphobia

The information for agoraphobia is actually indirect. Recall that Jannoun, Oppenheimer, and Gelder selected their sample from a psychiatric outpatient clinic. Eight of the subjects also experienced agoraphobia which had not been relieved by anxiolytic medication. Results after AMT with these subjects showed reductions in both general anxiety and use of medication. Unfortunately, the gains for the agoraphobic patients alone were not reported. Therefore, at this point, the value of AMT for agoraphobia remains speculative. It is highly interesting to note the belief that elevated autonomic arousal is characteristic of agoraphobia (Kelly, 1980; Lader, Gelder, & Marks, 1967) and to pair this with findings that autonomic-oriented therapy (involving relaxation) is more effective with phobics who are physiological reactors rather than behavioral reactors (Ost, Jerremalm, & Johansson, 1981). Moreover, Foa and Kozak (1985) argue that desensitization has proven ineffective for agoraphobia because it minimizes anxiety arousal, while exposure therapies have been successful because anxiety induction is emphasized. In fact, they conclude that ". . . two conditions are required for the reduction of fear. First, a person must attend to fear-relevant information in a manner that will activate his/her own fear memory" (p. 435), a condition met by AMT. Putting all of these pieces together, it would not be unreasonable to attempt AMT with agoraphobics, in-asmuch as AMT includes both relaxation and anxiety induction. This is clearly an area demanding research or further clinical case study.

Post-Traumatic Stress Disorder

Although not published research, Borrego (personal communica-tion, 1988) and Rivas (personal communication, 1988) have each re-ported their clinical use of AMT over several years with Post-Traumatic Stress Disorder veterans. Illustrations of their casework will be pre-sented in later chapters.

Problems Secondary to Primary Anxiety

Although researchers have mainly aimed at proving the efficacy of AMT for anxiety states, a number of very important side discoveries have also been apparent. These involve improvements in other charac-teristics of the treated clients, including self-esteem, depression, physical complaints, and maladaptive cognitions. In a variety of studies, each of these characteristics showed favorable changes following AMT for the primary symptom of anxiety or stress. Why this should be so is open to discussion. One possiblity is that the anxiety was the basis for the low self-esteem or self-confidence, the depression, the somatic symptoms, or the negative thoughts. Once the anxiety is removed, then the secondary symptoms vanish. Another possibility for self-esteem and depression is that AMT increases positive self-efficacy due to the self-control which the clients are achieving, and this sense of mastery represents a turning point. Bandura (1982) has certainly demonstrated that mastery training increases self-efficacy, a strong argument for self-control treatment orientations.

Self-Esteem

The earliest reference is that of Nally (1975) who actually was more interested in changing the behaviors of delinquents. He postulated that anxiety was either blocking the youngsters' learning of prosocial be-haviors, or that the prosocial behaviors were available but prevented from appearing because of the anxiety. The subjects were 26 adjudicated delinquents sentenced to a home for delinquents, where they were ex-pected to remain until their 18th birthday. Those selected for the study had scored at about the 75th percentile on the IPAT (a raw score of 36–41 or higher), or on the Spielberger State Anxiety Inventory (a raw score of 42 or higher), or on the Spielberger Trait Anxiety Inventory (a raw score of 44 or higher). In addition to these measures, other scales administered were the Peterson Behavior Problem Checklist (Peterson, 1961), and the Miskimins Self-Goal-Other-Discrepancy Scale (Miskimins & Brauch, 1971). The Peterson Behavior Problem Checklist involved ratings by cottage counselors on prosocial behaviors. The Miskimins Self-Goal-Other-Discrepancy Scale provided information on self-esteem. Finally, Nally constructed a questionnaire, Analogous Social Rules, as a way of measuring the delinquent's knowledge of social rules and their willingness actually to behave in accordance with such rules. Rules covered respect for authority, courtesy, friendliness, and helpfulness. Follow-up testing was conducted one month later with the IPAT and Spielberger scales. The Peterson and Miskimins scales and the Analogous Social Rules scale were administered at pretest and four-week follow-up only. The AMT treatment covered four sessions, each being one hour, over four weeks. A control group involved time spent in other rap sessions or time spent in supervised recreation with the therapist.

AMT was found not only to reduce anxiety, but also did increase prosocial behaviors for the treated group as compared to a control. Thus the anxiety scores for the group were: AMT—IPAT pretest = 46.1, posttest = 33.5, follow-up = 34.1; trait pretest = 51.3, posttest = 37.3, follow-up = 39.2; state pretest = 52.9, posttest = 39.7, follow-up = 38.3; control—IPAT pretest = 47.6, posttest = 44.9, follow-up = 46.2; trait pretest = 51.9, posttest = 48.8, follow-up = 48.9; state pretest = 51.1, posttest = 45.4, follow-up = 48.9. Regarding prosocial behaviors, the counselors ratings of the AMT adolescents showed a decrease, indicating improvement, from 88.8 to 68.1, compared to the control group's scores of 85.8 and 80.6. On the hypothesis that reductions in anxiety levels would be associated with improvements in prosocial behaviors, correlations were calculated between the posttest anxiety test scores and the Peterson scores. All correlations were high and significant: prosocial conduct and IPAT = .54; prosocial conduct and trait anxiety = .44; prosocial conduct and state anxiety = .51. This pattern did not exist when correlations were computed between the pretest anxiety and pretest Peterson scores.

Self-esteem was also enhanced following treatment. The AMT treated group showed significant improvement in self-concept as measured by the Miskimins scale (pretest = 48.5, posttest = 31.1), compared to the control adolescents (pretest = 47.5, posttest = 40.8). Once again, correlations between anxiety postest scores and self-esteem scores were significant (IPAT = .50; trait = .32; state = .69) while pretest scores showed no such relationship. In understanding a possible reason for the improvements in self-esteem in Nally's work, we might consider the research of Hill and Pipes, which we cited earlier. They also found improvements in self-esteem following reductions in social anxiety. One wonders whether the improvement in self-esteem is connected with the fact that a key component of social anxiety is the discomfort over being evaluated (Amies, Gelder, & Shaw, 1983; Beck & Emery, 1985). In a sense, low self-esteem is simply another type of evaluation, of self by oneself; while social anxiety may reflect evaluation of self by others. Perhaps once a person is comfortable about other-evaluation, then self-evaluation also changes to a more comfortable level of positive self-regard.

Some time ago, Suinn (1961) proved that self-evaluation and evaluations of others were positively correlated among youths. Specifically, this study demonstrated that level of acceptance of a teacher or a parent was significantly predicted by level of self-acceptance. A person who experienced high self-regard was likely to hold the teacher or parent in high esteem. Although this study centered on self-esteem being the starting point, the correlation could imply a reverse relationship as well, that is that believing others as holding you in in low regard might lead to holding yourself in low regard as well. Applying this to social anxiety would mean interpreting social anxiety as a belief by a person that he/she is held in low regard by others, thus prompting anxiety about relating to others. Therefore reduction of the social anxiety might represent the client being able to feel accepted by others, which in turn could increase this client's level of self-esteem. Admittedly, this is all speculation, but there does seem to be some association between self-esteem and social anxiety intervention side effects.

Finally, returning to Nally's data, he also found that AMT treatment led to improvements on the Analogous Social Rules scores, indicating that the treated delinquents showed a higher sensitivity and awareness of social rules and were more willing to act in accordance with these than the control group. However, the correlations between anxiety scales and social rules scores were not significant and generally low.

Depression

As with self-esteem, effects of AMT on depression were already reported, in discussion of works of Jannoun, Oppenheimer, and Gelder. As will be recalled, depression was assessed through both self-report and by an observer. The self-report involved the Leeds Self-Assessment for Depression, while the judge-ratings involved use of the Hamilton Scales. The data were as follows: self-assessment of depression showed a decline from pretreatment of 6.5 to posttreatment of 4.4 to one-month follow-up of 4.2 and three-month follow-up of 3.7; judge's rating of depression showed a change in depressive symptoms from a score of 14.5 to 7.2 to 8.8 and 6.1 by three-month follow-up. Although the depression scores were substantially reduced, Jannoun *et al.*'s subjects were not initially clinically depressed. In contrast, Cragan and Deffenbacher (1984) did see a sample with initially high depression scores.

Cragan and Deffenbacher (1984) provided AMT to stressed medical outpatients from family practice physicians, observing that antidepressant medication is often prescribed. Fifty-five volunteers were solicited from a general medical outpatient clinic for a stress management program. Although the patients did not report a primary complaint of depression, their depression test results were equivalent to those of psychiatric patients, based upon norms on the Multiple Affect Adjective Checklist (Zuckerman & Lubin, 1965). In addition to determining whether AMT reduced depression, the study also had a variety of other objectives. One objective was to compare the results of AMT with an applied relaxation procedure. A second objective was to compare effects on anger/hostility outcomes.

A multi-measurement approach was taken in assessing anxiety. Among the measurements used were the Spielberger Trait Anxiety Inventory and the Multiple Affect Adjective Checklist as trait anxiety measures; the Spielberger State Anxiety Inventory and blood pressure as state measures; a rating scale on physiological symptoms specific to certain situations; and the anger and depression subscales of the Multiple Affect Adjective Checklist. Follow-up testing was also conducted four weeks after posttesting.

AMT treatment consisted of six sessions lasting 60 minutes over six weeks, with 9–10 subjects in each AMT treatment group. The applied relaxation treatment group was taught to use relaxation during *in vivo* stressful and nonstressful experiences. This procedure differed from AMT mainly in that subjects were not trained with the use of anxiety imagery during treatment sessions.

Regarding depression, results indicated that the two treatment groups showed significantly reduced depression scores when compared with the wait-list control group. Scores were reduced to a normal level (Figure 3.2). In fact, the Multiple Affect Adjective Checklist scores for the AMT and applied relaxation groups were nearly identical at pretest (AMT = 22.5, applied relaxation = 22.1), posttest (12.9, 15.4), and follow-up (13.2, 13.9). Trait anxiety scores on the Spielberger and the Multiple Affect Adjective Check list also showed substantial reductions for both treatment groups compared to nearly no changes in the control group. The AMT group showed significantly greater reductions on the Spielberger trait scale than the applied relaxation group at posttest; but these differences were eliminated by follow-up, as the two groups were

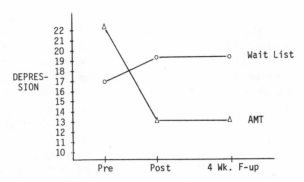

Figure 3.2. AMT for depression in general medical patients. (From Cragan & Deffenbacher, 1984.)

virtually identical by the four-week period. On the state anxiety scale both groups showed significant reductions compared to the control group.

Again, the two treatment groups were nearly identical in the level of reduction of state anxiety by follow-up. Blood pressure measurements showed no improvements for any of the groups, but blood pressure levels were well within the normal range for these subjects to begin with. On the other hand, the scale on physiological symptoms connected with specific situations did show significant reductions for the two treatment groups, and no changes to speak of for the control group. Finally, the anger/hostility measure showed a significant reduction for both the AMT and the applied relaxation subjects.

Two interesting additional findings were reported by Cragan and Deffenbacher. The first related to the perceived relative benefits of the two treatment approaches. Although the actual end results appeared almost identical in terms of depression, anxiety, anger/hostility, a higher percentage of the AMT subjects rated their treatment as having a significant impact on their lives than did the applied relaxation group. A second finding related to the information on the types of stress symptoms often experienced by the subjects. Tension in the neck and shoulder area was the most frequently identified (21.8%), followed by headaches (14.5%), stomach upset (13.6%), general shakiness (10.9%), and insomnia (6.4%). With such a high number of physically oriented symptoms that have similarity to stress symptoms, Cragan and Deffenbacher speculated that many of the reasons for such patients seeking help from a family practice physician may actually be traceable to stress-connected symptoms, rather than true medical complaints. Therefore, they conclude that stress-management programs could be a useful referral service for outpatient general medical practitioners, and a useful alternative to either pharmacological treatment or psychiatric referrals.

In passing, we should mention the report of Baskin (1980) which showed AMT to be more effective than control group not only on Type A behaviors, but also in lowering learned helplessness behaviors. Learned helplessness has been theorized as an important source of depression (Seligman, 1983), and training to improve self-control appears to decrease depression (Miller & Norman, 1981). Baskin's results would seem, therefore, to fit the premise that AMT's effects on depression may be due to the self-control components of AMT.

Physical Complaints

We had previously summarized the data on physical problems associated with anxiety, such as hypertension, ulcers, and so forth. Two other studies relate to somatic symptoms, but did not quite fit this prior category. The Cragan and Deffenbacher study just cited evaluated physical symptoms such as neck/shoulder tension, headaches, stomach distress, and insomnia. AMT as well as applied relaxation treatments both helped in the significant reduction of these symptoms, including during follow-up. In addition, the study reconfirmed that such treatment was of substantial aid in these patients handling major daily sources of personal stress, including those of high intensity.

Deffenbacher and Craun (1985) also dealt with medical outpatients, this time involving those stressed patients seeing a gynecologist. Since AMT appeared useful with dysmenorrhea, its use with a broader range of gynecological symptoms was studied. The participants were 16 gynecology patients from the health service of a university. Patients were asked to identify their most serious gynecological symptom and to rate the severity of this symptom. In addition, general anxiety was measured with the Spielberger Trait Anxiety Inventory, situational anxiety was measured with a rating scale on physiological symptoms in specific situations (the same scale used by Cragan and Deffenbacher), and physiological symptoms were also assessed with the Anxiety Symptom Checklist (Edie, 1973). Stress symptoms unique to the individual subject, called person-specific symptoms, were assessed by having each subject identify the symptoms which most characterized their stress reactions, such as headaches, nausea, back pain, and so forth. Follow-up was also obtained three months and two years later. Anxiety Management Training consisted of six sessions once a week. No control groups were used.

AMT was found valuable in reducing the severity of gynecological complaints such as premenstrual tension and depression, dysmenorrhea, and vaginal infections (ratings decreased from 74.0 at pretest to

38.4 at posttreatment, to 33.3 at three-month, and 35.3 at two-year follow-up). As with other studies, AMT reduced levels of trait or general anxiety, with the patients dropping from the 83rd percentile on level of anxiety to the 48th percentile at posttest and the 30th percentile by three-month and two-year follow-up. Data also confirmed significant reductions in situation-specific anxiety symptoms, physiological stress symptoms, and person-specific stress symptoms. All gains were maintained through both the three-month and the two-year follow-up, with a general trend for the anxiety levels to continue a downward progress across time. As an illustration, physiological symptoms reduced from a score of 232.1 at pretreatment, to 190.3 at posttreatment, 182.8 at three-month follow-up and 178.1 at two-year follow-up. As with the Cragan and Deffenbacher study, the most frequent person-specific stress symptoms were generally somatic, including headaches, nausea, back pain, insomnia, and shoulder pain as the most frequently cited. This study, although lacking a control group, is notable in the highly significant confirmation of prior studies showing the continuing gains possible on follow-up by AMT clients. These patients showed substantial and continuing reductions at the end of therapy, at three months, and at two years in general anxiety, physiological reactivity to stress, personal stress symptoms, and severity of gynecological symptoms.

Emotionality and Anger

Initially, AMT was conceived of as being only an anxiety management procedure. In rethinking the process, it is my belief that what we have is an *arousal* management procedure. In effect, any condition in which emotional arousal is a component could be considered reasonable for AMT to be tried. General emotionality was characteristic of the single case reported earlier in our discussion of general anxiety. Anger and possibly lack of impulse control or low frustration tolerance might also be examples.

Anger

Recent findings which associate anger and hostility with Type A behavior and risk of cardiovascular disease place a new spotlight on the importance of anger management (Matthews, 1982; Williams, 1982). Hart, of course, had the earliest example of AMT for control of anger, with persons selected on the basis of their Type A characteristics. Cragan and Deffenbacher examined the effects of AMT on anger and hostility with a group also selected on the basis of their other characteristics, i.e., their gynecological symptoms. Their results confirmed that although the AMT sessions focused on anxiety, apparently the skills generalized such that the patients also experienced significant reductions in anger/hostility feelings.

More recently, Deffenbacher and his students (Deffenbacher, Demm, & Brandon, 1986) have tested my new conceptualization by treating persons who were specifically selected for being in the upper quartile on the Spielberger State-Trait Anger Scale (Spielberger, Jacobs, Russell, & Crane, 1983). The high anger subjects were 29 university students whose high anger scores suggested a history of negative consequences for their anger, including property damage and legal difficulties. Instruments used in the study included the Spielberger anger scale, the Anger Inventory (Novaco, 1975a), pulse rate after imagining an anger arousal scene, the Spielberger Trait Anxiety Inventory, ratings of physiological symptoms associated with anger (person-specific anger symptoms), and the Coping Questionnaire (Novaco, 1975b) which classifies anger responses as verbal antagonism, physical antagonism and constructive action. Follow-up was obtained five weeks and one year after treatment. Thirteen of the subjects formed a treatment group, with 16 being a control group. AMT was revised[1] to provide the use of relaxation control to eliminate anger arousal generated through anger imagery. The training covered six one-hour AMT sessions meeting once a week with subjects in groups of six or seven persons. A more detailed description of the AMT method for anger control will be found in Chapter 12, with a case history illustration found in Chapter 5.

The results showed the AMT treated subjects as exhibiting significantly lower general anger on posttest as measured by both the Spielberger anger scale and the Anger Inventory. By one-year follow-up the Spielberger measured level of anger was reduced to the level of normal subjects. These gains in the two scales' scores were maintained over the one-year period (AMT group: Spielberger anger pretest = 28.0, posttest = 20.0; one-year follow-up = 17.9; Anger Inventory pretest = 320.9, posttest = 262.1, one-year follow-up = 263.2; control group: Spielberger anger pretest = 25.0, posttest = 24.1, one-year follow-up = 24.3; Anger Inventory pretest = 301.5, posttest = 316.7; one-year follow-up = 319.9). Heart rate decreased slightly for the AMT group but not to a significant level; however, the physiological symptoms of anger did reduce significantly as did state anger. Regarding coping behaviors, the AMT-treated group showed decreased tendencies to react to anger with verbal antagonism or physical antagonism, and increased

---

[1]Deffenbacher now uses the term "Affect Management" to refer to the use of the AMT procedure with anger.

tendency to cope through constructive action, as compared to the control group. Again, these gains for the treated subjects were maintained over time.

In this study, AMT was used to target anger control, with anxiety problems not discussed during the AMT sessions. Hence, any reductions in anxiety would be considered a result of the AMT-for-anger training generalizing to anxiety situations. As it turned out, scores on the trait anxiety scale showed a reduction in levels for the AMT group which were maintained through the one-year follow-up, such that the AMT subjects were significantly lower than control subjects (AMT trait scores went from 50.44 to 41.2 to 37.1 at follow-up; control subjects scores were 47.6 at pretest, 46.1 at posttest, and 49.6 at one-year follow-up). The fact that the initial reductions in trait anxiety after treatment failed to reach statistical significance (although they were reduced) led Deffenbacher *et al.* to the conservative recommendation that AMT "for anger reduction might be enhanced even more by giving direct attention to general anxiety. . . (since it) appears to covary significantly with the anger" (p. 489). This hypothesis has yet to be tested in research although it has clinical implications.

Hazaleus and Deffenbacher's (1986) subjects had experienced serious problems in anger control, for example, subjects were being prosecuted for disorderly conduct due to anger outbursts, or had been involved in property damage amounting to thousands of dollars, or had been involved in physical assault, or had experienced serious somatic reactions from anger, such as vomiting and headaches. These subjects had been selected by reason of scoring above the 75th percentile on the Spielberger Trait Anger Scale and had volunteered for an anger management program at the university. The eventual sample was composed of 21 placed in an AMT group, 20 in a cognitive therapy group, and 19 in a no-treatment group. AMT (now called Affect Modification) consisted of six one-hour sessions meeting once a week and composed of nine to 11 group members. Cognitive therapy involved a combination of Stress Inoculation Training (Meichenbaum, 1977) and Systematic Rational Restructuring (Goldfried, Decenteceo, & Weinberg, 1974) and involved preparing for and confronting anger provocations through adaptive cognitions. As with the Deffenbacher *et al.* (1986) study, instruments used included the Spielberger Trait Anxiety Scale, the Anger Inventory, ratings of physical symptoms associated with anger, pulse rates during an anger imagery, the Coping Questionnaire, the Spielberger Trait Anxiety Inventory, and the Beck Depression Inventory (Beck, 1967). A four-week follow-up was also conducted. Clinically, the sample proved to have significantly higher trait anger scores (as measured by the Spielberger and Anger Inventory scales) than norms, although depression scores were within a normal range.

Both treatment groups achieved results similar to the Deffenbacher *et al.* study in reductions of anger, physical symptoms asssociated with anger, and inclination to respond with verbal antagonism to anger provocation. These significant improvements were maintained through the one month follow-up, and were significantly lower than scores for the control group. No differences in heart rate were obtained between the control group and the two treatment groups. However, the failure to obtain changes might relate to the fact that the subjects showed initially low pulse rates anyway on pretesting, a low level which also characterized the subjects in the Deffenbacher *et al.* study.

Regarding cognitive therapy effects, the cognitive-treated persons showed a significant increase in constructive coping; the AMT group also showed improvements, but these did not reach significance. Unlike the AMT group, the cognitive therapy group showed significant reduction in state anger; however, by follow-up, both treatment groups showed similar gains. The cognitive therapy group also showed significantly less trait anxiety at follow-up. The AMT group also showed some reductions in trait anxiety scores but this failed to reach a statistical level of significance, particularly since the control subjects also showed reductions over time. Scores on depression did not show substantive changes for any of the groups. Hazaleus and Deffenbacher concluded that both types of interventions "could effectively reduce anger and maintain this reduction and. . . could be delivered cost-effectively in groups" (p. 226). However, they were again recommending that AMT involve both direct treatment of anger as well as direct treatment of anxiety, for subjects who have both high initial levels of anger and anxiety.

Finally, we should mention the individual casework of Hsi (personal communication, 1981). She conducted a workshop for six minority adolescents on stress management as part of a summer enrichment program. She targeted three types of circumstances, based upon my reconceptualizing of AMT as an impulse-control or arousal-control procedure: anxiety control, impulse control relating to frustration, and anger control. The workshop actually involved AMT sessions; for the anxiety control the scenes were anxiety arousal scenes; for the impulse control the scenes involved frustrating situations; for the anger control the scenes involved anger-arousal situations. Individual case reporting was obtained on self-ratings of arousal for each of these types of conditions. Although the sample was too small for reasonable analyses, the youngsters did appear to improve in their ratings of reaction to anxiety-, frustration-, or anger-provoking situations (Figure 3.3).

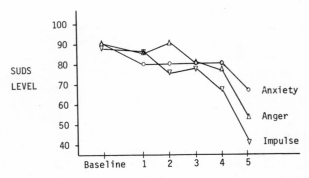

Figure 3.3. AMT for anxiety, anger, or impulse control. (From Hsi & Suinn, 1981.)

Cognitive/Intellective Performance

Anxiety has also been considered as a major hindrance to activities involving information processing, such as academic work or vocational decision making. Thompson, Griebstein, and Kuhlenschmidt (1980) matched university students on scholastic aptitude and anxiety prior to providing either AMT alone, AMT augmented by biofeedback training, stress management training alone, or stress management training augmented by biofeedback. The subjects were 30 college freshmen from a small liberal arts college, selected on the basis of academic anxiety. Academic anxiety was defined as represented in scores on the Achievement Anxiety Test (Alpert & Haber, 1960), with scores falling above the first quartile on norms on the inhibitory anxiety subscale. This instrument was used only as a selection procedure; actual outcome measures involved the Spielberger Trait Anxiety Inventory, the Spielberger State Anxiety Inventory, a checklist on somatic/cognitive anxiety symptoms, and grade point average. Follow-up was also conducted three months later. The primary hypothesis was that anxiety reduction would lead to improvements in intellectual performance as exhibited in grades.

The treatment groups were formed basically around either an AMT approach or a stress management training approach, either with or without biofeedback. The stress management training approach used the AMT procedures, but provided subjects with more alternative relaxation methods, such as progressive relaxation, autogenic exercises, cue-controlled relaxation. Treatment was conducted over six weeks and involved two half-hour sessions each week; the first half-hour session was a group session of about five subjects, while the second half-hour session was an individual session. The group sessions were conducted directly by a therapist, while the individual sessions used audiotapes. Biofeedback training involved electromyographic feedback from the forearm with feedback provided visually through a meter. There were 20 subjects in the treatment group condition and 10 in a no-treatment control group condition.

In results, analyses showed that the AMT alone and the stress management alone groups were significantly higher in grade point average than the control group for the Fall semester grades. For the Winter grades, the AMT augmented by biofeedback group was significantly higher than the control group, although the AMT alone and stress management alone groups approached significance. To capture an overall sense for the various levels of academic grades, the authors rank-ordered the grade point averages. In the Fall, the AMT-alone and stress-management-alone groups both achieved a mean grade point average of 3.0, followed by the augmented AMT group with a grade point of 2.85; then the control with 2.64 and, finally, the augmented stress management with 2.44. In the Winter, the augmented AMT group achieved a grade point average of 3.24, followed by the stress management alone of 2.98, then the AMT alone with 2.94, then the control group of 2.72, and finally the augmented stress management group with 2.61. Ten of the total group of 30 students achieved a grade point average higher than 3.0; of these, nine were from a treatment condition, and only one came from the control condition. It is difficult to know why the augmented stress management group did as poorly as they did; the authors offered the speculation that the relaxation training of the stress management approach might have been too difficult, for example, the autogenic training procedure. This might explain the results if one also assumes that the biofeedback took away the time needed to master the relaxation techniques; but where there was sufficient time, then the stress management training was effective (as shown by the higher grade average of the stress-management-alone group).

In terms of anxiety data, the trait anxiety mean for all treatment subjects combined was reduced from the 70th percentile to the 54th percentile, while the state anxiety mean dropped from the 66th to the 25th percentile. The control subjects' posttest mean scores fell at the 54th percentile on trait anxiety and the 70th percentile on state anxiety. The fact that the posttesting was done during midterm examinations was taken to mean that the treatment had special value "in preventing the increases in state anxiety associated with classroom examinations" (p. 100). On the somatic/cognitive anxiety scale, all of the treatment groups were significantly lower than the control group at posttest. The median values for the treated subjects combined was 2.6 for somatic anxiety and 2.7 for cognitive anxiety, compared to scores for the control group of 3.2 and 3.3. By follow-up, the treated group mean was 2.8 for somatic and

2.5 for cognitive anxiety, contrasted to values for the control subjects of 2.9 and 3.0.

In addition to the observation that control over anxiety does appear to have some impact on intellectual achievement, Thompson *et al.* (1980) also call attention to the reductions which occurred in cognitive anxiety. Their interesting comments were as follows: "Why these two noncognitive approaches would produce decreases in cognitive anxiety is worthy of speculation. One possible explanation is that relaxation self-control procedures reduce cognitive anxiety by encouraging *in vivo* desensitization and/or covert positive reinforcement. An alternative explanation is that somatic and cognitive symptoms interact in a reciprocal fashion and that a decrease in either produces a general reduction in both" (p. 103). It is my sense that even *in vivo* desensitization or the use of contingent reinforcement would not have direct effects on cognitive anxiety, and therefore the second explanation seems more viable. It is my contention that there can be several pathways opened up when stress is precipitated: a somatic path seen in persons who react first with somatic symptoms of anxiety, an autonomic path seen in those where the initial onset shows up with autonomic symptoms, and a cognitive path exhibited in those whose initial response to a stressor is a cognitive one. In addition, no matter where the initial response occurs, this response itself can trigger off another pathway in a chain of events.

In other words, a stressor might first precipitate an autonomic response, which in turn might trigger a cognition, which in turn might lead to a behavioral/somatic disruption. By breaking up the initial anxiety response through Anxiety Management Training, the later events in the chain can therefore be prevented. Hence it is theoretically plausible that AMT would lead to reductions in cognitive anxiety. However, to be even more certain of such benefits, AMT has been revised in procedures to include cognitive components, a procedure we shall outline in more detail in Chapters 6 and 7.

Vocational indecision was considered by Mendonca and Siess (1976) as being hampered by anxiety. Several groups were formed: an AMT only, a problem-solving training group, a combined AMT and problem-solving, and a placebo group. The AMT group was actually a combination of some basic AMT procedures, such as using anxiety imagery to practice applying relaxation for stress reduction. Added to the traditional AMT procedures, however, was the use of self-talk (Meichenbaum, 1972). In self-talk, the individuals remind themselves to attend to specific tasks rather than anxiety cues; this is also rehearsed through imagery. The problem-solving group relied upon procedures by D'Zurilla and Goldfried (1971) in covering problem identification, formulation of goals, generating alternatives through brainstorming, examining consequences, and making final decisions for courses of action. Treatment sessions covered seven sessions over 18 days with each session running about one hour. The placebo session involved discussions on careers following viewing of documentary films and listening to tape recordings on vocational development. A no-treatment control group was also formed. Subjects were 32 undergraduates who had previously indicated concerns over vocational decisions. Measures included the IPAT Anxiety Scale, a checklist on vocational exploratory behaviors, a questionnaire tapping awareness of information on careers, and a test of problem-solving (with subscales on information gathering, generating alternatives, and choice activities).

The results showed no changes in levels of anxiety for the AMT, problem-solving, or no-treatment control groups, and a very slight and nonsignificant reduction for both the combined treatment group and the placebo control group. In spite of this lack of results on anxiety, there were rather interesting results on the vocational and problem-solving measures. On vocational measures, the AMT group and the combination group produced greater gains than the other groups, such as on frequency and variety of vocational exploratory behaviors and awareness of career information. On the problem-solving scale, the combined group, the AMT group, and the problem-solving group all performed better than the no-treatment control group.

Performance Enhancement through Anxiety Reduction

A final exciting area for which AMT has shown potential involves the enhancement of performance through anxiety reduction or anxiety prevention. Only one study is available so far, although a few of my own cases are illustrative of the potential for AMT. Mathis (1978) compared an AMT group with a control group of music majors experiencing performance anxiety. Subjects were all students in the Music Department of a university who reported experiencing performance anxiety. The 18 volunteers were assigned to either an AMT group or a wait-list control group. AMT was conducted over five weeks, once a week, each session 50 minutes. Instead of having different anxiety-evoking imagery for each subject, one scene was used for all subjects in the group sessions. This scene was as follows:

> It is your turn to perform before a jury. You get out of your seat and approach the area where you are to perform. You realize that you are to perform without any music. You feel yourself becoming anxious as you approach the area in which you are to perform. (p. 8)

Following the usual AMT instructions, subjects used this scene to prompt the return of anxiety; most subjects achieved the anxiety arousal in about seven seconds.

The instruments used for the study were the Concept Specific Anxiety Scale (Cole & Oetting, 1972) which measures anxiety, the Behavioral Anxiety Rating Scale designed by Mathis for judges to rate behaviors reflective of anxiety (such as shallow breathing, rigidity in body motions, disrupted tonal quality, etc.), and judge ratings of quality of an audiotape of music performance (on qualities such as phrasing, style, technique, artistic effect, and so forth). The Behavioral Anxiety Rating Scale was completed by advanced music majors; the audio performance ratings were done by a professor in the Music Department. Judges were blind about whether the persons they were rating were in a treatment or wait-list group.

The results indicated first that the AMT-treated subjects reduced their anxiety levels, while the control group remained anxious. On the Behavioral Rating Scale, the AMT group showed a reduction from an anxious state to a relaxed state, while the wait-list showed no such improvement. Regarding the audio performance ratings, no significant differences were obtained.

Related to Mathis' research are some results which I observed in my own practice. I had previously applied AMT for a musician who was concerned about a forthcoming solo, as well as for a dancer with a national touring company in a Broadway musical. In these cases, which I will present in more detail later, AMT proved helpful. AMT was also used during my consulting with the U.S. Modern Pentathlon National Team. In the pentathlon, the athletes must cope with different types of intense stress in five diverse events. AMT seemed an especially appropriate tool since one of its major characteristics is its generalizability to various new and varied stressors. I was especially pleased that the one athlete who sought AMT training had his best performance, and attributed his success to AMT.

Returning to research studies, AMT was used with athletes to determine its effects in improving physiological efficiency. Ziegler, Klinzing, and Williamson (1982) tested the premise that muscle tension involves the consumption of energy which would show up on physiological measures. One common measure involves the rate of oxygen consumed under a physical treadmill work task. The subjects were nine members of a university men's varsity cross-country team. The outcome measure was oxygen consumption under a standard work load, with the amount of effort being standardized for all subjects as 50% of their maximal work load. The AMT approach involved imagery relating to track competition that creates anxiety, such as flashbacks to a disastrous performance, prerace stress reactions, etc. In addition to the typical use of relaxation to control the anxiety, Ziegler *et al.* also instructed the subjects to use other methods, such as positive track images, or cognitive thought control. AMT was conducted in sessions meeting twice a week for no longer than one hour, spaced over five and one-half weeks. Electromyographic biofeedback was also used as an adjunct to relaxation training for the initial relaxation sessions of AMT. Two other groups were also formed: a Stress Inoculation Training and a no-treatment control group.

Findings demonstrated that the AMT and Stress Inoculation Training groups achieved a lower oxygen consumption than the control group during the first half of the posttest treadmill run. However, only the AMT group achieved a significantly lower oxygen consumption during the second half of the treadmill test. Athletes from the AMT treatment group reported "considerable change in their approach to warm-ups, precontest 'mental sets,' and their practice and race behaviors. . . an increased level in handling 'emergency stress' (and a view that). . . stress. . . can be dealt with through training, rather than stress as an expected reaction. . . that an athlete 'learns to live with'" (p. 288).

The Stress Inoculation Training group reported having "more confidence, ability to control stress so that 'little things' didn't get in the way of performance, increased appreciation for positive track experiences and how they can be used in stress management" (p. 288). Based upon the oxygen consumption data, Ziegler *et al.* concluded that "athletes can gain mastery over their physiological response via an effective mental training program" (p. 286).

A procedure quite similar to AMT was used by Crocker, Alderman, and Smith (1988) for reducing the adverse effects of competitive stress on athletic performance. The athletes were 31 volleyball players who had been invited to participate in a training camp for the 1987 Alberta, Canada Games Team. The AMT-type program covered eight one hour experiences in relaxation, anxiety arousal and control, and homework. Additionally, some cognitive components were involved, such as evaluating irrational thoughts and using self-talk to eliminate stress. These eight sessions was conducted a week apart. Sixteen athletes composed the treatment group, and eleven composed a no treatment control group. Several measures were used. Anxiety was assessed using the Competitive State Anxiety Inventory and the Sport Competition Anxiety Test (Martens, 1977; Martens, Burton, Vealey, Bump, & Smith, 1983). Thoughts were logged using thought listing (Cacioppo & Petty, 1981; Long, 1984).

Volleyball performance was rated using a five-point scale evaluating the quality of the player's passing abilities. For this task, one coach served

12 times to each player, with the athlete's task to pass the ball to the setter. Results found no differences in levels of anxiety across the two groups. However, the treated group had fewer negative thoughts and demonstrated significantly better volleyball performances than the control group. The superior level of the subjects chosen for this study (they were elite enough to be qualifying for the Canada Games) might have been a factor in the failure of results on the anxiety scales. On the other hand, the increase in volleyball performance did occur, leading the authors to conclude that some levels of stress were present, and that the treatment aided in removing the stress, freeing the athletes to perform at an improved level.

Summary

This chapter highlights the various applications of AMT to certain conditions where anxiety is an important underlying dimension. Following the series of scientific demonstrations that AMT does have major impact on presenting problems where anxiety and stress are the dominant symptoms, researchers and psychotherapists have extended the applications of AMT. As we cited earlier, one intended value of AMT was in its direct application to generalized anxiety disorder. In addition, another proposed value was in the use of AMT for disorders whereby anxiety appeared to be a major contributing factor. Such disorders include essential hypertension, ulcers, situational anxieties, and performance anxieties. A variety of reports have been published on these types of disorders, as well as on some conditions which theoretically might have an anxiety basis, such as certain cases of self-esteem, depression, Type A behaviors, dysmenorrhea, diabetes, physical complaints, and negative cognitions. Finally, studies have also been reported on the use of AMT for anger control and for removal of obstructions to intellective performance.

The behavioral medicine applications of AMT have been promising for certain disorders. Essential hypertension appeared to be responsive to AMT treatment in a variety of studies, with some hypertensive patients showing improvements of their blood pressure from hypertensive levels to normal levels. In one case report, AMT was selected as the treatment of choice and a deliberate alternative to drug treatment, because of potential health risk of the medication. Type A behaviors have received a good deal of attention, with AMT or AMT combined with other treatments being used with some success. An underlying rationale is that Type A persons experience stress as a result of their characteristics; further, that removal of the stress would enable such individuals to adopt more healthy, non-Type A alternatives. The majority of the studies confirmed that AMT treatment reduced Type A characteristics, such as impatience and competitiveness, and trait anxiety, and with occasional reductions in cholesterol levels. Although other treatment approaches showed similar efficacy, at least one researcher concluded that AMT was the "most popular of the behavioral approaches" and is "the short-term treatment of choice."

As might be expected, AMT has shown convincing applications to situational anxieties. Public-speaking anxiety has been successfully reduced not only immediately following AMT treatment, but also at long term follow-up. Combined with practice in slow speech, AMT also reduced speech dysfluencies. A few studies suggest the value of AMT for social anxiety, and other works or case studies are suggestive that AMT may be appropriate for agoraphobia and post-traumatic stress disorder; however, research is needed on these latter two conditions.

It is most interesting to note that two possibly related difficulties, low self-esteem and depression, may be responsive to AMT, provided that anxiety is involved. Either the anxiety is blocking positive self-evaluations from appearing, or anxiety is preventing the appearance of actions which in turn would be successful and receive social approval and instrumental gains (and consquently reinforce positive self-esteem). Another possible reason for the association between successful AMT treatment for anxiety and improved self-esteem or reduced depression is the increased self-efficacy deriving from the self-control skills developed through AMT. In some important ways, self-control over anxiety may aid in changing a client's attitude from one of learned helplessness to one of learned mastery or coping.

The appropriateness of AMT programs for patients in general medical practices or family practices has been demonstrated by Deffenbacher and his colleagues. Apparently a goodly number of patients seeking medical help for physical distress might actually be experiencing physical symptoms deriving from stress. In such cases, AMT was useful in reducing the stress with the consequence of reducing certain physical complaints, such as headaches, stomach distress, insomnia, nausea, and dysmenorrhea.

There is evidence for the value of AMT in removing levels and types of anxiety which interfere with intellective tasks. Cognitive anxiety can be reduced through AMT, possibly relating to some of the cognitive components of the AMT procedure. One type of obvious intellective task is shown in academic studies, and AMT appears to be helpful in improvements in academic work for students. Another type of intellective task involves decision making regarding vocational choice. AMT

appeared helpful in reducing vocational indecision and increasing vocational exploratory activities and awareness of career information.

Two studies represent efforts extending the application of AMT to
performance enhancement of normally functioning persons. One demonstrated the possible value of AMT for musical peformance, while the
other demonstrated the value of AMT for improved athletic performance. In the former, music students appeared able to reduce their
levels of anxiety during performances before judges. Since anxiety can
be associated with loss of motor coordination, breathing dysfluencies,
and other such distress, these consequences can in turn create difficulties in performing. In the case of athletes, runners trained with AMT
were able to improve on their physiological efficiency, that is, in the level
of oxygen required to perform. For an endurance athlete, this improved
physiological efficiency can mean the difference between having energy
to finish well versus having no energy to complete the race.

Perhaps the most exciting extension of AMT is in the revision of our
conceptualization from AMT as an anxiety treatment method to AMT as
an arousal treatment method. This means that an arousal state, such as
anger, would be appropriate for AMT. Deffenbacher has spearheaded a
series of applications of AMT to anger control. AMT-treated persons
showed reduction in anger over one year follow-up, reduction in physical
symptoms of anger, and reduction in the tendency to respond with
verbal antagonism to anger provocation. It is interesting to note that the
anger-treated subjects reduced their anger levels through AMT, but trait
anxiety levels, although reduced, did not reach statistical significance
levels. On the other hand, in the study of musicians, AMT produced
reductions in anxiety levels, but not in quality of musical performance.
In two studies on Type A behaviors, AMT led to significant reductions in
trait anxiety, but not in Type A behaviors. In some cases, these failures of
changes to reach statistical significance hid the fact that improvements
did occur in the anticipated direction.

However, such findings do lead to some speculation. Deffenbacher,
in noting that AMT reduced anger when the AMT procedure focused
on anger but not anxiety, recommended that future anger clients receive
AMT using the anxiety-arousal/ anxiety reduction scenes (the traditional
AMT approach), as well as the anger-arousal/anger reduction scenes
(the revised AMT-for-anger approach). Similarly, one might speculate
that, in some cases, the removal of anxiety alone is sufficient to release
other behaviors which have been obstructed by the anxiety: for instance,
the increase in self-esteem and the release of pro-social behaviors in
Nally's research with delinquents; or the improved ability of patients in
psychotherapy to use psychotherapy insights in Van Hassel's work with

schizophrenics; or the improved openness and willingness to confront problems observed by Edie and Shoemaker.

However, for other cases, the desired adaptive behaviors may be absent due to skill deficiency. Hence, if AMT is to be successful in not only removing the anxiety, but also in enabling improved behaviors, then such behaviors must be addressed as part of a larger program. For instance, the Suinn, Brock and Edie study not only relied upon AMT to remove stress obstacles, but also employed a behavioral rehearsal component for practicing alternative behaviors to Type A behaviors. In this study, Type A behaviors appeared to be reduced.

Having provided the scientific evidence in support of the efficacy of AMT, we will turn in the next section to the clinical practice of AMT. This section, actually Part II, will start with an overview of the AMT sessions and outline the underlying principles. Case illustrations will provide a more personal feel for the AMT applications to client situations. This will be followed by a step-by-step description for the conducting of AMT, including recommendations on clinical problems, such as dealing with relaxation/imagery issues, and use of AMT in a group format.

III

THE CLINICAL
PRACTICE OF ANXIETY
MANAGEMENT
TRAINING

Overview of Anxiety Management Training

Basics of AMT

AMT was initially designed as a nonspecific behavior therapy that would be relevant for treating any condition where anxiety was a core issue. Most important, AMT was aimed at free-floating anxieties in which clients are unable specifically to identify the stimulus conditions that trigger their anxiety reactions. In order to accomplish this, we focused on the fact that although generalized anxiety disorder clients cannot concretely label their stressors, they certainly possess first hand acquaintance with their experience of anxiety itself. Such clients, with a little help, can describe in great detail how they experience their anxiety attacks, in terms of autonomic, somatic, or cognitive syptoms. They are aware of their feelings of anxiety whether these are autonomic/affective, such as "pounding in my chest as my heart races a mile a minute and I can't catch my breath," or somatic/behavioral, such as general restlessness or "the shakes," or cognitive, such as worries, negative self-dialogue, or "just knowing something bad is going to happen to me."

The basic premise of AMT is to take these concrete anxiety responses and train the clients in using them constructively rather than letting them precipitate more anxiety in a vicious cycle. Basically, AMT teaches clients to recognize these anxiety responses as they are building, and then to use them as cues for initiating the coping response of relaxation. Relaxation was chosen not only because of the simplicity in teaching clients this procedure, but because the relaxation response is inimical and contradictory to anxiety arousal responses, and therefore can be expected to eliminate the anxiety. Initially, clients are exposed to high anxiety arousal in order to practice gaining control over anxiety through the use of relaxation. As AMT sessions proceed, the clients then learn to become sensitive earlier to the signs that anxiety is beginning, and to initiate the relaxation at this earlier stage, in order to abort the anxiety before it reaches a high level. Our case experiences provide rather interesting data that some clients become so skilled that they automatically abort the arousal before it reaches a level of awareness, reporting instead that they "are never fearful anymore." Other clients, on the other hand, continue to sense when anxiety is starting up, and systematically employ the relaxation as a self-control procedure.

AMT can be covered in 6–8 basic sessions, proceeding more slowly or more rapidly depending upon the client's rate of learning and success in homework applications. In all sessions, imagery has been the standard method for anxiety arousal, through use of anxiety scenes from the clients' own lives in which anxiety was aroused. Homework, on the other hand, eventually involves real life application of relaxation to control stress experiences.

We will present the steps for group AMT treatment later; at present this and other chapters will focus on individual treatment. Although not counted as a true AMT session, an intake and assessment is always important. Furthermore, a brief post-session interview is always conducted at the end of each AMT session, and a pre-session interview is always planned for the start of the next AMT session. With this in mind, the following gives the essence of each session:

Intake session: Assessment and diagnosis.
Session 1: Rationale, relaxation scene development, relaxation training.
Session 2: High anxiety scene development, anxiety arousal through imagery followed by relaxation for anxiety control.
Session 3: Anxiety arousal with attention to identifying personal signs of anxiety arousal, relaxation control.
Session 4: Intense anxiety scene development, anxiety arousal followed by relaxation for anxiety control; alternation of high anxiety scene with intense anxiety scene for arousal and control. Client assumes responsibility for ending the anxiety scene and for initiating relaxation control. Time and situational monitoring are added.
Session 5: Anxiety arousal is followed by relaxation control under the control of the client. Client initiates relaxation control while remaining in the anxiety scene and visualizing the stressors.
Sessions 6–8: Format for Session 5 is repeated until full self-control is achieved.

This 6–8 session format represents the recommended AMT method and the method upon which the various research studies have been based.

Principles of AMT

Although the steps involved in each session of AMT are quite straightforward, these steps are founded on certain principles for achieving maximum behavioral change.

Principle 1

The best training for behavioral change must involve an active coping component. AMT is oriented toward having clients directly engage in experiencing high anxiety levels in order to gain experience in its control. In effect, AMT is an anxiety induction procedure that also includes training in an active coping method, specifically relaxation for anxiety reduction and control. The anxiety induction in treatment should derive from a treatment experience that replicates the real life environment. Although AMT sessions are not conducted as *in vivo* sessions, the scenes used in imagery to arouse anxiety represent real events in the clients' lives associated with anxiety.

Principle 2

Clients can progress more effectively when they are clearly taught the adaptive skills in a controlled environment. AMT relies upon guided imagery rehearsal to insure that the clients have clear directions in therapy. By using imagery and by having the instruction initially under the full control of the therapist, clients also have the reassurance that they will properly acquire the needed relaxation coping skill for use to control the anxiety induced.

Principle 3

Treatment should proceed at a systematic pace representing the client's ability to make gains. AMT involves direct observation by the therapist of the client's progress during each session, for instance, in gaining rapid control over the relaxation skill, and in gaining control following anxiety arousal. Furthermore, homework assignments are partly for further practice with AMT skills, as well as the means for gauging progress in real life. The pace of the AMT sessions is therefore always reflective of these evidences of client gains.

Principle 4

The best client gains are those which involve the client in self-control skills in order to avoid relapse and to promote continued gains following therapy. AMT involves a graduated fading out of therapist control through therapist instructions, and an increasing reliance on client control. Given that the pace of the sessions follows evidence of the client's gains in coping, this increase of client responsibility is also reasonably controlled.

Principle 5

The skills gained in therapy should be such as to generalize outside the therapy environment. AMT has built in the use of homework assignments, which increase in level of application as a reflection of the progress of the client. Each homework assignment therefore bridges the gap between the protected environment of the therapy hour and the real daily life circumstances.

Principle 6

Treatment for stress disorders increases in value with the addition of preventive components. AMT includes elements aimed at prevention, such as the training in identification of early signs of anxiety (cue discrimination), and in the procedures of time monitoring and situation monitoring.

Principle 7

Self-efficacy enhancement is a useful aspect of therapy. AMT appears to influence efficacy and self-esteem as a result of the self-control elements. Furthermore, AMT enables clients to experience directly their gains as they become aware of their ability to control their anxieties following anxiety induction in the sessions and through homework monitoring.

Principle 8

Anxiety therapy sessions which reduce anxiety arousal within the sessions have more reinforcing benefits than therapies relying solely upon anxiety induction. AMT provides clients concrete evidence of their behavioral change as they observe their increased control. Methods such as flooding/implosion which leave the client emotionally exhausted might not be perceived as clearly demonstrating to the client that control or change is occurring.

The Underlying Mechanisms of AMT

Each session of AMT was designed to implement certain underlying mechanisms which meet the principles we just discussed. These mechanisms involve: the use of a therapeutic rationale, guided rehearsal techniques, anxiety induction, cue-controlled relaxation, self-monitoring, fading, and homework assignments. Each of these has proven effective as positive therapeutic factors in influencing behavioral change. Each of these will be discussed next in the context of AMT. Since the detailed description of each AMT session will be presented in later chapters, illustrations of the way in which these mechanisms are reflected in the AMT sessions will be brief.

Therapeutic Rationale

At the beginning of any therapy, whether spoken or simply implied, all clients develop an understanding of the rationale for the treatment they are undertaking. This rationale can be extremely important, not because of its placebo or nonspecific effects, but because it can enhance or retard the clients' learning. If AMT is viewed as a form of skill training, and if the rationale is viewed as establishing a cognitive learning set, then we can readily see how the rationale can facilitate or inhibit this skill learning. The rationale basically states: Here is what the task is, here is what you will be expected to learn, here is what you need to pay attention to, here is what you should be doing in order to learn, and here are the conditions that will help your learning.

As we shall see in Chapter 7, the AMT method offers a rationale emphasizing that the therapy is really a form of skill acquisition and that this skill is learned through practice. Clients understand that, as with other skills, their active involvement is essential. In effect, therapy changes from becoming something that happens to clients, but becomes instead something that they do. Clients understand that anxiety doesn't simply disappear during therapy as if by magic; rather that the therapy enables them to learn a coping skill which not only has current use, but also future applications for different stressors in their lives. This shifts the concept of self-control to "something which a person *does* instead of something he or she *has*" (Mahoney & Arnkoff, 1978).

This type of rationale is particularly reassuring to clients who have lost confidence in themselves or who have been unable to achieve relief from their anxieties. It is also meaningful for clients who are unable to pinpoint the origins of their anxiety, or who are incapable of predicting the stress which triggers their tensional states. For these clients, the AMT therapist is fundamentally saying, "You do not have to know what is causing your anxiety, we can still teach you what to do about it and how to gain control over it."

Guided Rehearsal

The use of guided rehearsal, either through role playing or through imagery techniques, has become a well-known tool in psychotherapies. One major advantage is the fact that rehearsal methods permit clients to engage in actual practice of the desired behaviors. Knowledge alone of what is needed is often insufficient and fails to guarantee that the desired skills are of sufficient strength to be reliable. Rehearsal enables clients to strengthen these skills by practice until their skill deficit is overcome, for example, through rehearsing social skills until the shyness deficit is overcome. A second advantage of rehearsal methods is that it enables clients to engage in actual applications. Even where insights are achieved, clients must still act upon their insights to obtain gains. Thirdly, rehearsal methods can promote generalization through setting up different types of role play or imagery conditions.

Finally, guided rehearsal methods provide clients with a measure of safety, since the rehearsal is under the control of the therapist who guides each step. For AMT, the use of guided rehearsal is valuable, inasmuch as anxiety arousal is involved. Since the therapist in initial sessions assumes maximum control over guiding the session from anxiety induction through relaxation, clients are always assured that the anxiety arousal will remain in hand.

Of the guided rehearsal procedures possible, AMT relies upon imagery rehearsal. The main reason is the characteristic ability of imagery to achieve high levels of reality. Whereas role playing is still no more than 'playing' of roles, imagery can retrieve an experience so realistically as to be indistinguishable from the actual experience itself. I have used imagery for performance enhancement training with Olympic athletes. One primary goal was to find a procedure that could recreate a competition environment, such that the athlete could feel the same emotions, be able actually to experience the environment, and even engage in the competition itself.

Whereas role playing is still recognizable by the participant as an intellective experience, not unlike an athlete being on the practice field, imagery rehearsal is a "total sensory experience which replicates visual, tactile, proprioceptive, emotional, autonomic, and auditory sensations" (Suinn, 1984). Athletes report having intense emotional reactions, for instance, feeling the hurt of being hit by their boxing opponent, but also being able to practice new skills. In two case demonstrations I also discovered that what was happening in the imagery scenes was also replicated in muscle activity. Electromyographic (EMG) equipment can amplify and measure muscular activity. In both cases, EMG data replicated the type of muscle movements that would be expected of the athletic activity being visualized by the subjects in their imagery. Heart rate changes were also observed in both cases (Suinn, 1980).

The EMG data, the reports of athletes, and controlled research reports on imagery rehearsal for athletic performance enhancement as well as for imagery-based therapy, e.g., desensitization, all support the usefulness of imagery rehearsal (Suinn, 1986a). These are also consistent with our observation of our very first AMT study which confirmed that intense anxiety induction was feasible using imagery. Lang (1980, 1983) has conducted a sequence of experiments which support the contention that imagery scenes do lead to affect arousal resulting in physiological outcomes. In fact, Lang (1985) concludes that anxiety and phobic disorders are located in memory, and hence are cognitively based. AMT relies upon the guided rehearsal of imagery to gain anxiety arousal among clients. The ultimate purpose of this arousal is to provide clients with direct training in the use of relaxation to control this anxiety. As far as AMT theory is concerned, the type of scene that is used for anxiety induction really does not matter. What matters only is that the client becomes anxious during the session in order to practice the application of relaxation for self-regulation.

Anxiety Induction

The induction of anxiety is an essential step for AMT. The premise is that clients must have the opportunity to be actively involved in controlling their anxiety. In terms of social learning theory and our model of stress, the autonomic, somatic, or cognitive reactions to stressors represent the anxiety responses to the stress cues. Generalized anxiety disorder patients are unable specifically to identify these stress cues, either because they failed to encode them during initial exposure, or because retrieval of encoding is being disrupted, or because the number and variety of such cues has become so generalized that no single pattern can be identified. The AMT approach therefore basically ignores seeking to identify the external stress stimuli.

Instead, AMT seeks to induce the anxiety responses, and then to have these responses serve as the stimuli which prompt the next response, relaxation for coping. Under maladaptive conditions, the precipitating of the initial anxiety responses serves as stimuli for the release of even further anxiety responses, thereby intensifying the total stress reaction. The patient experiences a spiraling effect, as each increment of anxiety serves as the cue for triggering off either more intense anxiety reactions or reactions covering more subsystems. Hence a patient whose initial reaction to a stressor was an anxiety response in the autonomic subsystem might soon be reacting through the somatic or cognitive subsystems as well. AMT aims at breaking up this sequence of events by introducing the relaxation response. In conditioning terms, the old stimulus-response habit pattern of onset of anxiety triggering onset of further anxiety, is now replaced by the stimulus of anxiety onset prompting the coping response of relaxation activity. In self-control terms, clients are learning to initiate self-relaxation as the coping behavior upon the appearance of anxiety. Later, as part of prevention, the self-relaxation is initiated at an early enough stage so as to preempt any development of disruptive anxiety.

Relaxation

The initial premise was that a response was needed which would be strong enough to counter the anxiety arousal. Relaxation was viewed as one such response, since relaxation led to a lowering of arousal. The use of a competency scene in imagery was also attempted in the first AMT study on the belief that the competency scene would cue emotions that could successfully compete with the anxiety. As we said earlier, the relaxation procedures appeared so successful that the competency scene was quickly eliminated from the AMT procedure. In addition, it was questionable whether patients seeking therapy would be readily able to recall a recent competency experience.

Although the relaxation response as popularized by Benson (1975) has some positive outcomes, research has suggested that it is the active application of relaxation as a coping procedure that has the best outcomes. Clients who are only taught relaxation but do not use this skill to deal actively with stress show less gains. Goldfried and Trier (1974) found that speech anxious subjects receiving instruction on the active self-application of relaxation showed greater reductions in anxiety than a relaxation-only group. The gains for the relaxation-as-coping subjects also showed even more pronounced gains during follow-up. AMT relies solely upon relaxation as the anxiety coping method, not only because of it proven value, but because there are methods for conveniently and easily training clients in this skill. In addition, for an extremely active private practitioner, there are ancillary methods for relaxation training which do not require the presence of the therapist, such as the use of biofeedback equipment or audio training tapes. Finally, unlike the competency procedure, relaxation training appears to be more universally acquired.

Self-Monitoring

Self-monitoring is another procedure which appears not only to facilitate compliance and maintenance in behavioral change, but also can promote insight. Self-monitoring is no more than having clients do observations through recording their own behaviors (Kazdin, 1974). AMT begins self-monitoring during intake, whereby clients receive a simple form to record occurrence of anxiety incidents. Later self-monitoring forms are also used which correspond to the types of applications of anxiety control *in vivo* expected. Such forms also can be used to determine compliance and form the basis for a brief pre-therapy interview at the start of each AMT session.

An interesting side benefit of self-monitoring in AMT has been the development of insight by clients. For instance, since the first recording log has clients identify the situations as well as time of day in which anxiety was experienced, this can lead them to become aware of patterns, either in terms of the types of situations in which anxiety appears or even in terms of time. Self-monitoring can also prove a motivating force, since it provides a method for concretely assessing progress. As clients are able to perceive their movement in therapy and gains in control of anxiety, this provides reinforcement and encouragement. Such evidence of gains can also bolster confidence and increase self-efficacy. Finally, the monitoring can offer the therapist some information about possible larger changes. Logs can sometimes demonstrate that the frequency of anxiety incidents are decreasing. This type of information may well indicate progress by the client in the use of AMT as prevention. And certainly this information provides a clear method for deciding on when to terminate.

Beyond such uses of self-monitoring, this activity itself may also have its own value in behavioral change. In fact, Bellack and Lombardo (1984) commented that "A major problem in the application of self-monitoring to research is that it has *reactive* effects; behavior changes as a function of self-observation." What happens is that self-monitoring does tend to lead to changes, the direction being a function of the valence of the behavior or its expected consequences (Watson & Tharp, 1981). Undesirable behaviors tend to decrease while desired behaviors tend to increase (Komaki & Dore-Boyce, 1978; Nelson, Lipinski, & Black, 1976).

Fading

Fading derives from the standard procedure in human operant learning whereby stimulus control over an operant performance is gradually transferred to control by a different stimulus (Ferster, Culbertson, & Boren, 1975). For AMT, fading simply involves the notion that the transfer of control is shifted from the therapist as the stimulant for the relaxation control to clients as the initiators of their own relaxation to control anxiety. The value of the fading principle is that it insures errorless learning. For relaxation, the initial AMT session involves the development of relaxation under the direct instructions and guidance of the therapist, including the therapist's signaling when the relaxation is to begin and when it is to end. This same direct control by the therapist is employed for the onset of anxiety arousal, and the use of relaxation to terminate the arousal. With the third AMT Session, fading is used in having the client take more responsibility for initiating the relaxation that begins each session, but not the relaxation that is used following

Table 4.1. Fading of Therapist Control in Favor of Client Control

Session 1: Relaxation	Therapist initiates relaxation through guided directions
Session 2: Relaxation	Therapist initiates relaxation through abbreviated guided directions
Anxiety induction/ relaxation control	Therapist initiates scene for anxiety induction, termination of scene, and initiation of relaxation for anxiety control
Session 3: Relaxation	Client initiates self-relaxation
Anxiety induction/ relaxation control	Therapist initiates scene for anxiety induction, termination of scene, and initiation of relaxation for anxiety control
Session 4: Relaxation	Client initiates self-relaxation
Anxiety induction/ relaxation control	Therapist initiates scene for anxiety induction, client terminates scene and client initiates relaxation for anxiety control
Session 5: Relaxation	Client initiates self-relaxation
Anxiety induction/ relaxation control	Therapist initiates scene for anxiety induction, client initiates relaxation for anxiety control during anxiety scene, then client terminates anxiety scene following elimination of anxiety

anxiety arousal (for anxiety coping). As sessions proceed, more responsibility is transferred to the client. Table 4.1 illustrates the initial high control over instructions by the therapist, and the transfer from the therapist to the client. Although the typical client is usually able to proceed within four sessions to major self-control over anxiety induction and anxiety control, transferring this responsibility can be delayed if an individual client is slow in progressing.

This application of the fading concept provides a useful bridge between the gap of treatments which would rely solely upon therapist management and directions, versus treatments which would make the client responsible for his/her own self-management from the very start of therapy. In addition, as the therapist proceeds to the AMT session which requires more client responsibility, the therapist might also communicate, "From your homework reporting, and given your progress in our last session, I feel you are ready for the next step in AMT. Today, we'll have you on your own use more of the relaxation skills you've acquired." What this accomplishes is the acknowledgment that the client does have the required skills to accept more self-control.

Homework

Homework has now become recognized as a means of insuring compliance, as a mechanism for assuring continuity between treatment sessions, as a procedure for developing generalization of gains outside of the therapy session, as a means of obtaining information about progress for therapy planning, as a method for integrating the therapy into daily routines, and to provide personal meaning to the therapy process. Homework has been adopted into programs as diverse as marital therapy (Margolin, 1987), impulse control training for children (Kendall & Braswell, 1985), cognitive therapy for anxiety disorders and depression (Beck & Emery, 1985; Neimeyer, Twentyman, & Prezant, 1985), and asssertiveness training (Kazdin & Mascitelli, 1982).

All of these advantages of homework assignments are reasons for their importance in AMT. Also, just as the concept of fading forms the basis for changes in how each AMT session is conducted, in the same way there is a certain logic to homework assignments. What is required of the client is an extension of the learning which is being promoted in the session preceding the assignment (Table 4.2). Essentially the homework helps to consolidate the learning as well as transfer its application to real life, and, in some instances, to promote a further extension of the skills. To be specific, Table 4.2 shows the objectives of such assignments and the match to the training of each session.

The client's results from homework are always reviewed through

Table 4.2. Relevance of Homework to Progress in Sessions

Session 1:	Training is in relaxation in the controlled quiet setting of the therapy room.	Homework strengthens this skill through requiring practicing relaxation in quiet place at home.
Session 2:	Abbreviated relaxation instructions are used, including first use of anxiety induction/relaxation control.	Homework further consolidates relaxation skills by requiring practice in nonactive settings outside home, e.g., waiting in car.
Session 3:	Anxiety induction/control continues; attention to identifying early signs of the start of anxiety.	Homework focuses on applying relaxation control when client begins to notice early signs of stress.
Session 4:	Anxiety induction/control continues with client assuming more responsibility.	Homework emphasizes use of relaxation control for prevention, checking stress levels at specific times or conditions.
Session 5:	Anxiety induction/control continues with client assuming primary responsibility in dealing with anxiety.	Homework encourages application of relaxation control as a means of both prevention and control of anxiety experiences.

self-monitoring logs at the beginning of the next session. This review enables the therapist to gauge progress and hence to make a decision about the client's readiness for the next stage of AMT. In addition, the review insures compliance; it is for this function of compliance that such a review is essential. As Piasecki and Hollon (1987) warn, "In our experience, the leading cause of patient noncompliance is therapist inattention to what clients have already been assigned (in homework)" (pp. 130–131).

Comparison of AMT with Other Therapies

The development of various behavior therapy strategies were at a peak during the 1970s, with many proving their worth, and others seeming to lose popularity or becoming consolidated into other approaches. Anxiety Management Training can be compared to some of the more standard, currently visible therapies in terms of theoretical differences or differences in the procedures.

AMT and Desensitization

Since research has demonstrated the application of AMT to phobic disorders, one logical comparison is against desensitization, since desensitization was designed for treatment of phobias.

Theoretically, systematic desensitization (SD) is based upon counter-conditioning, with the belief that systematic desensitization substitutes the pairing of feared stimulus-relaxation for the initial phobic pairing of feared stimulus-fear response. This substitution occurs through the process of conditioning. We might point out that the individual need not be attentive to, consciously aware, or able to encode the stimulus events for conditioning to occur. We might call this form of conditioning *exteroceptive conditioning*. This type of learning represents the separation between emotional processing and emotional insight discussed by Rachman (1980). In desensitization therapy therefore, the client does not have to engage in an active role for the conditioning to occur. Essentially, the client's role is a passive one in that something happens *to* the client resulting from the instructions.

Procedurally, systematic desensitization requires that the client be able to identify the stimuli associated with the fear in order to construct an anxiety hierarchy, a list of phobic situations which arouse phobic reactions, ranging from very low to very high. The client learns relaxation, then, through imagery, visualizes the situations from the anxiety hierarchy, starting with the lowest. No anxiety arousal is permitted, and scenes are terminated if such occurs. If the client suffers from more than one phobia, then treatment begins anew with an anxiety hierarchy that matches the other phobia. Prevention or control of new anxieties or phobias are not part of the treatment goals.

AMT has both a different theoretical base as well as clearly different procedures and outcomes. Exteroceptive learning similar to desensitization can take place: Some clients will report that their anxiety scene (or phobic scene) is no longer able to elicit anxiety arousal. This may in fact reflect a type of desensitization taking place, whereby the relaxation replaces the anxiety. On the other hand, the basic premise of AMT is that it is a self-control training procedure, whereby clients learn to use relaxation as an active coping method. In this sense, and along with the training in becoming aware of early signs of anxiety arousal, AMT is more a form of what we might call *interoceptive conditioning*. Interoceptive learning involves the activity of encoding as the person is aware of the learning experience, and therefore differs from exteroceptive learning in this regard. Hence, in comparing desensitization with AMT, both desensitization and AMT might involve some form of exteroceptive learning, but AMT also clearly includes some training aimed at interoceptive learning.

Procedurally, AMT does not require the identification of a hierarchy, nor actual identification of the specific phobic stimuli. Instead, all that is needed is for clients to recall an incident in their lives associated with high anxiety and to describe their anxiety reactions and the setting in order to reexperience the anxiety arousal. Relaxation is taught gener-

Table 4.3. Comparison of Desensitization and AMT

	Desensitization	Anxiety Management Training
Orientation	Anxiety passively replaced	Anxiety coping skill learned
Method	Guided imagery, includes relaxation	Guided imagery, includes relaxation
Scenes	Stimulus-specific (emphasizes specific phobic stimuli)	Response-specific (emphasizes the anxiety responses)
Hierarchy	Stepwise and graduated from low to high	Two high-anxiety scenes, fundamentally no hierarchy
If patient becomes anxious	Considered not acceptable	Considered important to learn coping

ally through the same procedures used with systematic desensitization. For multiple phobias, AMT does not require beginning all over, inasmuch as the self-coping approach of AMT promotes generalization. Furthermore, AMT does have prevention and transfer of learning as objectives. Finally, AMT typically covers a briefer number of sessions than systematic desensitization. Table 4.3 highlights some of these comparisons.

As we saw in the earlier chapter on research, AMT and systematic desensitization have similar outcomes immediately at the end of therapy for the targeted phobia being treated. However, at follow-up, AMT clients appear to show continued gains. Further, AMT clients show generalization of coping skills to other anxieties or phobias, while systematic desensitization clients do not.

AMT and Implosion/Flooding

These two therapies can both be classified as anxiety induction or exposure approaches, whereby the clients are faced with their anxieties. However, their differences more than outweigh similarities in both theory and procedures.

Implosion and flooding both rely upon the technique of exposing clients to their anxiety-provoking stimuli, either imaginally or in real life (Last, 1985; Michelson, 1985). Both have as their theoretical foundation the two-factor theory of learning, which includes the role of avoidance behaviors in preventing extinction. These techniques therefore emphasize extinction as the process, and the promotion of extinction through preventing the avoidance behaviors. The two differ in theory in terms of their beliefs about the underlying origins of the fear or anxieties. Implosion relies upon the hypothesis that the origins represent the early psychodynamic history of the client, whereas flooding is more atheoretical or neutral on this idea.

The technique of implosion involves presenting clients imaginally with phobic stimuli in order to arouse anxiety over an extended duration. No relaxation is involved, inasmuch as the entire purpose is to achieve anxiety induction without permitting relief, escape, or avoidance. Consistent with its psychodynamic foundations, implosive imaginal scenes include elaborated description of psychodynamic material associated with the anxiety stimuli. These imaginal scenes are presented hierarchically involving increasingly higher approaches to psychodynamic issues. In contrast, flooding involves exposure, either imaginally or *in vivo* to anxiety stimuli, but without the hierarchical approach or psychodynamic content of implosion. Both implosion and flooding can be completed in a shorter time frame than AMT.

AMT differs theoretically in being based upon a self-coping model rather than a conditioning/extinction model and, like flooding, has no premises about psychodynamic interpretations of stressors. While implosion and flooding emphasize preventing the maladaptive responses of escape or avoidance, AMT focuses instead upon the learning of adaptive or coping behaviors for anxiety control and early recognition of anxiety arousal. Flooding has been applied entirely *in vivo* and implosion has been applied entirely in imaginal presentations; on the other hand, AMT provides continuity between the imaginal and real life through the use of imagery in the sessions and real life applications via homework assignments. There have been almost no comparisons between AMT and implosion or flooding in the research literature, other than the work of Shoemaker (1976) with community mental health clients diagnosed as anxiety neurotics. He reported that AMT led to significant reductions in

Table 4.4. Comparison of Implosion and Flooding with AMT

	Implosion/flooding	Anxiety Management Training
Orientation	Anxiety passively extinguished	Anxiety coping skill learned
Method	Guided imagery for implosion; imagery *in vivo* for flooding	Guided imagery plus homework for *in vivo* application
Scenes	Stimulus-specific but can rely mainly on anxiety response; psychodynamic for implosion, not for flooding	Anxiety response-specific; no psychodynamic material
Hierarchy	Psychodynamic hierarchy for implosion; basically none for flooding	Basically no hierarchy
If patient becomes anxious	Considered essential in order to prevent avoidance; anxiety prolonged in session	Considered essential to practice coping skill; anxiety eliminated in session through relaxation

anxiety on three measures of general anxiety, with AMT being superior to implosion and a placebo control. Implosion was no more effective than either the control or a relaxation-only group on two measures. On the measure of state anxiety, implosion was more effective than relaxation-only, but relaxation-only results were not significantly better than the control. Findings on the trait anxiety scale were previously illustrated in Figure 2.3.

Table 4.4 summarizes some salient comparisons of AMT with implosion and flooding.

AMT and Stress Inoculation Training

There are some aspects which AMT and Stress Inoculation Training (SIT) have in common (see Table 4.5), although Stress Inoculation Training is currently more a program of various optional techniques. The early version of Stress Inoculation Training focused on cognitive learning theory, but this therapy has since been revised and the interventions used expanded (Meichenbaum & Deffenbacher, 1988). The theory for Stress Inoculation Training identifies anxiety as not only involving heightened autonomic arousal, but also as being associated with anxiety-laden cognitions, such as thoughts or images. For Stress Inoculation Training theory, cognitive processes have always had an important place, as seen in discussion of internal self-dialogues, negative self-instructions, attributions, views about life, and appraisals. Procedurally, Stress Inocu-

Table 4.5. Stress Inoculation Training and AMT

	Stress Inoculation Training	Anxiety Management Training
Orientation	Anxiety coping with diverse interventions, e.g., applied relaxation, cognitive restructuring, humor, affect expression	Anxiety coping with active use of relaxation
Method	Diverse interventions, may include guided rehearsal, relaxation, homework, self-instruction, self-monitoring, problem solving	Guided rehearsal for anxiety induction and relaxation control
Hierarchy	Hierarchy used, anxiety induction used, imagery includes relaxation for coping as well as competency/coping imagery	No hierarchy, imagery involves applying relaxation for coping
If patient becomes anxious	Anxiety induction desirable	Anxiety induction desirable

lation Training is viewed as having three phases: conceptual, skills acquisition and rehearsal, and application and transfer of coping skills. Although early descriptions of Stress Inoculation Training appear to present the exact steps of Stress Inoculation Training in a more delineated way, the current eclectic programmatic approach seems more of a fluid process, with adaptions for individual cases. Briefly, the identifiable elements of each phase are as follows (Meichenbaum & Deffenbacher, 1988):

Conceptual Phase. Basically an intake assessment phase, whereby patient and therapist collaborate in understanding the nature of the anxiety and the types of interventions suitable, such as cognitive restructuring for thought-controlled anxieties, or relaxation for physiological tensions.

Skill Acquisition and Rehearsal Phase. Here a variety of alternative skills are considered, including cognitive restructuring, problem solving, information gathering, self-reinforcement, self-instruction, and applied relaxation. Generally, such skills are grouped as instrumental or problem-focused (information gathering, problem solving, social skills training) versus palliative or emotion-regulating (cognitive restructuring, applied relaxation, humor, expressing affect). Acquiring these skills is developed through differing strategies, such as self-monitoring, imagery rehearsal, role playing, homework assignments, etc. Meichenbaum considers several skills as helpful to most anxious clients, namely, applied relaxation (similar to AMT), self-reinforcement, and cognitive skills such as cognitive restructuring, self-instruction, and positive self-statements.

Application and Transfer Phase. Aims at transfer to daily life through homework, modeling, graduated *in vivo* exposure, and imagery rehearsal. These phases can overlap as the therapist and client collaborate in identifying and clarifying cognitive issues, as gains are made or failures open up new understanding, or skill strengths produce earlier applications.

Conceptually, the current Stress Inoculation Training appears to be a therapy representing the generalist or eclectic therapist, while AMT represents more of the specialist model. In a sense, Stress Inoculation Training is an armory of interventions representing differing armaments, awaiting selection for the unique target at hand. Depending upon the conceptualization of the client's problem by client and therapist, autonomic induction methods might be used, or cognitive therapy methods, or operant practice methods. In contrast, AMT remains clearly delineated as an anxiety induction approach. When Stress Inoculation

Training selects anxiety induction and applied relaxation, then the general approach is quite similar to AMT. However, the major distinction is in the degree to which each step for training in anxiety induction followed by anxiety control through relaxation is specified. Toward this end, AMT has been refined into steps based upon mechanisms of fading, fitting homework to each session, integrating self-monitoring, and, most important, describing the procedures for anxiety arousal and the subsequent control. Stress Inoculation Training instructions call attention to the general principles governing applied relaxation, such as the need for an active approach, reminders to use relaxation in anticipation of stressful events, and directions to "relax away" the anxiety during imagery rehearsal. In contrast, AMT offers guided training in the proper application of relaxation for coping.

If Stress Inoculation Training is more a general system for therapy, then AMT is more a systematic prescription for training. In one arena, Stress Inoculation Training is more detailed and prescriptive: recommendations on coping self-statements. Here Stress Inoculation Training analyzes the steps into: "preparing for the stressor," "confronting and handling stressors," "coping with feelings of being overwhelmed," and "evaluation of coping efforts and self-rewards"; examples are given for the types of thoughts or self-instructions of use to clients for each step (Meichenbaum, 1985). This emphasis on cognitive processes also distinguishes Stress Inoculation Training from AMT. If irrational cognitions are the origins of anxiety or a phobia, Stress Inoculation Training would arm the therapist with cognitive therapy for this battle, while AMT would be considered inappropriate. However, if cognitions acted as the cues for anxiety arousal, and if eliminating this relationship was a useful therapeutic objective, then AMT would be appropriate. AMT trains clients in coping with anxiety arousal if the arousal is triggered by external stressors or by internal stressors, including thoughts.

Both AMT and the earlier, simpler version of Stress Inoculation Training have each been studied and been independently demonstrated as effective with similar-symptom groups, such as test anxiety, speech anxiety, music performance, social anxiety, generalized anxiety disorder, and Type A patterns (Altmeier, Ross, Leary, & Thornbrough, 1982; Butler, Cullington, Mumby, Amies, & Gelder, 1984; Clark, Salkovskis, & Chalkey, 1985; Deffenbacher & Hahnloser, 1981; Levenkron, Cohen, Mueller, & Fisher, 1983). However, the two treatment approaches have rarely been compared in research. Hazaleus and Deffenbacher did complete one study on anger management, using both AMT and a cognitive therapy *based upon* Stress Inoculation Training including a strong cognitive restructuring component (see Systematic Rational Restructuring in the next section).

Results were equivalent for AMT and Stress Inoculation Training in reducing general anger, physiological arousal, response to provocations, and tendency to respond to provocation with verbal antagonism. At one-month follow-up, the Stress Inoculation Training plus restructuring group showed greater tendencies to cope constructively with anger than the AMT group; however, both treatment groups were equivalent on level of state anger. At one-year follow-up, Stress Inoculation Training subjects showed lower general anxiety than control subjects, while AMT subjects' levels were not significantly different from Stress Inoculation Training or controls. This is in contradiction to the finding of Deffenbacher, Demm, and Brandon that AMT subjects treated for anger showed a significantly lower general anxiety level than control subjects.

Kelly and Stone studied AMT, AMT combined with cognitive therapy based upon Stress Inoculation Training, and AMT combined with values clarification. All three treatments were found equally effective in reducing Type A behaviors, leading the authors to conclude that neither Stress Inoculation Training (SIT) nor values clarification added much to AMT treatment alone. On anxiety, however, both AMT/SIT and AMT/values showed lower reductions in anxiety levels than AMT alone.

Mygdal (1978) compared AMT, Stress Inoculation Training, placebo, and a control group in a study of anxious teachers. Results did not confirm any significant differences among the groups, although there was a trend for the two treatment groups to lead to lower anxiety on self-report scales, but not on behavioral or supervisor ratings.

Ziegler *et al.* compared AMT with Stress Inoculation Training with athletes and found that both methods led to significant improvements in physiological efficiency, measured by oxygen consumption and heart rate. These gains were superior to those of a control group.

In summary, there have not been many studies in which both AMT and SIT have been directly compared. The efficacy of each treatment approach has been independently studied, and found useful for symptoms such as test anxiety, speech anxiety, performance anxiety, and for persons suffering from generalized anxiety disorder or showing the Type A behavioral pattern. One study on anger comparing AMT and Stress Inoculation Training found both to be equally valuable for anger management, with Stress Inoculation Training being better on general anxiety reduction during follow-up. Another study comparing AMT and Stress Inoculation Training directly for Type A behaviors showed results leading the authors to conclude that a program which added Stress Inoculation Training to AMT did not add much to behavioral change outcomes. However, a combination of Stress Inoculation Training and AMT produced lower levels of anxiety.

AMT and Systematic Rational Restructuring

Among the various cognitive therapy approaches to anxiety or phobias is Systematic Rational Restructuring (SRR) which focuses on the major role of cognitions in anxiety (Goldfried, Decenteceo, & Weinberg, 1974). The theoretical foundation derives from Ellis' conclusions that irrational belief systems create negative emotions, and Lazarus' contention that stress derives from a person's appraisal of an event as threatening (Ellis, 1962; Lazarus, 1966). In Systematic Rational Restructuring, Goldfried adds that these individual beliefs or appraisals are ways of construing the environment, and reflect underlying basic schemas. Two basic schemas are said to be common: those reflecting the need for approval ("If I'm not liked, then I'm no good") and those reflecting a need for perfection ("If I don't do a perfect job, then I'm a failure in everything"). Systematic Rational Restructuring aims at helping clients discover their underlying schemas in their beliefs and view evidence which leads to changing such beliefs. An important characteristic of Systematic Rational Restructuring is its attempt to aid clients in learning how to change their perspectives by themselves, a self-management goal.

Systematic Rational Restructuring covers various procedures that are considered flexible and more "clinical guidelines" than hard and fast steps (Goldfried, 1988). The procedures involve:

- Enabling clients to accept that thoughts mediate emotions. In a way this establishes the rationale of therapy to the client.
- Eliciting from the client a realization that the belief is unrealistic. Systematic Rational Restructuring focuses on questioning how realistic the client's beliefs are, one method being through the therapist acting as a devil's advocate. The emphasis is that the therapist take a position such that the clients themselves offer arguments to refute their own irrational stance. During this stage, a schema similar to that being maintained by the client is discussed by the therapist but in an impersonal way, "Supposing I said I believed that everything I do must be perfect, and if I am less than perfect on even one task, then I'm a failure. What do you think of that?"
- Identifying the unrealistic beliefs mediating the client's anxiety. Through the prior discussions clients may see the relevance of the examples to their own anxieties and implicit beliefs. If not, then therapy proceeds to move toward a more personal set of examples which involves the clients' own situations. Initially focus is on the false assumptions or appraisals ("So you are figuring that you didn't carry off the interview as well. . . as well as what. . . how well did you figure you needed to do?"). Once the irrational com-

ponents are identified, then the clients are moved toward recognizing the more basic schema underlying the false assumptions ("Let's suppose you didn't do perfectly this time, why would that upset you so much?")

• Helping clients to reevaluate their unrealistic beliefs. This is the behavioral change phase during which clients' emotional reaction (anxiety) must now serve as a signal to stop and to question the reality of their assumptions, and to substitute a more adaptive appraisal. This goal is achieved through several techniques, including imaginal rehearsal, homework practice, or therapeutic techniques such as the two-chair exercise.

• Imagery rehearsal requires the client to visualize being in an anxiety situation, then to identify what thoughts they are having that cause the anxiety. They would "think out loud," and begin to analyze whether their thoughts are irrational, and then work at revising these thoughts to be more realistic. By monitoring their anxiety levels during this exercise, the clients can become aware of improved coping. A hierarchy of real-life anxiety-producing incidents are constructed, with successful coping at the one level determining progress to the next scene. To facilitate this style of thinking aloud and questioning, the therapist might model the process.

• Homework practice involves the assignment of trying out this self-coping/thinking process. This assignment is not specifically planned; however, the clients are encouraged to use life opportunities to practice, even though some incidents may prove difficult. Self-monitoring is required involving records of the situation, type of unrealistic thoughts, realistic reevaluation, and change in anxiety levels.

• The two-chair exercise is borrowed from Gestalt therapy and involves having the client engage in a self-dialogue, shifting from chair to chair to assume a different vantage point.

Systematic Rational Restructuring and AMT have very different theoretical foundations, with Systematic Rational Restructuring being firmly based upon cognitive theory. Whereas Systematic Rational Restructuring assumes that "changing the thought will lead to controlling the anxiety," AMT assumes that "coping with relaxation leads to controlling the anxiety." Whereas Systematic Rational Restructuring assumes that "false beliefs should be identified in order to serve as the signal for coping through realistic thoughts," AMT assumes that "anxiety reactions—autonomic, somatic, or cognitive—should be identified in order to serve as the signal for coping through relaxation."

As with many cognitive therapies, Systematic Rational Restructuring involves activities stressing verbal discussions, inquiries and questioning, and logical examination and refutation. In contrast, following the intake assessment, AMT tends to minimize such verbal interactions, and instead emphasizes training activities. Imagery may be used by Systematic Rational Restructuring and will involve hierarchical situations for the purpose of practicing realistic reappraisals. AMT relies heavily upon imagery, without a hierarchy, and also for the purpose of practice, but to gain skill in relaxation control. Homework in Systematic Rational Restructuring appears less systematically planned as a match for each treatment session; in AMT, homework systematically derives from the progress within each session. Self-monitoring is used by both treatments, with some similarity in the recording logs. However, Systematic Rational Restructuring records only thoughts, both unrealistic and realistic. AMT records early signs of anxiety onset, which might include thoughts, or somatic or autonomic symptoms; similar to Systematic Rational Restructuring, AMT also records level of change in anxiety following coping as well as descriptions of the situations faced. Table 4.6 summarizes these comparisons between Systematic Rational Restructuring and AMT.

Research reviews of Systematic Rational Restructuring have included studies on rational-emotive therapy (RET), since Systematic Rational Restructuring has a basis in RET theory and is similar in procedure (Goldfried, 1979). However, the focus of many studies on the Systematic Rational Restructuring model itself is more limited, and has

Table 4.6. Systematic Rational Restructuring and AMT

	Systematic Rational Restructuring	Anxiety Management Training
Orientation	Anxiety coping through actively changing cognitions	Anxiety coping through active use of relaxation
Method	General guidelines provided, diverse process, emphasis on cognitive change via self-evaluation, guided rehearsal, homework, modeling, Gestalt methods	Specific procedures provided, guided rehearsal, including for anxiety induction and relaxation control
Hierarchy	Hierarchy used when guided rehearsal is used	No hierarchy
If patient becomes anxious	Acceptable, client remains in scene until anxiety is reduced by relaxation or other coping	Anxiety induction desirable for learning relaxation coping

generally been on situation-specific anxieties, such as test anxiety, public speaking anxiety, and social/interpersonal anxiety (Goldfried, Linehan, & Smith, 1978; Kanter & Goldfried, 1979; Lent, Russell, & Zamostny, 1981). AMT and Systematic Rational Restructuring have not been directly compared. However, Hazaleus and Deffenbacher did treat one group for anger with AMT, and another group with a cognitive therapy based upon Stress Incolulation Training and Systematic Rational Restructuring. These results were reported in our summary of Stress Inoculation Training, and basically showed the equivalence of the methods, except for follow-up. The cognitive therapy group at follow-up showed greater use of constructive coping and less general anxiety than the AMT group.

Jenni and Wollersheim compared AMT against a cognitive therapy based upon rational-emotive therapy in the treatment of Type A behaviors. Using the Bortner scale as the measure of Type A, the cognitive therapy approach achieved significant changes, while the AMT group did not. On state anxiety, both treatment groups reached nearly the same level of post-therapy anxiety, a level significantly lower than that of a control group. On trait anxiety, both treatments showed significant pre- to post-therapy reductions; however, the post-therapy levels were not significantly different from those achieved by a control.

In summary, Systematic Rational Restructuring and AMT have not been directly compared in terms of treatment efficacy. However, both approaches have been independently studied and found helpful in reducing anxieties relating to testing, public speaking, and social/interpersonal situations. One study on anger compared AMT with a cognitive behavior therapy that combined features of Systematic Rational Restructuring and Stress Inoculation Training, and found that this cognitive approach had results equivalent to those when AMT was used. However, the cognitive therapy group showed greater reductions in general anxiety on follow-up than the AMT group. Another study also used a cognitive therapy based upon rational-emotive therapy with Type A persons, and found the behavior therapy to be effective, while AMT was not effective.

Summary

This chapter provides an overview on AMT, first by outlining the basics of each AMT session, and then stating the principles underlying AMT. There are fundamentally five AMT sessions, in addition to the usual intake interview. Further sessions beyond five are assigned as needed to strengthen the client's ability to manage anxiety, and where such sessions are used, the format follows the outline for session five. Typically, six to eight sessions are planned, with more or fewer sessions being conducted depending upon the individual needs of the client.

The principles underlying AMT reflect those principles most associated with facilitating behavioral change. These include: the need for active involvement by the client in acquiring coping behaviors, the need for acquiring such skills under a controlled therapeutic environment, the importance of pacing the therapeutic/training experience in a systematic way as skills build in a stepwise manner, the value of having conditions for skill acquisition which promote increased self-control and self-reliance by the client, the importance of encouraging generalization to settings outside the therapy setting, the need for preventive elements in the therapy, the value of improving self-efficacy, and the importance of both anxiety exposure experiences along with anxiety reduction experiences during the therapeutic session.

The AMT procedure implements certain psychological procedures, these being: attention to the therapeutic rationale, use of guided rehearsal, development of anxiety arousal through imagery, the application of relaxation for anxiety reduction, and the use of fading, self-monitoring, and homework.

The chapter also compares AMT with other behavior therapies, including systematic desensitization, implosion and flooding, Stress Inoculation Training, and Systematic Rational Restructuring. There are generally only a few studies which directly compared AMT against these other therapies. Where each of the treatment approaches have been studied independently, results appear to indicate that each of these treatment approaches have been successful in reducing situational anxieties, such as test anxiety. Further, AMT, Stress Inoculation Training, and Systematic Rational Restructuring (or a cognitive behavior therapy which has features in common with rational restructuring) have been found by different studies to be useful in reducing anger or Type A behaviors.

Although AMT has been found to be superior to desensitization when directly compared on follow-up data, and on generalized anxiety, a few studies have found Stress Inoculation Training or cognitive therapy better than AMT at follow-up on general anxiety or Type A behaviors. Because of the scarcity of such direct comparative studies, it is too early to tell from outcome data whether AMT, Stress Inoculation Training, or Systematic Rational Restructuring is truly the treatment of choice for certain symptoms or disorders. The most conservative conclusion is that each does seem to have treatment outcome effects greater than those achieved by no treatment. Hence, at this stage, the choice of which therapy to adopt must rest with the therapist's knowledge of the differences in procedures or theoretical foundations of the three behavior therapies. For instance, AMT would be preferred over desensitization where multiple phobias are present, since AMT is more efficient. AMT would also be the preferred mode of therapy over implosion or flooding, if the therapist prefers a self-control therapy model that teaches the client a skill which is available for resolving other current or future difficulties. Regarding AMT and Stress Inoculation Training, AMT might be preferred as a more systematically described method, while Stress Inoculation Training appears to have now evolved into a less structured, more general program of psychotherapy. AMT could be the treatment of choice instead of Systematic Rational Restructuring where the therapist is seeking an approach that involves not only cognitive but noncognitive factors in anxiety. Other procedural differences among the therapies would also play roles in the choice of therapy: for instance, whether the treatment approach can be administered in a group setting, how many total sessions need to be scheduled, whether *in vivo* sessions need to be designed, and what skills are required of the therapist.

5

When to Treat an Anxious Client with Anxiety Management Training
Case Illustrations

Anxiety Management Training has applications for a variety of anxiety-based problems, as confirmed by the outcomes in research studies. Briefly, AMT would be appropriate for the following:

- clients for whom anxiety is the primary symptom, such as generalized anxiety disorder, phobic disorder, panic disorder, or situation-specific anxiety states, such as test anxiety or mathematics anxiety;
- clients for whom the anxiety contributes substantively to the primary symptoms, as in essential hypertension, ulcers, or tension headaches;
- clients for whom the anxiety may be viewed as exacerbating the primary condition, as in dysmenorrhea or diabetes;
- clients for whom the anxiety is an obstacle to effective psychotherapy or counseling, such as patients at a plateau in insight therapy or clients in career counseling;
- clients for whom anxiety is severe enough to disrupt performance, such as athletes or musicians;
- clients for whom the anxiety may be a mediating factor in preventing adaptive changes, as in Type A behaviors;
- clients for whom emotional regulation is desired due to the immu-

tability of the stressors, such as irresolvable life stress or daily hassles;

- clients confronted with multiple stressors or anxieties, such as multiple phobias or multiple environmental stresses;
- clients for whom anxiety may be a mediating factor in another psychological symptom, such as depression or low self-esteem; and
- clients for whom anger or frustration management is a primary symptom, and possibly as a step in hyperactivity control.

Clients with Anxiety as Primary Symptom[1]

Generalized Anxiety Disorder (Jeff)

Jeff was being seen in a community mental health center initially for a complaint of malaise, loss of energy, constant tiredness, and fatigue. He had seen several physicians, including a specialist in blood diseases, and a nutritionist, and had extensive blood chemistry work. All reports had been negative, and no physical, biochemical, or dietary disorders were diagnosed. He was told that "stress" might be associated, and Jeff eventually made his way to a mental health center to seek stress management. The intake staff member convinced Jeff to agree to a series of short-term appointments with a social worker to obtain more detailed information on what was happening, inasmuch as the presenting complaints did not seem sufficient to confirm that stress was the underlying factor.

Jeff is a 30-year-old, plump accountant who had recently been divorced, and who was living by himself for the first time in his life. Prior to his marriage, he had lived at home, then with a roomate who was "a real homebody. . . knew how to shop, how to even bake, how to keep a budget. . . just everything." Following the divorce, Jeff managed gradually to learn the bare essentials for self-care, including some simple cooking. His work involved being one of five persons in an accounting firm, with rumors being that his work was so well regarded that he was one of two employees being considered for a partnership. In all, Jeff did not report any sense of distress about the divorce ("although I sometimes miss her. . . it was a good life, but she left and life goes on"), nor any sense of pressure or stress on the job. He described adapting "so-so" in his role as a single and commented, "At least I'm only responsible for myself, I don't have any kids to worry about."

[1]Some details of these cases have been altered in order to provide for anonymity of the clients.

Since discussions surrounding the malaise did not seem to be leading to any new information, the social worker encouraged him to talk about the divorce. It was a quiet one: one day his wife Jill simply announced that they had "grown apart," and she wanted to do other things with her life. Although Jeff did not want the divorce, he felt helpless in the decision—"She didn't ask me what I thought. . . she just left"—and made no attempts to stop her. Jill did not ask for any settlement or any form of support.

As Jeff described his marriage, he centered more and more on how idyllic it seemed to him, in terms of having little responsibility, being cared for, living an essentially passive life without many decisions. It seemed a haven as he came home from his daily responsibilities. Soon after these discussions, Jeff began to report nightmares, each around a theme of searching for his car, which he parked somewhere, needed to find to meet a deadline, but could not remember the location. After three weeks, he began reporting anxiety attacks, sometimes at work, more often at home. Attacks at work involved moments of trembling, confusion, waves of panic, increased heart rate. Since he had his own desk area closed off from the sight of others by dividers, none of the other coworkers ever noticed these attacks. Similar attacks occurred at home, at different times, seemingly not associated with any specific circumstances.

Now a fear was added that he was going crazy, or that some serious biochemical damage was occurring which caused the attacks. He soon became apprehensive about his vulnerability to such waves of anxiety, worrying about when the next one would develop. His sleep disruptions continued to occur, along with insomnia. His apprehensive state began to lead to more and more insomnia and sleep loss. Further in-depth discussions about his feelings regarding his loss of his idyllic marriage, feelings of passivity, and conflicts over his enforced independent living seemed authentic, but appeared to have no bearing on reducing his nightmares or his anxiety attacks. At this point, AMT was considered as an adjunct to psychotherapy to attempt to reduce the anxiety and clear up the sleep disturbance, before loss of sleep further complicated his symptom picture.

Comment. This case might conceivably have developed satisfactorily if the social work had been successful in enabling Jeff to see the relationship between his repressed conflicts over dependence/independence and the loss of his spouse, and his anxiety and malaise. However, although the discussion seemed meaningful to Jeff, the increased anxiety attacks, nightmares, and loss of sleep were becoming serious problems of their own accord. Possibly these were no more than signs that the repression was being released so that the deeper emotions were surfacing. However, since eight months of therapeutic discussions were not producing a decline of these anxiety symptoms, AMT was used as a focused intervention to control the anxiety.

As with cases of anxiety where the client is unable to pinpoint the exact stimuli precipitating the anxiety reactions, Jeff could only know that he experienced waves of anxiety at different times and places. Hence, to obtain a description of an anxiety situation needed for AMT treatment, the therapist used the following instruction: "Tell me about the last time you experienced an anxiety attack that was about a 60 level. . . on a scale from 0, meaning no anxiety, to 100, meaning panic." Jeff's reply was: "I was at work about one week ago. Then, without warning and for no good reason. . . I started to shake. . . is this what you want?" This was an appropriate start of a description, and since he was beginning to describe his anxiety symptoms, he was encouraged to continue: "Go on, that's good, tell me more." Jeff then responded:

> "Like I said, there was no warning. . . my hands just shook, it was scary. . . and I could feel the nervousness inside me that kind of kept pace with the trembling. . . the feeling you have when you're being scared by some horrible monster. . . goes up your throat. . . and I've had this before, but thought it would go away, but here it is again. . . I closed my door so no one would walk in on me, actually wobbled back to my desk, my legs felt weak. . . closed my eyes and tried to breath calmly. . . but my breathing was kind of sporadic, tight. I could still think and probably answered the telephone for a brief call, but I was really trembly and weak-kneed."

AMT requires that the client be able to identify and describe the details of a real life experience in which anxiety has been present. The reason is that this "anxiety scene" is then used in the AMT session to enable reexperiencing the anxiety arousal, in order for the client to have practice in eliminating this arousal through the use of relaxation. Having a precise description of his anxiety symptoms will help the therapist as the therapist reminds Jeff about these feelings during the use of the anxiety scene, thereby further enhancing Jeff's ability to experience the anxiety arousal in the session. In addition, it is important to have details that also describe the surroundings, details we call "scene-setting details," to further aid Jeff when he is asked to recall the experience in the AMT session. Hence, he was asked, "Expand a little more on describing the setting of the instance you just cited. . . so I can picture it myself, like what were the surroundings like that day, what were you doing, and so forth. . . as many details as you can so I can really picture myself there." Jeff's description was as follows:

> "I was doing the monthly billing for a business account we have, a laundry business. . . sitting at my desk, the door of my office was open, we have these

cubicles formed by dividers to make our offices. . . and I just had this attack, like once before here."

It is essential to have a very specific incident that is identified. Jeff appears to have had two such experiences in his office. If his description is left ambiguous, then when he is later instructed to recall the incident in order to experience anxiety arousal, he might mix the two events together, and have his recall disrupted. Hence it was necessary to obtain more precise information, and therefore Jeff was asked, "So you were at your desk, at work, doing the billing for the laundry business. . . you said this attack was similar to one you experienced before. . . so tell me some more descriptions of this particular day. . . what details can you give me that makes it clear that you are remembering this one occasion and not the other. . . for instance, do you recall the date, time?" Jeff became much more precise at this point:

"Oh, you want more details. . . yes, as I said, a week ago. . . exactly 10 a.m. . . .I know because I had looked at my watch to gauge how much time I had to complete this file. . . I had the file in my hands, opened and there were twenty bills and receipts attached. . . my door was open, did I tell you that?. . . and I was reading the first receipt, holding it in my hand when my hand started to tremble. . . "[T: "And how did this differ from the other occasion?"]. . . "the other time was in the afternoon, when I had just returned from lunch. . . I was getting ready to review a file, but it was another company. . . "[T: "So getting back to the morning with the laundry company, describe the setting more for me. . . are there other details you recall about your surroundings, what you were doing, thinking?"]"...no, I was reading this file. . . had a cup of coffee in front of me, my favorite mug with Garfield on it. . . there were some typing sounds from the secretary. . . my desk is cluttered, had a pen in my hand. . . "

AMT was conducted with the usual approach: Jeff was trained in muscle relaxation in the first session, then given the homework assignment to practice the relaxation before the next session in a week. At the next session, he was asked to close his eyes and go through the exercise in order to achieve relaxation. After being relaxed, Jeff was then instructed to "Switch on the anxiety scene you described before. . . the one of being in your office in the morning. . . 10 a.m. . . .the laundry file in your hand, reading the first receipt. . . really switch on this scene so that you are there again. . . actually allow yourself to be there. . . one week ago. . . coffee in front of you. . . your hands start to tremble, you're having this attack. . . you thought maybe it wouldn't happen again. . . but there it is. . . trembling, weakness in the knees. . . nervousness keeping beat with your trembling. . . sporadic tight breathing. . . let the anxiety return again. . . let yourself experience the anxiety" (the exact steps and instructions for AMT sessions will be outlined in Chapters 6, 7, and 8). Following this anxiety arousal, Jeff was given instructions for regaining the relaxation by turning off the anxiety scene and returning to muscle relaxation.

Fifteen AMT sessions were used, with anxiety arousal coming eventually from two scenes involving the anxiety attacks, one being a situation before sleep during which he became extremely apprehensive. Jeff experienced a dramatic reduction of his anxiety symptoms, expressed a sense of confidence of "being in control of my life. . . nothing can shake me now that I've proven I can manage the worst." His psychotherapy continued on the themes of dependence/independence and his personal feelings about potential increased responsibility as a partner.

Phobic Disorder (Jennifer)

Jennifer was a 16-year-old Asian-American student who was experiencing a great deal of anxiety over examinations. Her father had been raised in Japan, where the taking and passing of tests determined the individual's entire future, starting from the admission to the best secondary school to admission to the best university, and eventually offer of employment in the best firm. With the high significance attached to examination results, suicide among his friends had not been uncommon. Jennifer's father eventually emigrated to Hawaii as much to improve his job status as to protect his youngsters from the examination pressures. Nevertheless, Jennifer was brought up hearing all of these stories, in the context of being told how much better her life was without such stress. Further, she understood implicitly that she was expected to be an academic and life success, given that she lived under a freer environment, and should pass tests because she was a good student rather than because her future was dependent upon the examinatic n scores. By her junior high school year, Jennifer had been doing well, often being within the top three persons in her classes.

In the first year of junior high, however, she began to experience worries about examinations. This came as a sudden change, since she always took tests well and experienced no apprehensions. Now, starting with her first geography test, she found herself sweating, having difficulty swallowing and breathing, feeling a sense of doom ("I woke up knowing, just knowing that this was a bad day, kind of like an evil cloud hanging around; like I'm not superstitious, but I just knew something bad was going to happen"). In the middle of the 70-question examination, she suddenly went blank: "I couldn't remember anything. . . I couldn't read the items either, I'd just stare and stare, and they were just a jumble of. . . things that I could not decipher." Despite her own worse fears, her grade was still a low "C." Nevertheless, from this experience and onward, Jennifer continued to experience intense anxiety surrounding test-taking.

She often dreaded the time in school when the teachers would discuss their plans for the term, the assignments and expectations, because invariably the question of tests would be raised. In her anticipation, Jennifer would begin to feel her breath shorten, and she would have a feeling that she should leave the room before something happened. "It's not like I'm thinking, 'Oh, oh, we're going to talk about tests'; it's more a feeling, like your body is saying, 'Time to take a walk before the brick wall falls on you.' If you were to ask me why I was fidgeting, I wouldn't even be able to say." Even if examinations are casually mentioned in passing by the teacher, Jennifer's anxieties would remain, "It's like you opened up a coffin and all the bad moths came flying out and you can't shove them back in. I'm now only thinking about tests, how much I hate them, and there's this feeling in the pit of my stomach. . . and I'm not hearing what the teacher is saying anymore." Circumstances that trigger her anxiety include studying for an examination, hearing classmates talk about how they are preparing for an exam, waiting for the corrected tests to be returned, and even just seeing the word "test" in a workbook.

At this point in the intake, the therapist asked her to estimate her current level of anxiety as she was talking about her fears; her response was, "Right now? For awhile now. . . since we started on this. . . about testing. . . it's been difficult. . . using your scale, it's close to, about 90." Jennifer's grades have started to be erratic. Some teachers have been sympathetic and willing to follow up a written examination with an oral one immediately after in response to Jennifer's observation that "All the answers come back to me as soon as I walk out of the room. . . it's while I'm looking at the test questions that I go blank. . . but I know it all, and I can tell you anything right after." However, even this approach has not been fully successful, since Jennifer has also failed in such orals: "Maybe it depends on my mood. When I was tested by my history teacher, I just thought he *looked* grim and serious and like he was really judging me, and I didn't do well, I clutched. I didn't feel right. But I like my science teacher and she didn't try to sound like a judge or jury, we just talked for a while, and pretty soon I was answering some questions, just like we were having a conversation about. . . about, just about anything over dessert. I was in a really good mood then."

For nearly a year, Jennifer has felt her confidence in herself waning, and believed that her parents were more and more disappointed in her. "I feel that they're not saying anything directly, but they feel I'm being lazy and if I put my mind to it, I could do well. They don't understand it when I say I'm scared of exams. My father says, 'If you want to know being scared, you should have lived in Japan. How can you be scared in our American system?' Then they say, 'Don't worry about it, it'll pass, just do the best you can and make us proud of you.'" Jennifer was now becoming tense when seeing her father after school, and especially after an examination, "I'd come home and be all right. But he arrives home from work about 5:30 and then we have dinner, and the first thing. . . I just know. . . eventually he will casually ask, 'How's school today,' and meanwhile, while I'm waiting for this, I lose my appetite, I'm getting more and more nervous and fidgety. . . I don't want to look at him. . . look him in the eye, or talk about things."

Comment. Jennifer has not wanted to see anyone professionally about her difficulties, but her science teacher had arranged for her to see the school counselor, walking down with her for an appointment and sitting in on the first meeting. Although desensitization was given serious consideration, the counselor decided on starting with AMT because of the possibility of achieving noticeable gains more quickly and because of the possible generalization to the anxiety produced at dinner by the father's questions. The sense was also that AMT could return Jennifer's self-confidence since she would be learning a skill which she could apply in a variety of circumstances, during the examination, when studying for an examination, when overhearing classmates talk about the examination, when papers were being returned, and even during oral examinations; that is, she could use AMT skills under the various conditions which already appeared associated with her anxiety.

AMT generally relies upon the client identifying two anxiety incidents to be later used to obtain anxiety arousal in the sessions. One incident should be associated with a moderate level of anxiety, about a 60 intensity anxiety while the other should involve a very high level, about a 90 intensity. For her 60 level incident, she remembered and described the moments before being given the oral examination in history. The incident was as follows:

> "I was sitting in this testing room, a small room with chairs and tables. . . no one else was there except outside in the outer office was a testing office secretary. . . and I was waiting for Mr._____, my history teacher. . . I had studied well and felt pretty good. . . at least no written test. . . but then I felt that he sometimes looked angry, and he was O.K. as a teacher, but not real friendly, you know, not good with kids. . . and I wondered if this was going to be one where he would try to trick me. . . maybe he was late because he was put out about having to spend extra time with me. . . it was not like this was going to be a friendly conversation, or even like when my friends and I would review for tests by quizzing one another. . . this was going to be real, and he was going to be watching me and grading . . . on the other hand, this was better than those written things, with row after row of multiple guess questions. . . and the intense room, everyone quiet, pencils scribbling, erasing. . . all that thinking. . . this would be better. . . at least we would be alone. . . still, I was feeling the butterflies, breathing kind of hard. . . "

As it turned out, when the test began in earnest, and after the third question was asked orally, Jennifer begain to experience higher anxiety.

As she reported, "he looked grim. . . like he was judging me. . . I clutched." However, in assessing the level of intensity at this stage, Jennifer reported that it was still only up to 70 intensity. Furthermore, although she reported, "I didn't do well," she actually passed this oral exam at a B-minus level, a much better level than she had achieved on an earlier written history test. Using the 0–100 scale and obtaining exact information on her test performance were both useful in interpreting Jennifer's statements. Thus, even though her words "I clutched" implied high intensity anxiety, and "I didn't do well" implied doing poorly on the history exam, in actuality such implications would not have been accurate.

For her 90 intensity anxiety scene, used to achieve high intensity arousal in the AMT session, she described the geography test, in the middle of the 70-question written examination when she went blank, was confused, and experienced panic.

Within four weeks of AMT, meeting for a total of four sessions, she was experiencing reductions in anxiety and, by the sixth session, she was no longer experiencing test anxiety. However, she expressed concern that she would not be able to handle the final examination week, because of the number of examinations and the major significance of their being final examinations. Hence, the counselor agreed to a 'booster' session right before finals. Jennifer's case is therefore still not closed since finals week is still a month away.

Clients with Anxiety Contributing to Another Primary Symptom

Tension Headache (Sandra)

Sandra has become a success in her career experiences, having been a housewife and mother for 15 years of her life, then embarking on outside activities, initially as a volunteer in the community delivering groceries to elderly shut-ins. She soon moved on to being a volunteer clerk for a local attorney, whose disabled father she had been helping and who had become aware of Sandra's interest in expanding her efforts. She did so well for two years that the attorney offered her a position as clerk-typist when one of the secretaries resigned. Sandra was ecstatic about the employment and spent extra hours on her work, and in reading about law. The attorney later ran for office as state senator, was elected, and asked Sandra to remain on his staff. Since this did not entail a move (they were already in the state capitol), she readily agreed. Four years later, her state senator was supported by his party to seek a congressional seat in the U.S. House of Representatives, and was readily elected. Again he asked Sandra to be on his staff, this time as his personal executive secretary. By now, Sandra's children were on their own, but the major issue was whether her husband would agree to leaving their community and moving to Washington. As an auto mechanic, he had built a successful following, specializing in foreign cars. However, he decided that they had saved enough to protect themselves if he took the gamble on being able to attract a new clientele, and for the higher start-up costs in the nation's capitol. With a mixture of excitement and trepidation, Sandra accepted the new position.

The exposure to the sophistication of Washington, D.C. encouraged the growth of Sandra's social talents and intellect. She became the congressman's official "greeter," organized and often attended major social gatherings, and became more and more visible as the elegant right arm of the congressman. Some suggested that she should consider running for office herself, but Sandra always laughed this off, reaffirming her loyalty to her employer. However, as her own sophistication grew rapidly, her husband's did not. He remained disinterested in the social sphere of this major city, was content to concentrate on his now healthy business, and was soon spending as much time working late as did Sandra in her position. Although Sandra felt a growing distance between her interests and her husband's, they had few battles of conscience about their differences. Yet Sandra could sense some level of jealousy and perhaps even bitterness that he was no longer the major breadwinner and that Sandra had increased her self-confidence, and that in many ways she had become superior to him in status, in her knowledge of national affairs, and in her visibility. Still, their marriage seemed intact, and only minor spurts of disagreement intervened in their otherwise quiet marriage.

As the congressman entered his fourth term of office and his authority and power grew, Sandra's duties became more and more substantial. She was now taking on some of the functions of a legislative aide, doing background work on certain policy issues, and even preparing briefs on proposed legislation as well as offering opinions on the consequences of cosponsoring certain bills. The challenge of such expanded duties was satisfying, not only because it stimulated her intellect, but because she viewed it as confirmation of being recognized as a valued assistant. She was now working six and a half days a week, and taking no vacations. Her tension headaches soon began to appear. She could identify no specific causes, since their onset did not seem to be associated with an unusually heavy work schedule, or a particularly stressful deadline, although she felt that she was more subject to them if she had not been sleeping well. Taking sleeping pills helped some, but she was still having a tension headache at least once weekly, sometimes in the evenings, sometimes during the mornings. If she hadn't slept well, the headache was more likely to be a morning one.

Initially she worried about whether she had a brain tumor causing the headaches, but medical examinations quickly ruled this out. On the other hand, she was diagnosed by a physician as suffering from tension headaches, with all the classic features. For instance, her headaches were characterized by a dull pressure surrounding her forehead, with pain just above the neck. At its worst, the headache was accompanied by dizziness and the appearance of spots before her eyes. The pain was "similar to my having a steel band around my head that is tightening" rather than any throbbing. Once the headache appeared, it tended to last nearly all day, that is, seven hours. She was now having them on the average of six times each month. She also discovered that she was clenching her teeth while sleeping; her husband began reporting that she was disrupting his sleep because of the noise she made in grinding her teeth. They moved into separate bedrooms. Sandra also began to gain weight, but went on a strict dieting program in order to keep her figure, which she felt essential in her hostess duties. However, this resulted in another "minor" point of conflict with her husband, who intermittently complained about not having "real food" in the house.

Comment. Sandra was considered for AMT, although her physician recommended using Vanex, a major muscle relaxant and tranquilizer. She feared that she might become dependent on the medication. The initial obstacle during the early steps of AMT was her inability to identify experiences during which she felt anxious or stressed. "The thing is that I don't see myself as a person under stress. A hard worker, yes, a person with lots of daily activity, yes, but a person who is tense or stressed out, no." When asked what she felt to be the origins of her headache, she replied, "I'm told there is no organic cause, that it is due to stress, and I'm willing to believe that. . . even though I don't perceive myself as a tense person. I'm here to give it a shot, it can't harm me, and I might even be helped." In essence, Sandra showed characteristics similar to Type A persons who do not appraise themselves as being under pressure, but instead may even consider themselves as "challenged" or "stimulated" or "energized," and often take pride in their overload of work. Since her presenting problem was tension headaches, it was anticipated that the precipitating incidents would be found two- to four-hours prior to the headache onset, since the accumulation of muscle tension takes about that long to build into a headache.

The resolution to her being unable to select a life incident to describe that would clearly be anxiety-arousing, was to have her recall the last severe headache she experienced. She was then asked to identify what activities she had engaged in during the period of time before this headache appeared. Her memory, enhanced by looking at her appointment book, was that she had three major activities: a lengthy meeting with the aides of a junior congressperson involving negotiations over a bill, completion of typing on a brief reviewing a request from an environmental group to stop a proposal for the construction of a dam, and a telephone conversation with her husband regarding their weekend plans. In describing the telephone conversation, she remembered it to be a pleasant one, as they had planned to make the weekend into a short holiday, going to a concert, then spending the rest of the evening over a quiet dinner in their favorite restaurant. The call was to simply finalize whether to meet another couple or not. The issue of writing a brief was described as 'something of a chore' since the environmental group had not made their arguments very reasonably and failed to document their case—"It was full of rhetoric and claims, but not substance." The meeting with the other aides was "interesting.. I knew they were going to be tough, and I had very little leverage, and their congressperson wanted to make a name for herself. . . and they were saying they were going to oppose us." This meeting followed the brief-writing but was before the telephone call.

As Sandra was encouraged to offer more details on what happened during the meeting with the aides, what the others said, and how she responded it became evident that this event was a significant one. She described more dynamic interactions, a greater range of issues, a heightened focus of concentration on the topic, and a greater investment in the outcomes. She still described the situation more in terms of a normal part of her job, with not an unwarranted level of stress, "but it was one I had thought about beforehand in detail, because of its importance. . . we had a lot invested in this one. . . I imagine I wanted to have it turn out the way my congressman wanted. . . so I really put myself in it, in the negotiations. . . I had my whole mind into this one discussion. . . lost track of time for awhile."

However, the more she described her involvement, the more it became clear that, if she wasn't under stress, then she was at least in an intense interaction. To this comment she replied, after some thought, "Yes, it was intense. . . and if that kind of experience is a sign of stress, maybe I was feeling stress."

She was then asked, "What was going on in you as you were in this intense encounter?" Her response was, "As I said a moment ago, focused. . . I was concentrating, really hard. . . I wanted to hear every tone of their voice, every inflection, every bit that would tell me how this was going. . . I started off thinking that this was such a pain—'just think, a junior congressperson trying to pull a stunt like this'—but at the same time, I knew I had to be patient since we couldn't afford any enemies and needed all the votes. . . I remember leaning forward most of the time. . . and feeling at one time a mite angry at these upstarts, then focused on how to present our own arguments. . . what would be persuasive, what leverage they were offering that I could take. . . all the time, maintaining an attitude of being interested and under control. . . and when I figured they were giving a little, budging a little, I remember thinking 'yeah, yeah, I've got them now. . .' . . . but I had to be patient, and not push too fast, kind of lean back a little and let them think a little, and not seem too aggressive."

The therapist then observed, "Sounds like you were working to remain under control, at least outwardly to these folks. . . but inside, maybe you were churning around a bit, chomping at the bit to get this done?" This observation prompted Sandra's thoughtfulness and her ultimate reply, "Now that you say it in that way, yes. . . so is that an example of being stressed? I never paid much attention to those types of feelings. . . but if we're talking about situations which I consider intense, I can relate to that. The intensity feels like. . . "(Sandra now goes into details which essentially describe stress responses).

In order to adjust for her identifying stressful incidents as incidents involving "intensity," Stress Log 1 (see Appendix A) which is used by clients to estimate and report their daily levels of stress during each stress experience, was modified. She was asked to rate her level of 'intensity' ("which we will understand might well be what could also be your way of describing stress") during experiences which she would consider to be "intense experiences." Within two weeks, as the therapist discussed Sandra's written log descriptions of how she was feeling and reacting during these "intense experiences," Sandra became more able to comprehend that her actual experiences involved a high level of stress, particularly shown in muscle tensing. For instance, her posture of leaning forward was one evidence; her telling herself to 'not appear too aggressive, lighten up a little, don't appear too impatient' were other evidences of being under pressure. In logging, she was especially asked to write down intense experiences occurring two to four hours prior to a tension headache.

By the third week of AMT, Sandra was now talking in terms of "stress experiences" as she recognized her feelings as representing tension and stress, rather than explaining them away as feelings of "challenge" or "stimulation." There were still events that were activities which solely involved stimulation and not stress, such as writing some briefs, meetings with certain aids, specific social gatherings. However, Sandra was now more able to distinguish between "intense," stress-related events from such stimulating tasks. Her headaches were reduced to about one per month, and when they occurred, they were less severe. There was some inconsistency in her improvement, however, inasmuch as one month the number of headaches increased to about three per month and some were comparable in intensity to the level of pain prior to treatment. She has now been in AMT treatment for two months, or eight sessions.

The next step is to spend more time in evaluation of the logs to determine if she is still missing some situations that are stressful. Also, as a situation appears suspicious, session three of AMT (which uses the anxiety situation and asks her to pay attention to her cognitive/affective/behavioral cues) will be used to see if stress signs had appeared, which she had failed to notice. Session three has the client relax, then recall the anxiety incident: "Switch on the anxiety scene involving _____, and really be there again, so that you're into the scene, as realistically as possible." The added instruction in this session is to observe, to pay attention to bodily cues of stress while reexperiencing the incident: "Notice how you are feeling. . . what signs tell you that you are under stress. . . perhaps in parts of your body. . . or your thoughts. . . " In Sandra's case, the final step would be to adapt this session's procedure to cover later situations that she did not think were stressful, but which might in reality be producing stress of which she was unaware. Such a situation would be used, with Sandra then being asked to pay close attention to whether she was experiencing stress as identified through her intensity, bodily cues, and so forth.

Clients with Anxiety as an Obstacle to Psychotherapy

Obstruction of Insight Psychotherapy (Bill)

Bill has been diagnosed as suffering from a schizophrenic disorder of an undifferentiated type. He has been a student off and on for a number of years at different community colleges. He is easily identified in that he frequents the campuses' "soapbox" corners, often loudly discussing the relevance of philosophy and religion to the betterment of mankind's mental and physical well-being. He is generally well dressed, although there are a few days during which he may appear disheveled. He also will stand in front of the student cafeteria handing out copies of cartoons on political topics, cut from various newspapers. In psychology classes he will voluntarily stand up and state that he is a "recovering schizophrenic" and will readily discuss his background, his symptoms, and his prior hospitalizations.

He comes from a middle-class family background, with a private school education, and he perceives his family as having been extremely kind to him and supportive of his development. In his view, his parents were the closest thing to being the ideal. He believes that his symptoms derived from improper diet which he consumed during his first year of college—"I made the mistake of living by myself in an apartment instead of in a dormitory. So I had junk food for an entire twelve months, and the unique combination of junk food all coalesced into a disease, which has plagued me through destruction of certain nervous cells in the anterior portion of my brain."

The symptoms involved disinterest in school, a loss of ambition, and sleeping 17 hours a day. He also expressed fearfulness at losing any memories of material he had learned during elementary and high school, if he learned anything new, such as through reading a newspaper or magazine, being in a class, or listening to the radio newscasts. If the news was on television, he would instantly turn off the set. His agitation led him sometimes to leave the house during the late evenings (he was now living at home), walking around the neighborhood until three in the morning. He was once picked up by the police on suspicion of being a Peeping Tom, but was released when his parents vouched for him. He experienced auditory hallucinations, but would never admit their content, describing them instead as being "soft murmurs, too low to be understood, but very soothing."

Bill has never been hospitalized. During his worst period of sleeping for long hours, his father continued to deny that he was in need of help: "He's just burned out from all that schooling. He should have had a vacation after high school. Give him time, he needs more vitamins and his rest and he'll be all right." Bill's father always acquiesced in Bill's needs and wishes, and soon stopped subscription to the newspaper and turned the television off himself when the news program was due. When the police picked Bill up for wandering the neighborhood, the father explained this wandering as "he needed the quiet time to meditate about his future, he was probably thinking about his future plans for himself." Bill's father also denied that Bill hallucinated, arguing, "Bill has very sensitive hearing. He could hear the ocean in the seashell, and this is no different. It's probably some sort of ringing in the ears. Bill never said anyone was talking to him; it's everyone else in this family that says Bill hears voices. It's not voices, Bill has never said it was voices. He just has been put under too much stress with too many people planning his life for him, speaking for him, telling him what's wrong and what to do."

Bill was arrested by the police twice more, the second time on a complaint from a neighbor who was hopeful that a judge would see how seriously ill Bill was. The police chief spoke to Bill's father, agreeing to a release only if a contact was made with a local psychiatrist. Bill began a course of treatment that was continued mainly through the insistence of Bill's mother, who finally felt that she had a sufficient excuse to stand up to her husband's denials. She made sure that Bill kept his appointments, double-checked with the appointment secretary to determine each date, got Bill dressed, drove him to each appointment and sat in the waiting room to make sure that Bill in fact was being seen.

During early sessions, Bill's major topic of discussion was his disinterest, the meaninglessness of life, his despair at being a "speck in the universe." His late evening-early morning walks around the neighborhood increased for a week until the psychiatrist warned him that he could be involuntarily hospitalized for observation if he was arrested and another complaint was filed against him. Instead, Bill began to stay awake evenings pacing the hallway from his bedroom to the bathroom and back. As therapy progressed, he began to ask questions regarding whether he was being too controlled by "others"; when asked to identify his feelings and from whom the control was issuing, Bill would change the subject and become agitated. His pacing decreased under medication, and he began more and more to allude to issues of being controlled, and feeling a wish to break loose of the control, and to "live my own life, of pain or pleasure. . . it doesn't matter, at least it would be my decision."

The psychiatrist inquired whether the controlling force was associated with his family, to which Bill began pacing in the therapy room and seemed to be talking to hallucinatory voices: "No. . . no, the room is not warm. It's nice hearing your advice, but. . . you must listen to me for a change. . . speak louder, speaking softly. . . how can I pay attention, you're soft. . . you can't hear me. . . yes, it's warm, getting warm, warmer. . . "

Bill seemed desirous of talking about the sense of being restricted, being controlled, not possessing freedom, and would describe these feelings as bothersome, but never could offer details in discussions about identifying the source of these restrictions. Instead, his agitation would take over. Any attempts to discuss how Bill felt about his father's attitudes and prior actions to protect Bill tended to precipitate the hallucinatory behaviors. Bill now seemed genuinely interested in being in therapy, but at a standstill regarding progress beyond expression of his negative feelings about losing his freedom. He seemed to feel fearful of identifying his "owners, jailers, controlling forces-infield." On the other hand, his night wanderings and night pacing were now nearly absent, he was sleeping only 12 hours, and more animated at home, except when his father came home from work. At this point, Bill often became mute and withdrawn.

Comment. The psychiatrist decided to try AMT, referring Bill to a psychologist who was part of the private clinic and who was experienced with AMT. Sessions were scheduled during the period when Bill seemed to be in his most alert part of his sleep-wake cycle, which turned out daily to be a half hour before his father returned from work. This method of determining when to schedule Bill was selected in order to avoid Bill's falling asleep during the relaxation training, a possible outcome if he was seen during a time when he was normally sleeping.

Bill insisted on learning the relaxation using three repetitions of tensing with each muscle group, instead of the two normally practiced. Further, he insisted on having the office recliner face the doorway and that the psychologist promise always to start the relaxation training by saying, "Please," as, for instance, "Please sit back on the recliner and place yourself in a comfortable position." The anxiety scene which Bill identified for AMT use involved an examination which he recalled in college in an abnormal psychology course. He had been sleeping poorly, had not felt prepared for the examination, felt that he had crammed too heavily, and had missed two questions in a row. The next question provided a case description of a person who was hearing voices, experienced disruption of the sleep cycle, was losing contact with reality, and was described as being an "extremely shy" person. One possible answer was that this case represented a psychotic condition. Upon reading this, Bill felt himself become very anxious, frightened, almost panicked. He could not explain these feelings, but only somehow felt that the question was important, yet frightening. Bill denied having any detailed thoughts relating to the question, or relating the question to himself.

During AMT, when this scene was used for anxiety arousal, the psychologist used the description, "You are reading the question about psychosis, becoming very anxious, knowing only that somehow the question is important. . . even if you don't know why, you have no specific thoughts about why the question is important, but just reading it has raised this sense of panic, or fright, that pervades your entire body. . . please permit this anxiety to return again, allow yourself to reexperience the full level of this incident. . . be there again, with all the awful feelings. . . " Even though the psychologist suspected that Bill's anxiety and fear were because the test question raised Bill's own fearfulness that he might have cause to question his own mental and emotional stability, the AMT scene was described exactly as it happened (including the lack of thoughts about why the question was important).

Since AMT requires the identification of a second anxiety incident associated with intense anxiety, the psychologist later queried Bill for a second scene during their fourth AMT session. Bill described the following scene: "I was in the jail, after having spent the night because the police found me walking the neighborhood. My father was walking in with the police officer, approaching my cell, and I could hear them talking, but they couldn't see me yet. The police officer sounded like he didn't feel I should be "turned loose," and my father was explaining why it was all a mistake and a misunderstanding. . . his tone was like one uses with a. . . with a little kid; you know, you. . . patient, mild, simple. I could hear them coming closer and closer, and suddenly I had this explosive anxiety. . . skyrockets, electrical shocks through my nerves, my muscles were so tight that I was sore, like electricity was tightening them up. . . I had these confused thoughts shooting at me, voices yelling at me in my head: 'what if they won't let me go out of this prison,' 'a prison is a prison,' and. . . "

At this point Bill seemed to be so anxious that he was stuttering and losing coherence. Hence, the psychologist introduced a brief relaxation, and while Bill was relaxed, asked Bill to complete his scene description. Bill said, "The confusion was like I had this gut feeling that two jailers were walking down arguing over me. . . that was scary since I was looking forward to going home. I knew it was my father coming to take me home, and I would be safe. . . wouldn't stay forever in jail. . . it was a brief fear, but so high that I. . . it felt like a shock spell going through me, and I gripped the bed I was sitting. . . sitting on. . . " When this scene was used in the AMT session to insure retaining contact with reality aspects of the experience, the psychologist carefully avoided references to voices and was careful to clarify *feeling* that his father seemed like a jailer, versus actually seeing him in a jailer's uniform.

Hence the scene was described by the psychologist to Bill as: "All right, visualize yourself at that moment of being in the cell. . . you had been arrested, you were hearing your father and the police officer coming down the corridor, talking. . . whether you should be freed. . . the tone of your father's voice, the content, they're coming closer, you suddenly felt that burst of anxiety. . . muscles became tight, you were so anxious that your body was extremely tense. . . question of your being freed from the prison. . . you even thought of your father as a jailer, knowing he wasn't dressed like one, but the thought of his being a jailer and the real jailer increased your anxiety. . . you gripped the bed, you were so anxious. . . you had these thoughts going through your head, 'supposing they won't let you out of the prison,' these thoughts made you fearful. . . so let that anxiety build again, just the way it had been, be there again. . . in jail, thoughts about whether you would be released. . . the high anxiety and muscle tension. . . "

The use of relaxation and imagery did not appear to affect Bill's hold on reality, and his auditory hallucinations were not exacerbated. The psychologist stopped at the end of the first exposure to each of the two anxiety scenes, interviewed Bill about details, and confirmed that the scenes were exact replications of the real life experiences and did not involve hallucinatory fantasies. It was interesting to note that all signs pointed to the conflict as being Bill's feeling constrained by the overprotectiveness of his father and unwillingness to permit Bill to admit being in need of help. Yet, neither the psychiatrist nor the psychologists felt that Bill was ready to confront directly these feelings, especially since the anxiety was so easily triggered when such insight was approached. The second anxiety scene (with father as jailer) as well as the hallucinatory content (hearing his voices say, "warmer" when the psychiatrist asked about family could have been Bill's way of acknowledging, "You're getting warmer") suggested that the insight was very close to the surface, but still too dangerous to be confronted. The intense AMT scene involving the jail required four sessions of repetition before the control through relaxation could be achieved by Bill without the help of the psychologist.

Following this, the psychiatrist decided to determine if Bill could face the implications of his feeling that his father seemed like a jailer, and recommended that the psychologist explore this question at the next AMT session. This was done in the following way: As is usual with AMT, the session began with Bill initiating relaxation on his own, then the high-intensity anxiety scene was used to achieve anxiety arousal, after which Bill used relaxation to reduce the anxiety and return to a relaxed state. This procedure was repeated three times. Instead of ending the relaxation and then going into a post-session interview on how the session went, this time the psychologist permitted Bill to remain relaxed on the recliner with his eyes closed, and the psychologist raised the question, "While you are relaxed, I'd like for you to think about what it seems to mean to you now that you had thought of your father as a jailer during this incident, even though he was not in a police uniform."

Without any delay, Bill responded, "Oh, somehow the two of them seemed to make a pair. . . I mean even with my father talking to the policeman, it occurred to me that, that the two of them were a pair. . . what I'm saying, what I see now is that I felt that the cell. . . sleeping in the cell was no different than sleeping at home in my cell, except that the jailer came home at night, I mean my father came home at night and I was locked in myself. . . you see, I couldn't feel free even though I could do whatever I wanted at home. . . does that make sense?" With this opening development, Bill seemed able to expand on his feelings without either the anxiety or the hallucinatory symptoms. Instead, he appeared to be comfortably cooperative, and could talk more freely about what he associated to the notion of his father being restrictive and home being similar to a jail.

The psychologist arranged for a meeting with himself, Bill, and the psychiatrist, during which the psychologist encouraged Bill to repeat the content of the last AMT session. Following this joint session, Bill seemed to be able to progress past the plateau he had reached in psychotherapy. He continued in therapy weekly, has access to medication as needed, sleeps a more normal sleep pattern, and is discussing how to arrange to leave home.

Clients with Performance Disruptions from Anxiety

Sport Performance

A cross-country track and field team was divided into two groups, an experimental group and a control group in order to determine the effectiveness of AMT in improving physiological efficiency. Exercise physiologists have a procedure involving the use of a treadmill to determine each person's absolute physiological threshold. This procedure involves having the athlete run on a treadmill while heart rate and oxygen consumption are measured and monitored. (This is similar to the method used to measure a person's fitness level in cardiovascular fitness tests, and to identify potential risks for heart disease.) Once the physiological data indicate that the athlete has reached his/her ceiling, the test is terminated and the speed and gradient of the treadmill at that point becomes the reference point. This reference point identifies the level of effort or workload that is associated with the athlete's absolute threshold. By adjusting the workload to be, let's say, 75% of that athlete's absolute threshold, it is now possible to compare one athlete with another, since each is now working at a level comparable to the other. The effects of any variable can now be measured. If one athlete is exposed to this variable while the other is not, then the differences in oxygen consumption can be measured for the one versus the other, under the same workload. If one athlete shows less oxygen consumption, this is interpreted to reflect a more efficient state, and could be interpreted to represent the influence of the added variable.

The major hypothesis is that stress management can reduce muscle tension, which will therefore lead to greater efficiency in endurance activities. One presumes that muscle tenseness demands greater effort, for instance, of a runner as compared to the effort required when the runner is moving in a more muscularly relaxed or "smooth" style. It is often remarked that a boxer who is relaxed in the early rounds is more likely to remain fresh in later rounds, even with the same number and intensity of punches thrown. This is due to the lesser energy consumed in throwing a punch while relaxed, versus that in throwing the same punch when muscularly tight.

Since stress often appears associated with muscle tension, then AMT would be expected to be helpful. The major revision in applying AMT to training runners would be in using muscle activity as the cues for identifying tension. Hence, the runners are instructed to identify experiences during which they found their muscles 'tightening up,' "or a situation in which you were tense and not running smoothly; this could be a situation in which you were under pressure or trying too hard, or simply a situation in which you were tense, for whatever reason." Once this incident is identified, it is used instead of an anxiety situation in imagery.

The AMT training then involves relaxation training, then the tense-running scene is visualized and used to retrieve the muscular tenseness, then the relaxation is used to remove that tenseness and to smooth out the running style. The imagery can be extended so that the runner now visualizes him/herself running in this more relaxed, smoother style. Thus, the AMT instruction might be, "Now, switch on the scene of the time you were running in regional finals, and you found yourself tight and tense. Be there again; you were on the cross country course in California, two-thirds of the way in the race, and had been running smoothly so far. But you are in terrain difficult for you and you're struggling a bit. . . finding yourself tightening up, losing your rhythm, working too hard. . . the pressure is on for you to keep your pace, some-one is passing you, the runner from Southern California and you didn't expect that. . . O.K., notice that muscular tightness, the effects on your breathing, on your smoothness, on your stride. . . let all those problems return again as you're in this scene. . . . now, while you're still in this scene, retrieve the relaxation, that level of muscle relaxation that you've learned. . . allowing the relaxation to move quickly and instantly across your body. . . as this happens, letting your running become smooth, your stride more relaxed, your rhythm much more smooth and re-laxed. . . using the deep breaths to regain the relaxation. . . if you're tight in any parts of your body, just let the relaxation take over, so that your shoulders are more relaxed. . . your arms are swinging more free-ly. . . your stride is much smoother. . . whatever works best for your body as you regain the relaxation in running. . . " In this experiment.

both groups of runners were required to run steadily on the treadmill at 65% of their threshold; in other words, they were faced with a work load of 65% of their absolute tolerance. Both AMT-trained and untrained athletes ran on the treadmill for 10 minutes to establish a baseline on oxygen consumption. Then the AMT-trained group were instructed to run in the more relaxed, less tense style that they had learned to adopt from using the AMT imagery of running when under stress or tight. During baseline, both groups showed similar levels of oxygen consumption. However, during the final 10 minutes, when the trained group was running in the 'relaxed style', this group showed a reduction of oxygen consumption, of from 10% to 20%, while the untrained group showed no changes. These results strongly suggest that AMT can affect muscular tension, and this reduction in turn can mean improvements in physiological efficiency on an endurance task, under a high workload for individuals.

Clients with Anxiety Preventing Adaptive Changes

Type A Behaviors (Matt)

Matt is a successful mathematician in a major state university. He is impatient when at a stoplight, cuts others off in the middle of their comments, sets fast deadlines as goals for himself, speaks with emphatic and rapid bursts, seems always on the run, and is a risk for a heart attack. He is a person with a Type A behavioral pattern.

Matt always has been goal-directed. He disciplined himself in undergraduate school to set aside times devoted entirely to studying, with extended times prior to examinations. If the examinations interfered with a planned social gathering, he simply skipped the party in order to remain with his study schedule. He was systematic in his study method; writing down in a tablet questions deriving from lecture or readings, with the answers to these questions on the next page. He had one tablet for each course. In reviewing for a forthcoming examination, he read the questions he had written, and tried to come up with the answer. If he failed, he would turn to the next page for the answer, then later return to this question.

In graduate school, his discipline was maintained, although he discovered he had to extend his study hours to two o'clock in the morning. He graduated a half year earlier than others, was hired as an Assistant Professor. Although he had a heavy teaching load, his discipline paid off. He set himself deadlines to meet in course preparation, and frequently surpassed these deadlines; then he used the extra time to get ahead on other deadlines. He tends to be extremely impatient at things which "waste my time," such as standing in lines at the movies, sitting at a traffic light, waiting on the telephone for his call to go through, waiting for a travel agent to come up with alternative flight schedules. To resolve these, he only goes to a movie if there is a short line (otherwise he goes home), always hangs up if his telephone call fails to be answered in three rings, and has subscribed to an airlines flight schedule service so he can look up travel times himself.

Matt takes pride in his work habits, although he does become irritated with his inability to be more patient. He interrupts others before they can finish their sentences, since he is bright enough that he readily anticipates their thoughts, and is too impatient to be able to wait for them to finish. Matt's exercise activities are such that he also pushes himself. For instance, he started jogging every other day for a half hour, but has now pushed himself to covering greater distances in the half hour, and he now jogs or runs every day. He plays tennis with fierce competitiveness, although without great technique, and seems to experience more anger rather than pleasure from games.

Matt's life is always scheduled with something. He is an active person, very seldom seen at rest. The image that others have of him is as a tornado: forceful, always in motion, and something that one should not stand in the way of lest you be blown away. His speech is best described as explosive, as he punctuates his words and phrases with exclamation points. His sentences are more machine gun bursts aimed at you than simple words. Despite his always being on the go, Matt denies that he is a tense individual; instead he sees himself as challenged by life, and naturally impatient to achieve goals ("What's wrong with having a direction in life?") and as possessing the energy and discipline to achieve these goals.

Comment. Matt was a volunteer for a project on Type A behaviors and prevention of heart disease. He confessed volunteering more because he saw the risks of early death than because he felt the need to change his behaviors. In the early orientation with other Type A volunteers, the myth was challenged that success required Type A behaviors and that failure or loss of ambition are the natural consequences of elimination of Type A behaviors. The group engaged in a discussion of their views of their Type A behaviors, with many nodding their agreement that they felt their characteristics of high drive and impatience to be positive ones.

However, some grudgingly admitted that they were often fatigued at bedtime, and occasionally envisioned themselves on a treadmill that had no end. Most could suggest alternative ways of managing their schedules that allowed more "down time" to catch one's breath, while not losing their efficiency. Many agreed that they were sometimes less efficient in trying to accomplish so much by a self-imposed, short deadline, and that even such tasks that were accomplished did not foster any additional positive outcomes compared to meeting a later deadline. As part of the orientation meeting, information on the relationship between Type A behaviors and cardiovascular disease were presented, and reference made to programs offering stress management to executives. The presence of stress, sometimes in a "hidden" way, through the pressures of deadlines, high self-expectations, failure to take breaks, were discussed. Finally, the hidden expressions of stress, such as in fatigue or in increased heart rate and blood pressure during "challenges" or impatience were presented.

Following the orientation, Matt still did not feel that he was under pressure, although he agreed that he was sometimes easily angered or irritated by his environment. He also agreed to take his pulse and have his blood pressure taken, and was surprised that he was borderline hypertensive in blood pressure. For his AMT arousal scene, he selected a situation in which he was especially impatient: chairing meetings where the expectation was that consensus was needed involving ideas contributed by all participants. "I could come up with a solution in five minutes if everyone would simply accept my ideas; but no, we had to waste time in hearing everyone out, in talking incessantly about advantages and disadvantages, and finally, we would ultimately end up doing what I had been thinking about anyway. But I learned that you have to give everyone their chance, and if you raise your solution at the beginning, even if it's a good one, it would be ignored because people just want to talk, to feel that they participated."

His signs of arousal or activation (these terms was used instead of the phrase "signs of stress") turned out to be expressed in symptoms such as "feeling impatient to end it all, to just cut in and tell them what I think. . . I want to get up and pace, walk around, just get moving physically. . . a feeling that grows inside that is bottled up, that I have to bottle up." The situation which most recently characterized such impatience was at the university, in an all campus committee on remedial courses for freshmen in mathematics. This incident was used as the arousal scene for AMT training.

As a separate part of treatment, Matt's blood pressure was taken during his arousal/activation scene. Prior to the scene, during relaxation, his systolic pressure was 120 while his diastolic pressure was 90. During the committee meeting scene, his systolic pressure rose to 145 with his diastolic now being 97. Upon regaining relaxation, his blood pressure went down to 125 systolic and 95 diastolic. Upon having this experience with blood pressure changes repeated several times, Matt became more convinced that there were health benefits at learning to reduce the "activation."

In session three the clients are instructed to "Pay attention to how you experience the activation or tension. . . signs that let you know about the activation. . . could be in bodily signs, or thoughts you have, or feelings." By identifying these signs, they can be used later as "early warning signals" that enable the client to initiate the relaxation early enough to abort the stress response before it reaches too high a level. For Matt, while visualizing being in the committee meeting, he noticed that his early signal involved "clenching my hands. . . I'd be sitting there, feeling comfortable, but if I looked down at my hands, they would be fisted up."

Matt used the cue of whether his hands were clenched or relaxed in his practicing of stress prevention in his daily life, and continued to practice the relaxation on a daily basis. He also routinely took breaks, especially if he had just completed a difficult task or had been involved in a tense interaction with a student. His breaks involved deep breathing and relaxation, or a walk around the hallways. He uses the relaxation while waiting in lines or at traffic lights. He has also learned to reduce his tendency to set early deadlines, and now distributes his work more appropriately. His blood pressure has been steady within the normal range for some time.

Clients with Anxiety from Irresolvable Life Stresses: Clients with Anxiety from Multiple Sources

Irresolvable and Multiple Situational Stressors (Rosalie)

Rosalie is an only child whose mother is suffering more and more from the symptoms of Alzheimer's disease, and whose widowed uncle has been in need of various medical treatment for several months. Rosalie's mother has been living with her for three years, and had generally been in good health. Since Rosalie is married and has three teenage children, this arrangement has been a positive one, inasmuch as the youngsters have enjoyed their grandmother, Elsie. However, with the increased forgetfulness, irritability, moodiness, and unpredictableness of Elsie, the children have started to avoid her, causing Elsie to feel left out and rejected.

At this point in time, Rosalie is under pressure from her husband to consider a nursing home with Alzheimer's facilities, since Elsie's welcome is now beginning to wear thin, and conflicts are beginning to surface. Additionally, Rosalie's uncle is scheduled for back surgery, and he has been extremely frightened about being hospitalized. Rosalie has been spending many hours providing reassurance. Finally, Rosalie's two daughters represent different stresses. The oldest is deeply involved with a boyfriend of whom Rosalie's husband disapproves, because he is a high school dropout and has only intermittent employment. The other daughter has been experiencing academic problems, which have come on suddenly since her prior schoolwork has been at the "B" level.

Rosalie had spoken with the school counselor about the academic difficulties of her younger daughter, and the counselor noticed Rosalie's looking and sounding under stress. The counselor suggested that Rosalie seek stress management counseling, and Rosalie entered an AMT program as an individual client. Rosalie feels that she is strong enough to handle the problem solving aspects of each of the situations, but is exhausted from running from one problem to another: "It's draining, it's truly draining. . . I go from one crisis to another, one to another. . . it's like a nonstop trip down horror lane, you want to go screaming out the door. I do not have a moment that I don't think about what's going to happen next. . . my emotions are like raw wires, I'm strung out, strung up all the time."

Comment. The major goal of AMT was to aid her in keeping her emotional arousal low, or in returning her arousal level to a more normal point after each stress. It was recognized that none of the pressures would desist as long as each had certain origins that were not resolved. Rosalie would not be in a position to stop meeting with her uncle, could not terminate her daughter's relationship with the boy without creating still yet another crisis, would not be able to determine the source of her other daughter's academic problems right away, and would gradually have to come to some decision about her mother. Hence emotional management would be the major gain from AMT.

After relaxation training, which Rosalie learned quickly in spite of her heightened arousal level, Rosalie selected for her stress scene the incident of being in the midst of an argument at dinner table over her older daughter's boyfriend. Rosalie had just hung up the telephone after a conversation with her uncle, and was still a bit emotional from that experience. Her husband was yelling at the daughter about how 'intolerable' this boy was, and Elsie was mumbling about how no one seemed to care about serving her dinner. Rosalie was aware of her other daughter seeming distraught, although she had yet to speak up. Rosalie's description: "It was like being in the middle of a bad movie, where the director told everyone to become emotional. . . but on different wavelengths. I felt like the only common thread here. . . but I felt frazzled, fried, stretched like a rubber band across the table. . . grandma was pulling me, my husband was stretching me, my daughter was leaning on me, and my other daughter was tugging, and Uncle James was hovering in the background for the leftovers."

Rosalie was able to achieve maximum anxiety arousal with this scene, but was also readily able to reestablish relaxation and calm. She was encouraged to use the relaxation at home in a preventive as well as therapeutic fashion. As prevention she was to take a moment to relax before a potential stressful interaction, for example, before telephoning her uncle, or before sitting at the dinner table with the family. For therapy goals, she was to use relaxation when she noticed her anxiety level starting to increase, for instance, when her mother was becoming too demanding. Since Rosalie's life experiences were a constant flux of such stressors, she was never free of situations which acted as triggers. However, she found herself worrying less and having less residual emotionality after she had left a stressful situation and was in between stressful events. In contrast, in the past she would not be able to shake her level of arousal or tension even after the event ended. Furthermore, she was no longer as reactive to her daughter's academic difficulties, "because now I can allow myself to see that the school counselor is working with her and everything that can be done is being done." She still must actively engage in relaxation exercises after dinner arguments over the boyfriend or encounters with her mother's moods or demands.

Rosalie has discovered that reserving some time after these high stress events to be alone, and to be able to focus on relaxation has been extremely helpful. She is beginning to feel that the same "objective distance" which she achieved regarding her younger daughter is developing with regard to her older daughter's boyfriend: "I'm close to feeling that it is my husband's problem, and his yelling and her smart replies are their problem, and not mine. It's like I become an observer, rather than having my emotions all tied up in their argument."

Clients for Whom Anxiety Mediates Other Symptoms

Mild Depression (Shirl)

Although depression typically has its own origins independent of anxiety, for Shirl the two seemed associated. Shirl experienced rather mild depressions that she described more as "my moody periods. . . my low-down periods." These never seemed to be disruptive, but did lower her usual sense of enjoyment of living. They were expressed as the following symptoms: "I would question whether I could be considered to have accomplished anything in my life after I died; I would think that the dinner I prepared wasn't really good enough for my family; I would look at myself in the mirror and hate my body for all its flaws; I would feel dark and moody, rather sad and hopeless in life achievements. But I could usually break out of this state if I paid attention. My simplest solution would be to get up and do something, just get moving around, maybe pay some attention to preparing something extra at dinner and remind myself to ask my family how they liked the meal, because they are great eaters, and always say enthusiastic things. . . .and I could get caught up in their enthusiasm."

In waiting for her annual physical in her doctor's office, Shirl saw an announcement of an experiment needing volunteers, "people who sometimes experience sadness which doesn't readily go away, who sometimes feel on a downer." She decided to look into this, even though she did not see her depressive episodes as problematical. In the intake interview, it was determined that anxiety and depression seemed linked for Shirl. Whenever she felt threatened or was concerned about a life event, this tended to precipitate self-doubting thoughts, which in turn changed into depressive thoughts and feelings.

For instance, she had been preparing to give a talk as part of a toastmistress assignment; she had signed up with this group since she had always had trouble in speaking in public. This talk was her first major task and she had worked hard on the content. However, as the day came closer for her presentation, she became more and more anxious. Her fear and anxiety began to consume her thoughts and feelings. "I woke up thinking about how soon the date was and how little preparation time I had left; I found myself jumping at small sounds and I realized I was daydreaming about the talk; I even began to have trouble falling asleep nights."

Within a day of the onset of this anxiety, her thoughts began to shift. "I spent the morning literally shaking in my boots about the talk the next night, but I suddenly began to think that I was being so foolish, thinking that I could learn to speak properly before an audience. . . then, I started to scold myself for wasting so much time on such a trivial topic, public speaking. . . I scolded myself for thinking that there would be a reason for me to speak in public, what did I think, that I was going to win the Nobel Prize and had to give a public acceptance speech?. . . I felt a bit better then, and knew that I was going to resign from toastmistress, but then I felt worse again since I saw this as giving up. . . and wondered what the others in the group would think of me. . . I'd be letting them down by running away. . . by midafternoon I was feeling depressed. . . that I had got myself into this predicament was proof that I didn't reason properly, had the wrong values, was impulsive and self-centered. . . why did I ever believe that I could come up with a talk that would capture others' attention. . . I didn't have anything to say, I never have. . . in all my life, the main reason I didn't speak up was that I knew others were smarter, had more to say, were more interesting. . . then I remembered how I felt in junior high, that others were always prettier, more vivacious, more sought after by boys, had more friends among the girls. . . I recalled how I was always left out of the cliques of girls. . . and how sad those times were. . . " The rest of the day, she was gloomy and depressed.

Comment. In AMT, this incident was used as one of the scenes to precipitate the anxiety experience, but narrowed to the one period in the morning when she was "shaking in my boots." Although the anxiety seemed to be present upon awakening in the morning, and was spread across the day, AMT requires that the scene be a specific incident rather than a lengthy set of incidents stretched across time. Shirl never did have an experience with anxiety that was higher than 70, and hence a high intensity scene was never used in the training. However, she learned to monitor signs of becoming anxious, and was able to learn as well to use the relaxation for control over her tensions. The depressive reactions were never directly attacked in AMT sessions. However, at the termination of eight weeks of AMT, Shirl reported that her depressive episodes were now nearly nonexistent. Further, even when some did appear, her usual coping skills still served her well in eliminating the depression. She was much more alert and sensitive to the starting thoughts that signaled self-doubts and depression, and is now able to shift her attention so that these thoughts no longer automatically precipitate the depressive state.

Clients for Whom Anger Management Is Desired

Anger Management (Chuck)

Chuck was born in a rural community on a ranch. From the very beginning the freedom of the wide open spaces, the accountability to no one but family, and the independence from large city life were the main pleasures in his life. He was always remembered by his family as enjoying being around the animals more than being around people: "Them steers don't expect much of you, you can be just what you are. . . people have too many rules and too many expectations." He was required to go to the little local school as he was growing up, and was frequently sent home for fighting. At one point, the major controversy was whether he was going to be kicked out of school permanently because he took a swing at the teacher: "He told me I wasn't moving fast enough in returning to my seat; he was always telling me what to do, picking on me." However,

Chuck's father read him the riot act, making it clear that, like it or not, Chuck would behave himself and go to school, even if he barely squeaked by in grades.

On reaching adulthood, Chuck planned on remaining on the ranch. However, his father died after an extended illness, costing major medical and hospital bills. The ranch had to be sold to pay off accounts, and Chuck moved into the nearest town seeking work. He eventually discovered that he was suited only to construction labor, and that such jobs were available only in large cities where building was more active. His days were spent on the job, his evenings in a small cafe and bar, usually in an empty booth at the very end of the cafe. Conditions were uncertain, particularly since Chuck's life was full of marginal adjustments, threatened by his intermittent violent outbursts. He lost two jobs due to fights with the foreman because he didn't like being told that he needed to work faster. He spent one week in jail because he smashed three tables, five chairs, and 30 glasses in a bar: "I was sitting there feeling sorry for myself; feeling that I belonged in the country, that the city had too many dos and don'ts, and do this and do that. . . and I got more and more angry until I just had to bust up something to get back my senses."

He enlisted in the Marines and was nearly court-martialed during his first week for threatening to strike the drill sergeant; he was restrained by five members of his platoon before he actually landed a blow. Somehow he lasted through basic training, only after being taken into a boxing ring by the sergeant, who said, "You want to get back at me, here's your chance to do it legally;" after which the sergeant proceeded systematically to batter Chuck around the ring. Bruised and whipped, Chuck nevertheless felt better than he had ever felt; the boxing "lesson" offered him the opportunity to hit back, even if he didn't land many blows. He vowed to make it on the boxing team. For months, he sought out as many lessons as he could, and found that what he lacked in technique, he overcame with his power and willingness to take a blow in order to give a blow. Within months, he fought his way onto the team as a heavyweight, and went on to win 50% of his fights. His losses were bloody ones in which he gave a reasonable accounting of himself.

Upon discharge, he discovered he had some small savings, and began to dream about saving enough in the future to buy a small farm. However, his own skill was boxing. He entered enough amateur fights to impress a local manager, who then agreed to help Chuck turn professional. Chuck never fooled himself into thinking he could be other than on a preliminary card or a last minute substitute on a more major bout. He was content to be working, and to have a little left over for savings. He doggedly set about boxing as often as he could, living as cheaply as he could, and fighting with enough flare to be sought after by promoters.

The main jeopardy to Chuck's plans was his increased tendency to lose his temper outside the ring. He became involved in one scrape as he again broke up the furniture, this time in his room. On several other occasions, he was on the verge of a barroom fight until restrained by friends. His manager, who had now become a friend, took himself aside, pointing out the fact that he could be sued if he were in a public brawl, that his plans and savings would all be lost, that he risked being barred from his only source of a living unless he developed a tighter rein on his temper or frustrations. Chuck agreed to AMT, being seen by an advanced graduate student conducting a study in a nearby university on anger management.

Comment. When AMT was explained, Chuck's immediate question was whether the AMT experience would "take away my instincts. . . my aggressiveness. . . my fighting instinct in the ring. . . it's what I have that makes me a living." The therapist made it clear that the AMT training would provide a skill which he would have as a tool, to bring out and use when he needed it, but that his natural ring aggressiveness was keyed off by the situation of being in the boxing ring, and this would not change.

The initial problem arising in AMT was the seeming unwillingness of Chuck to be cooperative with the therapist; between the first and second sessions it became clear that Chuck had not completed his homework log, and also did not appear to have practiced the relaxation at home very systematically. The initial interview at the beginning of the second session was also characterized by resistance from Chuck and apparent reticence to talk much. Since he had not practiced the relaxation, this session was a repeat of session one, concentrating only on relaxation training. In supervision, the student-therapist and supervisor reviewed the videotape of the two sessions. It became clear that the student had been adopting a firm, instructional tone which Chuck probably interpreted as, "Do this, do that" and was resisting. The student-therapist also used a tone that implied that session two was being repeated as a form of punishment for not doing the homework assignment. This possibly made Chuck even more reactive. The student-therapist agreed to soften the directive tone of instructions, to adopt more of an attitude of being a collaborator seeking Chuck's cooperation, and to spend more time in explaining the reasons for each step and how AMT was similar to his early training sessions when he was acquiring and polishing his boxing skills.

Session three therefore was turned into a review of the rationale of AMT, and time was spent in emphasizing the skill-training component and comparing this to lessons in boxing, with the therapist serving more as a manager/coach pointing out what the next steps would be, but permitting Chuck to engage in asking as many questions as he wished, and even being asked to make any suggestions. For example, Chuck was asked how he relaxed the evening before a fight; Chuck replied that he used to drink all night in a bar, but soon realized that the drinking was unhealthy; besides, it cost him money he could be putting in savings. Therefore, he substituted drinking coffee and listening to music on the jukebox in the cafe/bar. He particularly enjoyed country western music, and his favorite singer was Dolly Parton. He remembered a particularly relaxing melody which she sang, and the special evening that he first heard her record in the cafe.

The therapist-student quickly suggested that this type of information was valuable, and discussed whether this incident could serve as the foundation for relaxation training. The therapist explained again how this scene could be added on to the relaxation exercise today to enhance the relaxation training. The therapist also inquired about what approach his manager had taken that facilitated Chuck's being able to acquire different boxing skills. Chuck responded by saying, "He always treated me with respect. . . even though he knew more than I did, and I sometimes felt awkward in trying something out, he took the time to explain the theory. . . and he always took the attitude, 'let's try it out and see; might work for you, might not, but then we can talk about it when we're done and you can tell me what you think'. . . I never felt that he was pushing me."

(From this session on, the therapist was sensitive to adopting a similar attitude, with the brief interviews at the start of the session and at the end covering feedback from Chuck on "How do you think it went? Is there some aspect we can improve on that seemed to help?" In addition, the steps in the session were always introduced as "typically what we would be doing today would be. . . ", along with an explanation of the reason and followed with the question, "What do you think, are you ready to try it out?")

The anger arousal using visualization of a prior incident in Chuck's life readily prompted anger activation in the first trial, as could be seen by Chuck's facial features and upper body tightening up, his heart rate and breathing increasing until he was breathing deeply through his mouth, his hands clenched into fists on the recliner, and his blood vessels standing out. He was slow in returning to relaxation, with the therapist going over relaxation instructions with 10 minutes of the muscle relaxation, another five minutes of the cafe scene listening to Dolly Parton, and another five minutes in again reviewing the relaxation of the muscle groups. Because he continued to be slow in being able to return to relaxation after anger arousal with the anger scene, it was decided that the next session would repeat the same steps. Furthermore, he was asked if he could figure a way to increase his daily relaxation exercise to twice a day.

He was soon able to progress to the AMT session where the high-intensity anger scene was developed and visualized. His scene, arousing about 95 intensity anger was as follows: "I was sitting in the Long Branch Cafe and listening to the fella in the next booth talking about how he told his kids to shape up in school. I was remembering how it was for me, always someone telling me to shape up, to do this, do that. . . I remembered how tough that basic training was, not physically, but gritting my teeth and doing what I was told, that was the hardest part. . . feeling that tension inside of me that I had to chain up. . . then the guy in the other booth yelled, 'Hey, quit playing that one song, will ya; I'm sick of hearing it, can't you play something else'. . . I about blew up. . . it was like his comment entered my thoughts at the very moment I was remembering gritting my teeth in basic. . . I was just in a lousy mood anyway. . . but his comment was the last straw, or the first straw, whatever. . . like a steam boiler in me, all the people in the world, in my life telling me what to do. . . putting a cage around my freedom. . . forcing me to do what they want. . . I felt this explosion inside me. . . getting ready to punch him out, everything out, break out of it, break the table to bits. . . and I just got out of control; I had enough sense to just bash the table in and to stay away from that guy. . . throw the chairs around, cussed him out. . . he ran outa there like a rabbit, but I was in a fit by now. . . crunched a couple more chairs. . . ...but, you know, somehow I stayed away from the jukebox, which was still playing along; I knew enough that I didn't want to harm the music. . . "

When this scene was used in AMT for anger arousal, the elements up to the actual violent behaviors were used, so that the scene in visualization was ended before the loss of control, before the table was bashed in, before the cursing, and so forth. Instead the scene described all the preliminaries, including, "You're on the verge of losing control, of being ready to let go and bash in the table. . . instead, let's have you switch off that scene, and take a deep breath and release the tension and the anger in your body. . . using the relaxation with first tensing up the right hand. . . and now relaxing it. . . focusing on the ability to let the tension release itself. . . "

Ordinarily, for most clients, by the session whereby the anxiety arousal through visualization is used, the relaxation is reintroduced without tensing of the muscles; instead, a simple review of muscles being relaxed is sufficient. For Chuck, because of the intensity of his anger arousal, and his prior slower ability to retrieve the relaxation, the relaxation retrieval method was revised to involve the tensing and relaxing of each muscle group (identical to the muscle relaxation training used in the very first AMT session). The use of the tensing provides a concrete sensation for Chuck to center his attention.

Prior to the termination of AMT, Chuck had another boxing match scheduled, and asked to skip further appointments until the fight was over, since he was still a bit fearful of the AMT reducing his aggressiveness in the ring. He reappeared six weeks later, reported that he had lost the fight, but that it had been very close. Although he knocked down his opponent in an early round, this had been ruled a slip, rather than a real knockdown. Chuck felt his ring aggressiveness was intact, "You were right, as soon as I got in the training ring in the gym, it was like fitting into a glove. . . it was all there. And when I heard the bell for round one, I forgot everything except this guy in front of me. . . I didn't lose any of my edge. . . shoulda won, but heck, he was good too."

AMT was completed and Chuck tested his newfound control by attending a wedding reception which he had initially planned on skipping. He felt that this wedding would be in a fancy church, with "tuxedoes and punch, and everyone being expected to conform and be nice." His sense was that this was what he was trying to leave in buying a farm, and he had been certain that he would get into at least a verbal fight with someone who represented "the established society." Instead, he was able to dress reasonably sensibly (he wore a suit, but with a bolo tie and boots); sat calmly during the ceremony although he had to remember Dolly Parton's singing a few times that he felt a mild irritation at the wedding march ritual; and kept himself relaxed enough during the reception actually to look around to find someone he could talk to ("I just picked the biggest and toughest guy I could find. . . turns out he is a football player, and was just as uncomfortable as I was. . . we went to a bar together later.")

Within a month, he called to report that he was even more certain that the "relaxation stuff" was working. He had arranged to talk to the bank about a possible loan for a down payment on a farm. The bank clerk was a friendly person, but treated Chuck "like a grade school kid" upon discovering that he was a boxer. This "jerk of a banker proceeded to tell me how I needed to save. . . how I had to consider whether boxing was really a good living, how I was a poor risk because boxing was not "real, steady employment," how I might look into career counseling, how the bank or 'volunteer aid' could help me with financial counseling, how my lack of education made me a poor risk for most jobs but that even construction work was better than boxing. . . ..I was really surprised at myself. . . I just looked at him. . . noticed that I was feeling the boiler start to heat up inside me, then just kind of. . . kind of thought, it's time to release the steam from the boiler before it cooks over. . . and I just kind of loosened up, kept looking, kept looking at this jerk. . . and you know. . . he kind of even seemed a nerd. . . I could imagine him falling off a horse, or running away from a cow. . . so I laughed, said, 'Thanks buddy for the advice,' and left. . . I didn't even go to a bar, just had lunch in Woolworth's and talked with the waitress."

Clients with Anxiety Exacerbating a Primary Condition

Dysmenorrhea (Martha)

Martha has suffered all her life from physical pain associated with her menstural cycle. In examining her case, it became clear that she had many of the symptoms of congestive dysmenorrhea. She always knew when her menstrual cycle was due even without looking at the calendar since she experienced a variety of physical changes beforehand. "The very first warning is a dull ache, kind of in my lower back. . . I used to ignore this as just due to running around in heels too much, or maybe too much aerobics, or lifting things. . . but now I've learned to know that this really tells me that my period is around the corner."

General discomforts also start to appear a few days before her period, including the physical symptoms of an ache around the abdominal areas, tenderness and soreness of the breasts, and sensations of feeling bloated. Along with the full, bloated feelings, she also notices that her weight becomes unstable as she gains a little. "I try to watch my diet, and I do exercise. . . I'm starting to wonder if I'm just storing more water since I feel puffed up." Psychological symptoms also develop and Martha has also learned to associate these with the dysmenorrhea. "I used to think I was getting flaky in my life. . . couldn't figure out why I would have these moody states. . . sometimes I'd be on a real downer for no good reason, and then I'd be irritable about the slightest thing, like I had a short fuse. . . boy, I'm a real nerd to be around. . . now that I see the pattern, I can take a little more patience to stay in control, so I'm better about this."

Martha had been referred to an AMT project that was under way, announced through a local family practice center. Martha had been in the doctor's office to inquire about her weight shifts, and whether hormone therapy would be useful for her dysmenorrhea. She was started on a pilot course of hormone treatment, but also told of the AMT project for stress. Given her irritability and her nervous tension, Martha thought she would at least find out what the AMT could do.

The AMT project was not appropriate for Martha's situation. However, she was seen as an individual client. It was explained that the AMT could be appropriate for her tension as an additional help to her own

method of 'just being more patient' as a coping method. The idea of
using AMT for pain control was also mentioned as an application of
AMT being explored. She was agreeable to "taking a shot at this AMT
stuff."

Comment. AMT sessions were divided into two stages: the first, a
traditional application to anxiety reduction for her tensions and irritability. The second stage involved revisions related to the menstrual
pain.

For the first stage, Martha was asked to identify two types of arousal
scenes. The first was to be "a situation, an event, that really happened to
you, which you remember. . . that involves the few days before your
menstrual period in which you were especially nervous and tense." Martha described the following incident:

> "O.K. It was six months ago. I had been shopping in the morning and was
> supposed to meet a friend for lunch. It was our Southern Star mall, and I was
> feeling a backache from walking with heels on the hard floors. Then I just felt
> rushed, a feeling inside. . . something that said, 'gotta finish, gotta rush.' I
> knew I had time before lunch, but it was just a feeling, and I was dis-
> tracted. . . what did I need to get done, which stores should I go to
> next. . . just a sense of hurry."

For the second type of arousal scene, the irritability was the target
rather than the nervousness. So Martha was asked to identify "a situation, an event, that again was a real one, that involves the few days before
your period in which you felt that irritability." Martha came up with the
following:

> "Well, a worse one was before I recognized that it was a pattern. . . but one
> that stands out was four months ago. It was our anniversary and Jason, my
> husband, had really gone out of his way to arrange a nice evening out. He
> came home a little early from work, and I had arranged to get off work
> too. . . and I was starting to get ready. . . but he kept fooling around, and
> then he poked through my jewelry box while I was searching for my pet
> earrings. . . and I just flew off the handle. . . told him to 'stop it!'. . . and
> slapped his hand away. . . I really shocked myself, then caught myself and
> remembered that my period was coming around the corner. . . so I thought
> 'you gotta stay cool, simmer down, it's just the period'. . . and apolo-
> gized. . . but I felt my mood kind of going like an elevator. . . the more I
> wanted to be patient, the more tense I was. . . then I'd feel depressed that
> this was ruining the evening, could ruin the evening. . . then I'd try to cheer
> up, get control, 'O.K. hang in there, be patient'. . . and. . . "

Given that this description seemed to be a long sequence, possibly
describing her moods throughout the night, the therapist said: "That's in
the direction of what I'm looking for. . . a specific incident. . . I wonder
if all of those mood shifts were things happening over the night, or all

part of that one moment when you slapped his hand and caught yourself?"

Her reply made it clear that the mood, the thoughts, the irritability were all closely clustered within a brief span:

> "It was like a frozen moment in a movie. . . but it was all happening, you know how you have this rush of things, of emotions. . . thoughts, feelings, all the same time? I had hit his hand, said "Oh!", realized what was happening. . . tried to calm down. . . felt moody. . . thought about the evening being ruined. . . all within a few seconds. . . or at least it felt that way to me. . . Oh, and it did, because after all of these internal things, Jason then said, "Hey, no sweat. . . I deserved that."

This scene was therefore adopted for AMT, and AMT session five revised somewhat to attempt to combine the AMT effects with strengthening her cognitive coping as follows:

> T: O.K., now that you're comfortably relaxed, the next thing we'll do is to have you turn on your irritability scene just as we did the last time. But this time, you'll stay in that scene, and while you're still in that scene, I want you to do two things. First, while you're in the scene and experiencing that irritation and moodiness, use your relaxation technique to calm yourself, to regain a sense of controlled relaxation. . . calmness. Second, as you notice gaining control and being relaxed again, remember your thoughts. . . those thoughts about, "stay cool. . . it's just the period making you jumpy, irritable. . . be patient". . . And for signaling, as before. . . hand up to indicate your experiencing the irritability and hold it up as long as you are retaining that feeling. . . then lower the hand when you are relaxed.

This first stage was carried through six sessions, with the anxiety scene being used for AMT sessions two and three, and both the anxiety and irritability scene being used for the remaining sessions, alternating each scene for arousal and relaxation control throughout each session. By the sixth session, which carried Martha through one menstrual cycle, she had reported great improvements in retaining her ability to remain resistant to nervous tension and irritability. She marked off her calendar, made it a point to practice relaxation three times daily just prior to her menstrual cycle, and wrote "Be patient" as a reminder on her calendar.

After the sixth session, the AMT procedure was modified to fit the dysmenorrhea problem. Martha was given the homework following session four to take warm baths and to soak and to pay attention to the soothing sensations. Also, she was instructed to close her eyes, relax her body and imagine the warm water flowing over her stomach and around the back, and to picture this warm flow as loosening up muscle tensions.

For the seventh AMT session, she was told that the dysmenorrheic discomfort would now be the focus of the next sessions. The explanation was given:

"You've been doing really well with managing the nervous tension and irritability. The next thing we want to do is to use the relaxation method for managing the pain and discomfort of the dysmenorrhea. Sometimes we find that the pain is made worse because of being muscularly tense. So we're going to focus the relaxation at those areas you've had the most discomfort. . . the stomach and back. I've had you doing the warm baths to facilitate this process."

In this seventh session, the procedure involved the following sequence: relaxation, relaxation scene involving the bath and flowing the relaxation around the back and stomach, menstrual scene of feeling backaches and stomach pains, return to relaxation scene with the bath using the warm water flowing as a focus of attention across the back and stomach. This sequence was repeated throughout the session. The menstrual scene was described as follows:

"Switch on that menstrual cycle scene right now. . . it's last month, you had just wakened in the morning. . . about six in the morning, you notice the light coming through the window. . . Jason was already downstairs since this was the day he had a little extra work to do first. . . you have this ache, the aches around the stomach area. . . the feelings of being bloated there. . . and the aches in the back, the type of ache that gets worse with wearing heels. . . there is this dull aching pain in the lower part of your stomach, you're feeling heavy. . . you have been expecting this since your menstrual cycle is due. . . just let that pain appear again, let yourself be there as it was on that morning. . . the dull aching, the bloated feeling, the back. . . it's all there again, the signs of the dysmenorrhea. . . "

The menstrual scene was then terminated and the relaxation scene initiated as follows:

"O.K., turn off that menstrual cycle scene, and instead let's have you switch on the relaxation scene to remove that discomfort. . . you're in the warm bath. . . flowing the warmth across the muscles. . . using whatever technique in addition works for you in gaining muscle relaxation. . . the warm bath flowing the relaxation across the entire body. . . especially across the stomach, and the lower stomach. . . soothing and relaxing the muscles. . . and as you are in the scene, let yourself again feel the water as it flows around the back, loosening those tight muscles. . . and as this happens, let all of the feelings of pain, of aches, or tightness be replaced with the warm relaxation. . . just notice the relaxed muscles. . . how this relaxation can be retrieved and replaces the aches. . . "

Since she was again approaching a menstrual period shortly, an eighth session and ninth session were scheduled during the same week, one day apart. She was then asked to call in when she began to notice backache symptoms related to her menstrual period and to arrange to come in for another AMT session. During this session, the same process was used, with muscle relaxation, but without a menstrual scene. Instead, her actual backache or stomach sensations were acknowledged, and the bath relaxation scene used to reduce the pain sensations, as follows:

> "All right, now that we have completed the muscle relaxation exercise, I want you to pay attention to any pains in your back or stomach. . . (30 second pause). . . If there are any, we'll be relaxing them away using your relaxation scene of being in the bath. . . so right now, switch on your relaxation scene. . . in that warm bath. . . the warm sensations of the water are soothing, releasing your muscle tension. . . and you can feel that warmth as the water flows around the stomach, letting any tension release itself. . . using the feelings of warmth release and loosen any tightness around the stomach or around the back. You have been experiencing some of those aches today, and the relaxation from that warm bath, plus your skill in eliminating tension through relaxing should be applied. . . use this relaxation to eliminate the muscle tension, and along with the muscle tension, eliminate the aches and pains. . . relaxation around the stomach area. . . and substitution of the relaxation for the aches in that areas. . . (10 seconds). . . then relaxation includes the back area. . . and have that relaxation substitute for the aches in the back area. . . releasing the tension, and as that occurs, noticing the relaxation as it replaces the tension and the aches. . . (10 seconds). . . all right, let's have you switch off the relaxation scene, but retain the total sense of relaxation. . . of eliminating the aches by being involved in the muscle relaxation. . . and in a moment we'll have you open your eyes. . . all the time maintaining the relaxation in the stomach, back, entire body. . . so let's have you open your eyes right now."

Through this session, Martha was able to reduce substantially the pain sensations, saying, "I feel generally relaxed. . . and calm. . . there are some little signs of aches, but I just don't need to pay attention, they're little enough that I just am thinking about the warm, relaxed feelings. . . and those little signs kind of fade into the background." The nervous tensions and irritability were now also well under control.

6

The Intake Interview Process

Introduction to the AMT Method

Anxiety Management Training is an anxiety self-control procedure that is highly specific in identifying steps for each session, along with integration of the homework assignments. AMT is also highly specific in being designed to be directly appropriate for treating anxiety states or conditions associated with stress or anxiety. For these reasons, AMT is an especially valuable therapy technique not only for the practicing clinician, but also for the researcher interested in being able to replicate studies. A major advantage of the exactness of the steps in AMT is the clarity it brings to the practicing therapist who is interested in learning the AMT procedures. Unlike some therapies which identify theoretical intentions and describe the treatment procedures in more general principles, AMT offers a very systematic and concrete set of instructions, along with theory and principles. Such clarity of principles also permits the researcher to design research studies that test AMT hypotheses and the AMT method itself in a standardized way. One problem with less well-defined therapy techniques is the difficulty in knowing whether the therapist or researchers are actually conducting a session in a manner intended by the major proponents of the technique.

AMT is highly specific in that it is focused on the anxiety states. The major advantage of therapy techniques with a specific focus is that they make available to any therapist, without regard for theoretical orientation, a proven intervention for a particular problem area. Given that

179

anxiety problems represent a common disorder in the general population, the singular appropriateness of AMT for the management of anxiety makes AMT an especially valuable disorder-focused technique. In addition, AMT has value inasmuch as anxiety often has an important mediating role with respect to other disorders, such as being the basis for certain psychophysiological complaints, being at the source of obstructions to performance, and exacerbating other conditions such as depression or maladaptive cognitions. Having a specialized therapy for anxiety provides the same advantage to a therapist that a specific medication for a specific medical complaint has for a physician.

On the other hand, although AMT covers a highly specific series of steps in its application, it also provides for the flexibility needed for fitting the progress in training to the individual characteristics of each client. The means for deciding where the client is in the therapy process is readily defined, to enable therapeutic decisions about the readiness to proceed onto the next step, through clear observations of client responsiveness within each session, evaluations of homework activities, and interviews at the start and end of each session. This chapter and the next two will provide detailed descriptions of the conduct of AMT sessions. The current chapter will focus on the intake process, while the next two chapters will cover the specific steps in the actual AMT sessions.

Intake Interview

Although the intake interview is not counted as one of the AMT sessions, a detailed assessment session is as essential for AMT as it is for other therapies. The most useful assessment interview is one that combines a supportive relationship with a productive method of inquiry. The relationship basically sets the stage for enabling the client to be viewed with respect, and to feel a valued collaborator in the process, thereby to become a more complete source of information. Clients tend to evaluate the atmosphere in the intake by the interest, understanding, and acceptance demonstrated by the therapist. Such characteristics are associated with therapists who engage in appropriate listening and attending, accurate summaries, as well as meaningful guidance of the interview. In the initial part of the intake, a more open approach to inquiry is desirable where a more neutral orientation is assumed by the therapist. This precludes the therapist becoming so one-sided as to steer unconsciously the information in incorrect directions, while signaling to the client the importance of client participation. However, as the intake progresses, it is helpful for the process to receive more guidance from the therapist to insure comprehensiveness and to avoid misunderstanding.

In addition to the atmosphere established for the assessment session, the method of inquiry can be a constructive factor. One approach which I have found valuable is the "topic-incident-cycle" method of inquiry. This approach relies upon a particular flow in the interview as follows: beginning with an open-ended inquiry, moving to the identification of a topic, progressing to the elaboration through an incident, and ending with a summary to cross-check for accuracy and understanding. Once a cycle is complete, then a new cycle is repeated, but with another topic. The following illustrates this process:

> T: Good morning. Would you start with telling me something about what brings you here, the problem which is concerning you? (Open inquiry).

> C: I'm a nervous person, a very, very nervous person. . . I have these periods when I'm all tensed up. . . it's like an attack, affects my stomach, and I have this feeling something very bad is going to happen, I don't know what, but it'll be bad. . . and I get fidgety and restless and can't sit still, and yet I forget what I'm doing. I thought it would go away with time, but I've been like this for almost a year now. . . it's getting so I can't function.

> T: I can understand your concern. Tell me something about the anxiety, what is this like for you? (The topic identified is the anxiety itself.)

> C: It comes suddenly. . . like all of a sudden, I'm tense. . . and I feel my heart beating like crazy. . . I don't tremble or anything. . . and it builds up pretty fast, one moment I'm all right, but the next moment I'm all caught up. . . I also have this feeling that something dreadful is going to happen, maybe to me, maybe to someone else..and it takes over. . . can last for quite a while, but I'm not good for doing anything in the meantime.

> T: So you have these sudden experiences. . . tension, heart racing, a sense of something dreadful, that interferes with you. Would you share with me an example of an incident when you experienced such anxiety? (Elaboration through an incident).

> C: Happened last night. . . I was home, sitting in the living room since I already had dinner ready to go, waiting and watching the news, my husband was a little late. . . and then suddenly, boom, I have this surge inside me. . . like my stomach suddenly is filling with this force, tightening me up. . . and it moves up my chest until my heart starts to go real fast. . . and then my throat gets choked up. . . I stand up, and start to move, but then I don't know where to go. . . I stop. . . I have this sense that something bad is around the corner, I'm by the door and I start to think about things like accidents. . . Actually, it's not really thinking, more like flashes of thought, or like flashes, like images. . . an accident. . . or I see my husband at the door and he looks like something bad is going on, maybe he's going to tell me something, like leave me or something, but there's no good reason for this, we're fine, but still there's this feeling.

> T: So the anxiety comes suddenly, these powerful feelings in the stomach and heart, and then the images of something bad flash through. This all happened last night. I wonder how this experience compares with other times when you've become anxious to this degree? What would be another example? (Topic of the anxiety symptoms continues to be pursued, with elaboration through another incident.)

We will skip further statements from the client. Instead, the process of further inquiry by the therapist will be listed to illustrate the sequential progress of this interview approach.

> T: So there are great similarities in how you experience the anxiety, and the body feelings seem to be first. You feel this wave, stomach tightens, your heart rate suddenly goes high, reaches your throat, and you become restless and have to move around, but you don't have a direction. It's like you forgot what you were doing, and don't have a real direction. Then, you will have these thoughts that are more like images flashing. These change, so sometimes they are about your husband, sometimes they aren't really personal, it's just that they all involve a feeling of dread, something bad. Does this capture it? (Summary and check for understanding.)

> T: Now, I'd like to not miss anything. So can we just stand back a bit. You've given me several good examples of times when you were anxious and what that was like. So I've a good sense for how you feel the anxiety. Are there other circumstances when you've been anxious where your anxiety reaction was different from the ones we've gone over? (Topic is still anxiety symptoms, but with an open invitation to elaborate if there is need.)

> T: Good, I feel I have a good grasp of the anxiety that brings you in, and how difficult it is for you. We haven't yet gone over what you've been doing about getting these feelings under control. What do you do? (Open inquiry for a new topic, which will then repeat the same interview cycle.)

> T: I understand. So we've been talking about how you experience the anxiety and the various ways you've tried to deal with it, none of which worked for you. Earlier you mentioned that this has been going on for about a year. Let's talk a little about that. (Open inquiry for a new topic; interview cycle repeats format.)

> T: We've really been focusing on the anxiety. At this point, I'm wondering if there are any other topics we should cover? Anything else I should know? (Open inquiry.)

The topical cycle format in interviewing can be adapted for use with any initial intake. When it is used specifically as intake for anxiety disorders prior to AMT, the therapist should organize his/her intake to cover some specific topics. Among the topics deserving coverage are: information on the anxiety experience, information on the settings in which anxiety is experienced, and information on prior coping attempts.

Interview Information on the Anxiety Experience

It is important to obtain concrete descriptions of how the client experiences anxiety. This information serves as the basis for gauging the level of severity of the anxiety (a topic we will describe later), as well as for understanding the client's unique characteristics. In my thinking an individual client's anxiety characteristics can be understood in terms of different stress responses, with three response subsystems or channels: affective-autonomic, somatic-behavioral, and cognitive. If a client shows intense levels of symptoms in all three subsystems, this is one indication of a more severe level of disturbance. Additionally, in interviewing for information on the response subsystems, it is important to be aware of sequences, that is, whether the most immediate response to a stressor for a particular client is first in a cognitive channel, which in turn prompts autonomic and somatic symptoms. For another client, the sequence might be a primary response that is autonomic, which then leads to certain cognitions being prompted, which in turn leads to blockages in behavioral performance. The following are illustrations of client descriptions which offer different client stress profiles:

Affective/Autonomic-Dominant Stress Response

"I feel that my nerves are breaking up inside of me; I'm just one nervous wreck all the time."

"I can't breathe. . . I find myself struggling for oxygen. . . it's like suddenly there is a tight band across my chest."

"When I'm waiting for my number to be called to start the race, my mind is blank, but I sometimes get sick to my stomach. . . more than butterflies in the stomach, BIG butterflies that make me want to throw up."

"My hands suddenly get cold; it's like all the blood drained out of me and along with it, the heat. . . I shake my arms, put on extra clothes, but I'm still cold."

Somatic/Behavioral-Dominant Stress Response

"Yes, I knew in my head that there was nothing to fear and that I was completely safe, but my head was listening and my knees were not paying any attention. . . they were wobbling and shaking."

"I was at that critical juncture on the rock climb, where you have to commit yourself to letting go from the handhold in order to reach the next one. . . I knew it was simple to do, and I've climbed a lot in my life, but somehow I felt glued to the spot, I couldn't get my body to move."

"I can't sit still. . . I wind up pacing. . . moving around. . . not with anything in mind, just to be moving. . . I guess you would say aimlessly, but it's like my motor is wound up."

"It's like I lost control over my body. . . no, no not complete control, I still do things, but for example, I stutter over words. . . and I'm not as smooth in my movements. . . just a little bit off. . . you know what it's like to be a little tight in your muscles, and you can't always predict where the ball will go when you throw it?"

Cognitive-Dominant Stress Response

"I just know the worse thing is happening to me. . . I'm not going to survive the experience. . . I'm sure my whole life is going to fall apart right now, and I can't do anything about it - I know these thoughts are not rational, but I can't stop them."

"I find that I can't think straight. . . it's like my mind is racing at a pace so fast, I can't keep up. . . everything blurs around me."

"I discover that I'm trying to concentrate on just one thing, just one thing, but my mind keeps wandering. . . I can't keep focused. . . I hear someone talking nearby, and I'm paying attention to them. . . and then there is something else on the other side that I start thinking about or looking at. . . it's like I'm stumbling around inside my head."

"I worry, I just worry. . . I think about all the things that could go wrong. . . I'm not ready. . . or maybe I'll forget something. . . like you know how you leave your house and you worry about whether you turned off the stove; you know you did but you worry anyway. . . I know I shouldn't worry, because it makes things seem worse, but I can't stop."

Sequence of Responding

Cognitions primary: "I walk in the exam room and it hits me. I start to think about what the exam is going to be like. Up until this point, I'm O.K., comfortable, relaxed, confident. But as soon as I sit down, I start to worry. Did I spend too much time studying one chapter and not enough on another? I listen to others talking about what they studied, and I just know that they did it right and I did it wrong. I pick up my book and start to skim, but I'm now so anxious that I can't understand what I'm seeing, I can't really understand what I'm reading, so I read one sentence over and over again, but nothing sinks in, and I panic more. Pretty soon I start pacing and I notice my hands sweating, and I notice that I'm very tense, and I can't relax. I dread the teacher coming in the room with the exam. I'm absolutely sure I'm going to fail the exam, that I'm so stupid, I don't belong here in school."

(For this client, the thoughts appear stimulated by the examination room, with the worrisome thoughts leading to other symptoms such as distractibility and inability to process information. Then autonomic and behavioral symptoms are triggered by the thoughts, which in turn exacerbate the worries.)

Autonomic primary: "I hear my flight being called for boarding, and suddenly I break out in sweat. . . I can feel my heart beat, like it's going so fast it'll just come out of my chest. . . it's so loud too, it's booming in my ears. . . I just know that I must look a wreck, that other passengers must be aware that I'm scared to death, and that they are looking at me. . . and thinking it's funny, because there's nothing to be afraid of, everyone flies all the time. . . but that doesn't stop me from being anxious, from having those sensations that I'm sick inside. . . maybe I'm so sick that I shouldn't get on the plane, what happens if I have a heart attack and we're in the air. . . my hands are shaking and I don't want to get on the airplane, my mind is going a mile a minute, and I'm feeling faint. . . "

(The fear of flying is prompted by the signal for boarding, which precipitates the autonomic stress reaction for this client. Soon after the physiological reactions, the client begins to have cognitive symptoms, including interpreting the autonomic symptoms as possible signs of a physical disorder. Somatic-behavioral symptoms also emerge.)

Somatic-behavioral primary: "I tremble, I can't talk straight. I look down at my hands and they are shaking, so I grip my hands real tight to stop the shaking, but I can't. I know I'm not going to be able to walk either, because my legs feel like anchors. . . no, they're more like separated from me, like

I'm in the control booth but the wires are disconnected to my legs. At the
same time, I feel weak, like my knees and legs are water. . . does that make
sense, first I say I feel disconnected, but then I still have these sensations?. . . I reach for some water because I'm suddenly thirsty, and knock
over the glass. . . I feel so apologetic and embarassed, like 'what a klutz',
but I can't help it, something just goes wrong with my coordination, my
wires are mixed up, or too tight or something. . . and sometimes I feel
dizzy. . . but it's funny, you asked about my heart rate, and it's fine, I never
have a fast heart beat, my pulse stays o.k., or at least I don't notice it. . . "
(This client has a very clearly dominant behavioral response under stress.
Some autonomic and some cognitive reactions also appear, but to a minor
degree.)

Interview Information on the Anxiety Setting

As an aid to understanding the life stresses of any one client, the
interview should also cover details of the situations under which the
stress responses occur. The interview would begin with the open-ended
approach described in our interviewing model, with attentiveness to the
possible initial origins of the disturbance. For instance, the various
categories of stressors might serve as the guidelines for understanding
the background of the current anxieties, these categories being biophysiological, environmental, social, psychogenic, and cognitive. The
way in which these stressor experiences have led to the development of
current symptoms also needs to be explored. This history taking enables
initial decisions on whether the current complaints require interventions
other than or in addition to AMT.

For instance, if environmental factors are the major and continuing
source of stress symptoms (such as tension headaches), and if environmental intervention is feasible such as moving to a less crowded living
area, then AMT would not be needed. If cognitive overload due to poor
scheduling of work assignments is a primary source of the stress, than
better calendar management, rearranging deadlines, or learning the
skills needed to decline more work might be preferable. As a final illustration, if the social problems from ethnic minority status are associated with the stresses of poverty to create distress, then career planning,
employment training, financial counseling, and other such services
might be useful. In essence, the early part of the intake interview is
aimed at determining whether a more central contributing factor to
stress continues to play a current major role, so that the most effective
intervention would be one that aimed at resolving these key variables.

As this background information has been identified, there may still
be reason to recommend AMT. For example, the client may need help in
controlling immediate stress reactions while in training for improved
employment. Or, a client might still experience the precipitation of anx-

iety even though the initial sources of stress, such as the rape trauma, have been removed, because of the residual interoceptive or exteroceptive conditioning that has yet to be extinguished. Certainly, AMT would be appropriate where the anxiety state represents the immediate concerns of the client as the primary symptomatology, as in phobic disorders, generalized anxiety disorder, and so forth. At this point, where the decision has been tentatively made to rely upon AMT, then the interview should narrow its direction to obtaining concrete examples of specific times during which the anxiety was experienced. The following case illustrates how such an interview might progress:

T: Give me a sense for the conditions which seem to be related to your anxiety.

C: Well, I really get anxious when I feel I'm put on the spot. . . I mean, when I feel I have to kind of be assertive. . . assert myself. . . argue with someone over something.

T: O.K., so one situation involves settings when you have to asssert yourself, are there are other circumstances that bring on the anxiety?

C: Yeah, well, the main reason I came in was because I keep having these neck pains, and my doctor thought it was due to stress. I clench my teeth a lot too.

T: Do you have a feeling about what is associated with the neck pains or the teeth clenching? I mean, do you have any ideas about what these might connect up to?

C: Well, it has always seemed to me that I get a pain in the neck, the right side, when my spouse keeps talking about something, but doesn't give me a chance to reply, and she just keeps going and makes me feel I did something wrong, but she won't listen to me. . . and I know that, so I shut down, waiting for my chance to say something, even though I know she won't hear me. . .

T: So maybe another situation has to do, has something to do with arguments with your spouse?

C: Not exactly arguments, I wouldn't call them arguments. . . it's more like she wants some information, about whether we're going to a movie this week, and I can't tell her right away because I don't know my schedule yet, and she makes it seem that I'm not being cooperative because I don't know my schedule right off the bat. If I had to label it, it's more like those types of discussions where I'm kind of feeling on the defensive with her. It's only her.

T: Is this sort of, kind of related to the assertiveness bit too? Maybe you are anxious when you need to be assertive, to assert yourself in both cases? Or you're feeling defensive in both cases?

C: No, no. The assertive thing. . . I don't feel defensive, I know that i'm right and that they have to listen to me. It's just that it's not my style to be demanding or to complain. No, I don't think the two are similar at all. The assertive thing is one of those where I know I don't want to do it, makes me anxious and nervous and I have to talk myself into being assertive, but I'm anxious all the time, and it never turns out well.

The thing with my wife, I'm not anxious, not the same anxiety, just that it gives me a pain when I'm waiting. . . so maybe, now that I think of it, maybe the pain is the kind that comes from being tensed up. . . but it's still different from the anxiety with asserting myself. . . in that situation, I'm really anxious and know it. . . with my spouse, it's like I'm stressed out and it doesn't seem the same. . .

T: So what we have are two types of situations which seem to bring on the anxiety and tension. Let's go back and start with the first one, the assertiveness situations, give me an example of a time in which you were having to be assertive and describe what went on.

C: Ummm. O.K., O.K., I have this film, you see. . . and I just had it developed, and I walked out of the store, and I'm in my car, and I notice that they charged me for a second set of prints, and I didn't want a second set. . . so I think I oughta go back and get a refund. . . but I become anxious thinking about this. . . you know, the feelings I mentioned before when we were talking about my anxieties. . . anyway, I start to think about going in and then I feel I don't want to go through with it. . . I figure, it's only a few bucks, and besides, anyway I could use the extra prints, I might need them for someone. . . then I think, I'm just trying to avoid going back in. . . but I don't feel comfortable, what if I'm wrong, and the clerk tells me they don't give refunds. . . then I'm committed, I'll have to argue, because I can't back down now. . . and I think what if the clerk is aggressive and tells me I should have caught the mistake when I checked out. . . eventually I talked myself into going back, but I'm feeling like I don't want to do this. . . so I went back and the clerk is busy talking to another customer, so this makes it worse on my part, I'm waiting around and thinking about what I'm going to say, but I can't get the right words together. . . then the other person left, and I kind of stuttered it all out, in one burst. . . and she was real nice, she told me it was store policy to return any prints that were a mistake, and so she gave me a refund! Wow, was I relieved. . . I wanted to get out as fast as I could. I didn't even count my change.

T: So it sounds like you were anxious even though you knew you were right, and there were all these thoughts. . . you also knew you were anxious, and the thoughts didn't make it better. . . actually, it made it worse. I couldn't get a sense for the very first reaction you had when you found out you ought to go back and ask for a refund. . . you mentioned your thoughts, you mentioned your feelings, your anxious feelings. . . uh. . .

C: Yeh, I see, O.K., aah, it was the feeling first. . . like in my gut. . . I knew I was anxious. . . and then all those thoughts came instantly as I began trying to figure out what to do next, to go in or go home. . .

T: So you were all right until you saw the mistake, and the anxiety started when you knew you had to decide on going back in. If we use that scale of 0 to 100, how would you describe your anxiety at different moments in this circumstance?

C: You mean when I had the film, outside. . . yeh, well, it was about 60 when I knew I had to decide. . . when I knew an error was made. . . and while I was kind of struggling with myself about going back, it was like 65, when I was thinking about being wrong, or the clerk being aggressive or things like that. . . and the worst was standing there waiting, like about 70–75.

T: So was there anything else that was going on that influenced, that contributed to your being anxious. . . it seemed to be first the knowing you had to go inside and be assertive, and also all those thoughts. . .

C: Umm. . . no, it was pretty straightforward.

T: Give me another example of an assertiveness situation.

C: That made me anxious? Ummm. . . well, I needed to pay for a tie I was trying to buy, and was in a rush and I tried to pay. . . this was last week, in this men's shop. . . . .

T: So then what happened?

C: I went to the salesman, but he was talking, talking to a friend, another salesman. . . and so I waited to be noticed. . . but it made me nervous.

T: How did you sense you were nervous?

C: Again, it's like before. . . when I'm nervous, I have this feeling in my gut. . . like knotted. . . and I want to get away, don't want to deal with the situation.

T: So is this what happened in the store this time as well, or was the anxiety different?

C: No, it was the same; I had the feeling in the gut. . . and I wanted to put the tie back and just leave, but it was a nice tie, and it was a nice sale. . . and I knew it was something I wanted. . . but I also knew I had to do something to get their attention. . .

T: So you were anxious by now? About how high on the scale?

C: Yeh, like I said, I was feeling the gut anxiety. . . about 65.

T: Then, what happened next. . . you were standing, thinking you had to get his attention.

C: I paced around a little, I thought maybe they would see me. . . I thought. . . I knew though I would have to say something, because they didn't care. . . I had to just barge right up there and. . . but then what should I say, should I be nasty or polite, "Excuse me. . . "

T: And your anxiety now?

C: Oh, high. . . like 75–80.

T: Then what happened next?

C: Well, I finally walked around, pretending like I was looking at other things, about five more minutes. . . then I kind of got up steam and walked straight up, and said, "I want to buy this."

T: Then what happened?

C: There was this horrible moment. They stopped talking and just looked at me for a moment. . . and I thought, "My God, I interrupted them". . .but then he smiled, took the tie, and my money.

T: So with this moment, he's looking at you, staring, not saying anything, what were you experiencing?

C: Actually nothing. Just the thought, but it went so fast. . . he took the tie, smiled. . . all over; I didn't have the time to have a reaction, just the thought. That's it.

T: Then what happened.

C: What do you mean. . . I took my package, and left. . . I was O.K. . . .kind of relieved it was over. . . just left.

T: So in both of these circumstances, you just made up your mind and kind of. . . just walked over and kind of did it. Were you doing anything that helped you make up your mind, or helped you control the anxiety?

C: You mean, did I do something to become less anxious? No. . . I was still anxious during it all. . . I just then did it. . . but I was anxious all the way. . . only when I was leaving the store did I calm down.

T: All right, so now recall for me a situation involving your spouse. Describe that for me.

C: Well, that one about the movie. . . do you want to hear about that one?

T: If that was an incident that caused you anxiety that you felt important.

C: Yeh, well, she says, "Well, are we going to the movie or not this Thursday." And I didn't know yet, but this made me anxious.

T: Tell me a bit more about this situation, what was going on, the setting. . . like where was this happening?

C: Oh, O.K. . . . .I came home for dinner, and was washing up, and she was in the kitchen, and yelled at me, "Are we going to the movies?" And it seemed O.K. since we had been planning this, so I said, "Yeah, as soon as I get my schedule tomorrow." But then she said, "Don't you know yet? So are we not going. . . I thought we were planning on this Thursday." And I said, "Yeah, I think so, but I have to check my schedule." And she says, "Well, are we going to the movie or not this Thursday?"

T: So at what point were you feeling the anxiety?

C: Well, it was not until she started in on me, started in pushing, like "Are we going or not." When she first asked, I was O.K., I didn't see it coming. But once she started in pushing, when I couldn't do anything. . . like I couldn't get my schedule until tomorrow, so how could I answer her. . . and I had the feeling that she was blaming me.

T: That's when the anxiety first appears?

C: Yeah. . . O.K. you wanna know how high, right? Like 0 before, then all of a sudden, when she starts in pushing, I jump to 90.

T: And what were those feelings like?

C: Same. . . I get the gut sensation, tied up, feel it inside me. I'm clear otherwise, I'm thinking, not confused. . . I know what's happening, and I can still figure out what's going on. . . but I want to leave the kitchen, get out of sight. . .

T: So the feelings were in the gut, also wanting to be out of there. And about 90, pretty high. . . then what happened next.

C: Well it all sorta ended.

T: In what way did it end. . . what did you actually do, or what did she actually do?

C: It's what I did. . . I stood it as long as I could, and could see that she was going to keep asking, so I just kind of hitched up and said, "I gotta go upstairs and change"...and I kind of got out of there, and hid away upstairs for awhile.

T: So you left, went upstairs. And what about the anxiety?

C: It stayed about 90 for another hour. . .

T: What was happening to you during this hour?

C: I was changing, sitting around, thinking about not wanting to face her again. . . figuring she was going to raise the topic again, or maybe harp again on my schedule.

T: So what was that anxiety connected to during this hour?

C: Some of it was left over from that talking downstairs with her. . . some were. . . everything I'd think about going down and facing her. . . thinking about her raising the topic again. . . knowing for sure if I came down, she would raise the topic. . .

T: So the anxiety kept high as you kind of thought about her still raising the topic, kind of picturing her in the kitchen and her mood? Was there anything else making the anxiety stay?

C: Didn't need anything else.

T: So then what happened. . . how did the anxiety disappear. . . what did you do about it?

C: Nothing. . . just sat around upstairs for about an hour, and I could hear her doing the cooking. . . and then she called me down for dinner. . . helped that it was a pleasant voice. . . and I came down, kind of waited to see what she was going to say. . . and she seemed to have forgotten. . . so I lost my anxiety.

T: So actually it was hearing her sound pleasant and seeing her. . . was it one or the other than helped reduce the anxiety?

C: Well, the voice was a little help. . . like it allowed me to come down and face her. . . maybe dropped my anxiety to 80. . . but when I found she was not continuing the topic, it really dropped.

T: About how long ago did this occur?

C: Just last night.

T: And the one about the ties?

C: About three years ago.

T: And the film?

C: About a month ago.

T: Of the two, about the ties and film, which seemed to you to be the one you recall the clearest, made the most impression on you?

C: The one with the ties. . . no, the film, because I can still see the clerk with that other customer. . . I even remember what pictures I had.

This illustration of an interview that focused on several real events arousing anxiety points out helpful areas to review through obtaining specific examples of life incidents: the nature of the anxiety symptoms, similarities or differences in symptoms associated with different situations, the level of the anxiety experienced, the nature of variables that influenced the level of anxiety, time and location of the situations, what coping behaviors were used and with what success, the level of clarity of detail of each incident in the client's memory, and the sequence of events.

For this client, the anxiety symptoms appear to be experienced in pretty much the same way in a variety of situations, the two major situations being on the theme of assertiveness and blame/helplessness encounters with the spouse. The autonomic stress response seems an early sign, but closely followed by negative thoughts that exacerbate the anxiety and cause higher levels and maintain the high levels in a dominant way. The assertiveness situations appear to be associated with a lower level of anxiety than the spouse encounters (but this conclusion should be followed up in the interview, as the therapist asks for another example of a spouse-encounter incident, and then may directly ask if assertiveness tends to precipitate a moderately high level, while spouse encounter prompts an intense level of anxiety).

The triggering events seem to be cognitive, such as realizing that assertiveness is going to be required, or recognizing that the spouse is engaging in confrontative behaviors. The tendency of the client is to show maladaptive avoidance behaviors, but he still has enough self-control and psychological strength to force himself into active behaviors, even though these are avoidance behaviors in the case of spouse encounters. However, his behaviors of making himself "just do it" or of leaving his spouse and hiding away are not at all successful in controlling the anxiety.

The anxiety level decreases as a result of the other person's actions, which changes his appraisals (he sees that his spouse is dropping the topic) or as a result of the stressful incident coming to an end (he obtains his refund or pays for his tie). Although it may have been possible that the older incident could have been more clearly recalled, in this case, the more recent one had more impact on his memory. Finally, it would appear that the sequence appears to be the onset of a stressor, followed by anxiety of a moderately high level, increased to a higher level by thoughts, followed by indecision and a desire to avoid the situation, and in some instances an actual avoidance, but no evidence of appropriate coping. Instead, as the thoughts continue, the anxiety maintains itself, even in the absence of the direct stressor.

For AMT, the following parts of the interview information were of immediate value. The client had learned the use of a scale from 0 to 100 to gauge his level of anxiety. The consistent high ratings confirmed that a high level of stress is being experienced, such that AMT treatment would be warranted. It was helpful to note that two major themes emerged, since this would make it easier to identify anxiety arousal scenes for AMT treatment in sessions two and four, and would permit identifying situations for the client later to test his progress in anxiety control. The fact that the anxiety was associated with more than one type of life event, however, also suggested a more serious difficulty than if the anxiety were more narrowly associated with only a single type of life situation.

The anxiety experience itself appeared constant, in that an early sign was the gut feelings. For AMT session three, clients are encouraged to identify their early signs that signal the possible onset of anxiety, in order to use the relaxation coping method to abort the anxiety before it escalates. For this client, the gut feelings, or possibly even the neck pains, could serve as the early warning signs. AMT requires by session two that the client identify an anxiety experience from real life which represents a moderately high level of anxiety, and in session four an event which was associated with a high level of anxiety. The interviewer questioned which of the two assertiveness situations was the most clearly recalled, and would later also identify which of the spouse confrontation situations was better recalled. By this inquiry, it would be possible to decide later which life events could be the ones used for anxiety arousal in AMT sessions, given their clarity. Although it is preferable to have an event that was recent, the scene used for AMT anxiety arousal would be the one with the greatest clarity in the client's recall, since the sole purpose for such recall in AMT is to prompt anxiety arousal.

Further, as we shall see later, using a prior life event that is clear and detailed precludes problems developing in AMT sessions, such as a lack of anxiety arousal due to the client being unable to reexperience the details of the life event. I should quickly note here that the actual life event selected for use in AMT sessions to prompt anxiety arousal might be a life experience other than those obtained during the intake, if the client later remembers a situation that was even more salient, or, if the client experiences a new situation in between AMT sessions that appears more meaningful.

During AMT session two, in which a life event associated with a moderately high level of anxiety is used to arouse anxiety, the therapist will use instructions involving describing the situation, as well as the nature of the anxiety experience. Such descriptions provide the client with help in recalling the experience, through a reminder of what the situation entailed, as well as through emphasizing the elements of the experience that were most associated with anxiety arousal. For this client, the assertiveness incident with the film refund emphasized the circumstance of having to wait while another customer was served, the many thoughts going through the client's head, and the gut feeling. For the higher intensity experience of spouse encounter, again the gut feeling and thoughts appear extremely salient features that, when re-described, would prompt return of the anxiety experience.

Information on the time and location of the life examples being pursued is another way of assuring the therapist that the client is describing an actual life event. Having the client describe, rather than interpret an experience that was associated with the anxiety condition enables the therapist to decide for him/herself how to interpret what is happening with the client. For instance, if a client were asked, "What kinds of circumstances do you feel cause your anxiety?", and the client responds, "It's arguments with my wife," this response represents an interpretation by the client that all such encounters are argumentative, and may mislead the therapist also to infer that such spouse encounters involved intense disagreement, anger, or even possibly hostility. On the other hand, when the actual incident is described, as with this client, it appears that the anxiety could be aroused with a minor disagreement from the wife, since the client had become so sensitive to early cues of implied blame that his thought processes would intensify his anxiety level.

Obtaining information, such as on time and location, also enables confirmation that the description is a description and again not the client's interpretation. For instance, a reply that involves the client interpreting events might be, "Well, an example would be any time my wife and I got into arguments. Generally, it would be in the kitchen right after I came home. She would put the pressure on me, blaming me for something I could not control, and that would invariably trigger anxiety in my gut." This reply is really not a description of a single event, but an interpretation by the client, deriving from his view of what happened across a series of events; he is generalizing and drawing his own conclusions as he interprets several events. If the client were asked whether he was describing a particular incident, and if so, to date the incident, it would become quite clear very quickly that this client's response is based upon several events.

Interview Information on Prior Coping

As a final important topic for the intake interview, the client's past coping behaviors or attempts can be important, as well as information on possible skills which may serve as the foundation for AMT sessions. The following case involving anger illustrates the direction of such an interview:

> T: So another example of a situation when your anger was out of control involved feeling frustrated when you were asked to move up your deadline on your assignment, and you felt this was unreasonable. Tell me more details about what happened next.
>
> C: As I said, I had been called in to see my boss, and he said I had to move up the date. I said, "Why?" and he said, "I don't need to tell you why, things have moved up everywhere, so you have to get your job done one week earlier." Then I said, "I need the extra week, we're working as fast as we can," but he just stared, he just stared at me, and looked away, like I was nothing. . . I mean like I was dust. . . and I knew he wasn't going to give me the extra week. I started to get real tense, like I could feel my hands

bunching up. . . like I was going to hit him, my insides were swelling up, like a huge balloon. . . I felt frustrated, like he was in my way. . . and now I was staring at him, really focused, he was the only thing I could think of. . . just like it was a TV screen and he suddenly filled it up. . . .and I had the little thought, "Don't do something dumb"...but I knew I was beyond control. . . started to feel the blood, red blood rush to my head. . . saw red all over. . . and man, was I angry. . .

T: So then what happened?

C: I did it, I just did it again. . . stupid, really dumb. . . I just hauled off and told him off. . . I called him every kind of name, said he was stupid, told him he could take the job and shove it, that he could do it himself, that I wasn't going to do it, that he better get someone else that could take his shit, that I didn't want to work anymore, and I kept yelling and screaming until he stopped me. . .

T: How did he do that?

C: He stood up and told me I was fired, and then told me to get out.

T: Then what happened?

C: Nothing. I suddenly came back to earth. What could I do, I was fired. I wasn't about ready to beg. So I turned around and left. . . went to the bar and had a few. . . went home and had a few more.

T: In all these incidents, it seems like there were times in which you kind of said to yourself, "Don't do it." How well did this work?

C: Nothing. Never did. . . like there's a little voice, but it's so little. . . when I get angry, it's all over. . . even a loud voice I wouldn't hear. . . no, nothing.

T: Are there other types of things you've done either during such angry situations, or before or after, which gave you better control?

C: Nothing. . . well, on a few times, if I knew I was already a little irritated going into the situation. . . going in. . . if I took a few deep breaths, it would sometimes help, I'd be a little better. . . actually it worked once, but I never really did it more than once.

T: Tell me about this one time, describe that situation.

C: I played football, second string tackle. . . that day I missed an assignment that cost us the game. . . we were walking back into the locker. . . I was a tackle. . . I knew my ass was going to be chewed out. . . I dunno. . . I dunno, but for some reason, I took a couple of deep breaths, maybe I was already so tired and down that I figured it wasn't worth it. . . took a few, felt better. . . and was chewed out, but it was like I was able to keep my anger down. . . it wasn't that I wasn't wrong, I just missed it. . . but usually I would fight back, even when I was wrong. . . that's my trouble, temper, no thought. . . just temper, right or wrong.

T: So tell me about these deep breaths.

C: I read about it when I was playing. . . and some of the other guys in other sports talked about it. . . like soothes you, calms you. . . so I tried it couple times. . .

T: And how did you feel?

C: Actually, it had possibilities. . . but I never got into it enough.

T: You mention your friends talking about it, did you ever have any training in deep breathing or muscle relaxation techniques?

C: Not really.

T: We will be teaching you a method for muscle relaxation in our sessions, as a method for giving you control over the anger. Do you have any thoughts about this?

C: About learning relaxation? No problem. . . anything that will stop my thick head from going off the deep end all the time. . .

This client showed such severe problems with anger that he had lost several construction jobs because of his temper. Although he remembered the one incident in which he did control his feelings, this may have been due to a combination of fatigue and the deep breathing. At any rate, coping never seemed to be available, nor did he appear to have any well-developed skills in the deep breathing. On the other hand, he did appear open to the AMT training approach since it was related to his prior experimenting with the deep breathing.

Another client actually did have skills in relaxing. She was the spouse of a high level executive, and they had many opportunities to travel abroad. However, she was deathly afraid of flying, and had to force herself to join her husband on trips. She could only board if she drank several glasses of alcohol to deaden her senses. Even then, she would still experience enough fear that she relaxed only when she was again on the ground. As it turned out, she was a daily exerciser, swimming in a lake off her backyard.

T: Tell me about this swimming, sounds rather relaxing for you.

C: Oh yes, definitely. I keep fit, but the best thing is that I really feel good, I mean relaxed. My friends say the hot tub is the very best, but for me, I can be alone, and I lose all my cares. . . I swim very slowly, breast stroke. . . it's usually comfortable. . . and I count my strokes, each one. . . and I slowly move around the lake, counting each stroke, and my mind is calm and my body is in this rhythm. . . slowly, stroke by stroke. . . it's great. . . takes me about an hour.

T: So the swimming helps you relax. . . what seems to be the main things you are doing when you swim. Describe the last time you were in the lake.

C: Well, as I said, I swim slowly. . . yesterday, about four in the afternoon, was pretty warm out, so the lake was soothing, comfortable temperature. . . I started out where I usually do, off the dock. . . then I went to the right, my usual. . . and started in, counting each stroke. . . keeping a slow, steady rhythm. . . and I could feel myself immediately relaxing. . . then I went left after about fifteen minutes, towards the tennis courts on the other side. . . counting all the time.

T: So the rhythm and the counting and the slow movements?

C: Yes, exactly.

At this point, since we had covered the major features of the intake already, I asked her to close her eyes, and recall yesterday's swimming, with special attention to the rhythm, and counting each stroke. . . then remembering the temperature of the water. . . but focused on counting and each stroke. Within five minutes, she appeared to relax, as her facial area became smoother, her jaw dropped a little, her breathing slowed, her shoulders dropped, there was little eye movement under the eyelids, her muscle tone seemed lessened. I then asked her to open her eyes and proceeded:

> T: So what happened?
>
> C: Oh, marvelous. I was back there again, and I was really calm and in the water. . . can't tell you how great it feels to swim, and be relaxed. I was swimming, counting the strokes, nothing around me but the lake, the water.
>
> T: That works so well for you, we really should rely upon it for our training as well.

Instead of the standard muscle relaxation training exercise, for this client, we used her visualizing herself swimming. Since this worked so well, the time between the first AMT session, which is devoted to relaxation training and a week's homework in relaxation practice, was shortened. Within a few weeks she was able to control her fears of flying. In one month, she boarded a plane to Europe, did not consume any alcoholic drinks, used the relaxation from visualizing herself swimming and counting to control her initial symptoms of anxiety arousal, and sent me a pleasant postcard from Belgium.

Alternative Interview Approaches

Perhaps the major advantage of this intake interview approach is that it combines an open-ended format which treats the client as a valued collaborator and observer, with a structured inquiry involving guidance from the therapist. This structure, relying upon incidents to make the interview more concrete, can be reassuring to the anxious client. The structured interview enables the client to assume a more impersonal perspective, somewhat like a participant observer. Occasionally, the elaborations from different incidents, the comparisons across such incidents, and the identification of the sequence of experiences will promote a greater level of understanding on the part of the client.

Other examples of structured interviews include a broad approach for organizing clinical interviews by Peterson (1968) and a structured format specifically applicable for anxiety disorders by DiNardo, Barlow, Cerny, Vermilyea, Vermilyea, Himadi, and Waddell (1985).

Peterson's Clinical Interview

Peterson separates the clinical interview into a phase involving the definition of the client's problem, and a phase involving identification of the determinants of the problem behaviors. Within the first phase, he emphasizes the need to determine how the client perceives or defines the presenting problem, the severity of the problem, and the generality of the problem. Within the second phase, he examines the conditions that intensify the problem, alleviate the problem, that might be the origins of the problem, as well as other antecedants, specific consequences, and suggested interventions, as well as new topics. Some specific types of interview questions associated with this organizational approach are shown next:

A. Definition of problem behavior:[1]
   1. Nature of the problem as defined by client:
      "As I understand it, you came here because. . . " (discuss reasons for contact as stated by referral agency or other source of information) "I would like you to tell me more about this. What is the problem as you see it?" (Probe as needed to determine client's view of his own problem behavior, i.e., what he is doing, or failing to do, which he or somebody else defines as a problem.)
   2. Severity of the problem:
      (a) "How serious a problem is this as far as you are concerned?" (Probe to determine perceived severity of problem.)
      (b) "How often do you. . . ?" (Exhibit problem behavior if a disorder of commission, or have occasion to exhibit desired behavior if a problem of omission. The goal is to obtain information regarding frequency of response.)
   3. Generality of the problem:
      (a) Duration: "How long has this been going on?"
      (b) Extent: "Where does the problem usually come up?" (Probe to determine situations in which problem behavior occurs, e.g., "Do you feel that way at work? How about at home?")
B. Determinants of problem behavior:
   1. Conditions which intensify problem behavior: "Now I want you to think about the times when. . . (the problem) is worst. What sort of things are going on then?"
   2. Conditions which alleviate problem behavior: "What about the times when. . . (the problem) gets better? What sorts of things are going on then?"
   3. Perceived origins: "What do you think is causing. . . (the problem)?"
   4. Specific antecedents:
      "Think back to the last time. . . (the problem occurred). What was going on at that time?"

[1]From Peterson (1968).

As needed:
(a) Social influences: "Were any other people around? Who? What were they doing?"
(b) Personal influences: "What were you thinking about at the time? How did you feel?"
5. Specific consequences:
"What happened after. . . (the problem behavior occurred)?"
As needed:
(a) Social consequences: "What did. . . (significant others identified above) do?"
(b) Personal consequences: "How did that make you feel?"
6. Suggested changes:
"You have thought a lot about. . . (the problem). What do you think might be done to. . . (improve) the situation?"
7. Suggested leads for further inquiry:
"What else do you think I should find out about to help you with this problem?"

The Anxiety Disorders Interview Schedule-Revised

The Anxiety Disorders Interview Schedule-Revised (ADIS-R) was developed by Di Nardo *et al.* as a means of obtaining interview data for differential diagnosis of the various anxiety disorders. Unlike the Peterson approach, the ADIS-R provides for more precise structure, specifying not only the questions to be asked, but also providing choice points guiding the interviewer's next question, based upon the nature of the client's answers. Among the topics covered are the content of the client's anxiety, duration/frequency/latency information, severity, level of interference with life activities, and presence of specific symptoms. Also included in the ADIS-R is the Hamilton Anxiety Rating Scale. The ADIS-R structured interview offers a different set of interview questions that are tailored to different DSM-III-R disorders. Hence, there is a set of questions for generalized anxiety disorder, and a set for panic disorder. Some illustrative questions relevant to generalized anxiety disorder are shown next:

1. a. What kinds of things do you worry about?

_____

_____

If patient identifies anxiety or tension which is anticipatory to panics or exposures to phobic situations—e.g., "I worry about having an attack; I worry whenever I know I will have to cross a bridge"—as a major source of anxiety:

1. Are there things other than _____ which make you feel tense, anxious, or worried?

   Yes _____   No _____

   If Yes, what are they?

   _____

   _____

   b. During the last 6 months, have you been bothered by these worries more days than not?

   Yes _____   No _____

2. On an average day over the last month, what percentage or how much of the day do you feel tense, anxious, worried?

   _____%

3. Last time you experienced an increase in tension, anxiety, or worry, aside from panics or phobic exposures, what was happening/what were you thinking?

   When _____

   Situation _____

   Thoughts _____

4. Generalized Anxiety Disorder Symptom Rating
   Persistent symptoms (continuous for at least 6 months). Do not include symptoms present only during panic.
   Inquire about each symptom listed in each category:
   During the past 6 months, have you often been bothered by _____ when you are anxious?
   How severe is it?

0	1	2	3	4
Not at all	Mild	Moderate	Severe	Very severe/ grossly disabling

   a. *Motor tension*
      Trembling, twitching, or feeling shaky _____   Restlessness _____
      Muscle tension, aches, or soreness _____   Easy fatigability _____
   b. *Autonomic hyperactivity*
      Shortness of breath or smothering sensations _____   Nausea, diarrhea, or other abdominal distress _____

Palpitations or acceler- ated heart rate	___	Flushes (hot flashes) or chills	___
Sweating or cold clam- my hands	___	Frequent urina- tion	___
Dry mouth	___	Trouble swallow-	
Dizziness or light- headedness	___	ing or lump in throat	___

c. *Vigilance, scanning*

Feeling keyed up or on edge	___	Difficulty con- centrating or	
Exaggerated startle response	___	mind going blank because	
Trouble falling or stay- ing asleep	___	of anxiety	___
		Irritability	___

5. How much does this interfere with your life, work, social activities, family, and the like?

0 ——————— 1 ——————— 2 ——————— 3 ——————— 4
Not at all   Mild   Moderately   Severely   Very severely/
                                                                grossly disabling

Modes of Assessment of Anxiety

In addition to the interview process, diagnoses about anxiety states may be achieved through a variety of other procedures. Such procedures all seek some means for quantifying the anxiety to enable making some judgment regarding the initial severity of the complaint, to measure progress during treatment, or to determine the client's readiness for termination of therapy. The various procedures can be divided into three categories: who quantifies the anxiety, the way in which the anxiety is observed, and the method for assigning a value to the observation. Regarding who quantifies the anxiety, there are two categories: self-assessment, or assessment by others. Regarding the situations under which the anxiety is observed, these include: verbal recall, as during an assessment interview, or behavioral sampling, as during a direct observation. Regarding the means for assigning a value to the observation, there are again two approaches: psychometric, as through a score calculated on a psychological instrument, or physiological, as through a measurement of heart rate or blood pressure. These categories of procedures, of course, intersect. For instance, during the interview, the therapist might ask the client to estimate the level of anxiety he or she experienced during the most recent anxiety attack, using a scale of from 0 to 100, thus utilizing a self-rating with a psychological scale in a verbal recall situation. Or, a client's spouse might be enlisted to measure blood pressure changes during the client's next telephone sales contact, thereby using a physiological measurement by another person during a behavioral situation. Some of these categories of assessment procedures deserve further discussion.

Self-Ratings

A highly popular procedure involves the subjective units of disturbance scale (SUDS) (Wolpe, 1973; Wolpe & Lazarus, 1966) which simply asks the client to rate his or her level of distress using a scale of from 0 to 100. On this scale, 0 would indicate a level that is free of tension or anxiety, while 100 is indicative of a level of extremely high anxiety or tension. The advantage of the SUDS approach is its applicability to a variety of situations. A SUDS rating can be used to obtain a state anxiety estimate, through the instruction, "Tell me your SUDS level that represents how you are feeling right now." Or a SUDS rating can be used to obtain a trait anxiety estimate, through the instruction, "Tell me your SUDS level that represents the level of tension that is generally characteristic of you." Or a SUDS rating can be used to obtain a level specific to one situation, through the instruction, "Tell me the SUDS level that represents how anxious you are made when you are being evaluated (or making a speech, or confronted with open spaces, or faced with a spider, etc.)."

Self-efficacy has also been assessed using a self-rating scaling similar to the SUDS and illustrates that the 0 to 100 scaling system is really a generic approach adaptable to nearly any variable. Bandura simply asked clients two questions: "Do you think you are able to. . . (carry out the target behavior)" Yes/No; and "How confident are you about what you just said?" 0%——————100% (Bandura, 1977a). Research by Bandura has confirmed that subjects' self-ratings turned out to be accurate a very high percentage (82%) of the time as predictors of actual behaviors (Bandura, 1977a, 1977b, 1978).

One difficulty with this approach is that it is truly subjective. Occasionally the therapist needs to be aware that a particular client may be relying upon a highly individualistic frame of reference. For instance, one client who had experienced a severely traumatic event never reported any current anxieties as being higher than 50 SUDS. Yet this client had been self-referred for complaints of having his daily life seriously disrupted by episodes of anxiety. As it turned out, the client considered the one traumatic event as 75 SUDS and that he was reserving 100 for a potentially more catastrophic event that probably would never happen. However, since there was even a small possibility, then the client believed that it was proper to save the 100 SUDS designation for that eventuality. Naturally, this meant that anything less than the original trauma could only receive a SUDS lower than 75. And of course, this meant that the client was assigning even disruptive events a value of 50 SUDS. As will be seen later, such individualistic use of the SUDS approach can create problems for Anxiety Management Training.

Observer Ratings

Instead of having a client rate him/herself, another approach would be to have a professional, such as the therapist, rate the client's characteristics. One common rating scale for anxiety is the Hamilton Rating Scale (HAR, Hamilton, 1959). Hamilton also published a rating scale for depression (HRSD, Hamilton, 1960). Although these two original scales showed equivocal results in identifying anxiety versus depressive disorders, Riskind, Beck, Brown, and Steer (1987) revised the scales. The revisions were accomplished through selecting items which loaded on the proper factor in a factor analysis (either anxiety or depression), and which showed negative correlations with the other disorder. Hence the revised HARS was composed of 14 items with high factor loadings on anxiety and negative correlations with depression, while the revised HRSD was composed of 17 items with high loadings on depression and negative correlations with anxiety.

Sample items from the revised HARS include: "anxious mood," "somatic tension," "fears," "insomnia," "gastrointestinal symptoms," "general behavior in the interview." Sample items from the revised HRSD include: "depressed mood," "feelings of guilt," "suicide," "loss of weight," "retardation," "agitation." The observer rates the client in terms of the intensity and severity of each of these observed characterstics, and assigns a value on a four-point scale. Values for the HARS range from 0 to 56; values on the HRSD range from 0 to 68. These revised rating scales appear a useful means for preliminary diagnosis of generalized anxiety disorder, or to distinguish between symptoms of generalized anxiety disorder versus major depression.

Behavioral Sampling

Behavioral observations are an extremely valuable additional source of information. The interview method is subject to accuracy of recall by the client and the subjective interpretation by the client of his or her reactions. On the other hand, direct observations permit greater accuracy and more objectivity. Yet such observations are by no means perfect.

Anxiety is inferred and hence the accuracy of the observer as to the presence of anxiety is influenced by the accuracy of the inferential data. Furthermore, depending upon how the observations are obtained, there may well be some element of artificiality in the setting. For instance, role playing would be clearly more subject to this problem than naturalistic observations. Finally, there is evidence that observations may lead to some reactivity. Even when the observer is the client him/herself, as in self-monitoring, the very nature of being observed can introduce an artificial variable, such that the observation process itself can produce changes in the behaviors (Kazdin, 1974; Kopel & Arkowitz, 1974).

Keefe, Kopel, and Gordon (1978) offer two suggestions for improving on the reliability of observations: "First, clients should be provided with a thorough explanation of the reasons for observation (to) lessen defensiveness and anxiety about the procedures. Second, observations can be conducted over long time periods so that clients habituate to the novelty of the process" (p. 87). Several types of behavioral sampling methods might be considered for use: role-playing, simulations, and naturalistic observations.

Role-playing is a flexible approach inasmuch as there is no limit to the types of circumstances which can be role-played. Typically, the therapist obtains from the client as accurate a description of the setting as possible, including the environment, the personal characteristics of the significant persons who are involved, the feelings of the client, as well as the words and actions that are occurring. Clients will differ in the degree to which they can put themselves into the role, but for many, this approach can provide useful information. One means for increasing the level of reality of the experience has been the introduction of videotape stimuli. Such prerecorded stimuli have generally been used to assess the client's level of behavioral deficit, but can also be used to identify signs of anxiety. For instance, behavioral role playing testing has been used to identify levels of deficit in assertive behaviors among clients (Hollon & Beck, 1986; Linehan, Goldfried, & Goldfried, 1979; McFall, 1982). In such videotapes, the client views interpersonal situations in which the context is explained by a narrator, and an actor or actress is viewed, making a statement. The client must then offer a personal response.

For instance, in the Behavioral Assertiveness Test (Eisler, Miller, & Hersen, 1973) one scene is as follows: *Narrator*: You're in a crowded grocery store and in a hurry. You pick one small item and get in line to pay for it. You're really trying to hurry because you're already late for an appointment. Then, a woman with a shopping cart full of groceries cuts in line in front of you. *Woman*: "You don't mind if I cut in here do you? I'm in a hurry."

With the availability of portable videocamcorders, developing tailor-made tapes can be readily achieved. For example, where a client's main anxiety relates to evaluations, the following scene might be filmed: *Narrator*: You are recently on the job in a company that requires that your supervisor meet with you every two weeks to report on your work. This is your first such meeting, and although you think you're not doing well, you also suspect that every new person has the same problems. *Supervisor*: "Well, I don't think much about our being required to have these meetings, so let's get it over with. I hear you're not doing so well so far, what do you have to say for yourself?"

Simulations provide the next more realistic type of settings for direct observations. As with role playing, there is an assumption that there is a basic continuity between the responses of the client under a simulated condition and the responses that would be shown under the real condition itself. Bernstein and Beatty (1971) placed an airplane-phobic client in a Link airplane trainer to simulate the noise, movement, and visual characteristics of a real plane. Although such equipment is usually not readily available, another way of achieving simulation is via the use of imagery rehearsal. There is some evidence that the combining of relaxation followed by imagery seems to reproduce an experience that is very close to reality (Suinn, 1976). In fact, reports confirm that the imagery includes visual, kinesthetic, physiological, tactile, emotional, and auditory features—in effect, it closely simulates real life. A major step of AMT involves the use of imagery in order to present the client with an opportunity to apply and strengthen coping skills. However, this same procedure for initiating anxiety arousal (see Chapter 7) can also be a method for obtaining initial anxiety level self-ratings, using the SUDS approach we described earlier.

Naturalistic observations certainly can provide the most accurate information on clients, but vary in the ease of availability. As with all behavioral assessments of anxiety, a first step is identifying what is to be observed and coded as evidences of anxiety (Mash & Terdal, 1976). The setting should reflect the types of environment that are associated with anxiety arousal. For an agoraphobic person, this could be any open space area that it outside the client's safety areas. Some therapists and clinics have: "standardized behavioral walks" which is a preset course, divided into equidistant units or stations (Barlow, O'Brien, & Last, 1984; Vermilyea *et al.*, 1984; Williams & Rappoport, 1983). Clients are instructed to walk as far as they can. Measures can include counting the number of stations completed, as well as self-ratings of level of anxiety, duration of the walk, and even heart rate. Standardized behavioral walks can be designed and incorporated into nearly everyone's professional practice.

The next step is to define what is being observed, coded, or rated.

As we commented earlier, anxiety is typically inferred through observing other actions. For instance, Mahl (1956) infers that high anxiety shows up in disruption of speech. Hence a speech-dysfluency ratio is coded, that is, the proportion of non "ah" dysfluencies (such as stammers, speech blocks, omissions, repetitions) to total words spoken. In public speaking anxiety, or interpersonal anxiety, speech rate or latency before speaking can be representative of anxiety. Sometimes a client shows a well-developed behavioral ritual that is triggered by the presence of anxiety—for instance, a client who reaches for a cigarette when under tension. In this case, counting the number of "reaches" can be used as an index of anxiety.

Occasionally, anxiety or stress might be hypothesized as a precipitating factor for another response, which in turn has its own overt manifestations. For example, Type A persons are those persons considered to be high risk for cardiovascular disease, and who are characterized as being impatient and tense when having to wait. Hence, such impatience might be observable when the client is standing in a waiting line, or sitting in the driver's seat in his or her car at a stoplight. Such impatience might be manifested through foot tapping, finger tapping, or other such behavioral signs. A final step is the training of the observers who must record or code the observations. Typically, the best method for achieving high observer accuracy is by defining the behaviors to be recorded in clear, concrete terms. The number of finger taps is easier to observe and record than whether a person is "being cooperative."

Psychometric Scaling

The primary advantage of using psychological tests is the standardization they provide, along with the use of normative information for interpreting results. Across the years, a number of instruments have attracted the attention of practitioners and researchers. Some representative psychological instruments are briefly described next.

The State-Trait Personality Inventory offers a combination in one form of six subscales: state anxiety, trait anxiety, state anger, trait anger, state curiosity, and trait curiosity (Spielberger, Barker, Russell, DeCrane, Westberry, Knight, & Marks, 1979). Consistent with the earlier State Trait Anxiety Inventory (STAI, Spielberger, 1970) state anxiety is assessed by having the client rate him/herself for feelings "right now." On the other hand, trait anxiety is represented by answers indicative of how the client "generally feels." This same format for directions is used for items involving anger as well as curiosity in the STPI. The total scale involves 60 items, with 20 referring to anxiety, 20 to anger, and 20 to curiosity. Clients are to use a four point rating scale to indicate the level or frequency of the anxiety/anger/ curiosity. Scores can range from a minimum of 10 to a maximum of 40 for each subscale.

The Taylor Manifest Anxiety Scale is another instrument that has received usage over time (Taylor, 1953). The scale is composed of 50 items which are answered in a true-false format. Some questions are scored as indicative of anxiety if answered true, for example, "I am a very nervous person." Other questions are scored as indicative of anxiety if answered false, for example, "I am usually calm and not easily upset." Scores can range from 0 (low anxiety) to 50 (high anxiety). The continued use of this scale might be attributed to the fact that it was an early measure of anxiety used in research both on clinical and experimental studies. Hence there is a well-established literature on the Taylor scale.

The Multiple Affect Adjective Check List (MAACL) is basically 132 adjectives which clients use as a checklist to indicate whether the adjective describes them or not (Zuckerman & Lubin, 1965). The instrument is self-administered and can be given under state instructions ("how you feel now—today") or trait instructions ("how you generally feel"). There are three subscales, anxiety, depression, and hostility. The range of scores for anxiety is 0 to 21, while the range for depression is from 0 to 40, and 2 to 28 for hostility. Scoring keys are provided for obtaining the raw scores, which in turn are converted to T scores for use with the norms.

The Beck Anxiety Inventory is a 21-item, self-report scale which derived from an initial pool of items from three checklists, the Anxiety Checklist (Beck, Steer, & Brown, 1985), the PDR Checklist (Beck, 1978), and the Situational Anxiety Checklist (Beck, 1982). The client uses a four point rating, ranging from 0 (not at all) to 3 (severely, "I could barely stand it"), to rate the various symptoms represented in the items. Total scores can range from 0 to 63. In a validation study, the scale differentiated between 93 clients suffering from anxiety disorders and 67 clients suffering from depressive or other nonanxiety disorders.

The S-R Inventory of Anxiousness was designed to represent a multidimensional approach to trait anxiety. The four dimensions represent: interpersonal anxiety, physical danger, anxiety in ambiguous or novel situations, and anxiety in routine, innocuous situations. In this test, a total score is calculated. However, since this single score confounds the multidimensional intent of the scale, the S-R Inventory of General Trait Anxiousness was developed as a revision. The four dimensions are retained; clients are asked to rate their reactions using nine "response modes": seeking experiences like this, perspiring, having an uneasy feeling, feeling exhilarated, having fluttering feelings, feeling tense, enjoying the situation, heart beats faster, and feeling anxious. Through a factor analysis, the scale has been determined to provide a measure of anxiety in two situations (interpersonal and physical danger), and to provide an estimate of two types of responses (physiological distress and approach) (Endler & Okada, 1975; Endler, Hunt, & Rosenstein, 1962).

The Cognitive-Somatic Anxiety Questionnaire (CSAQ) was designed on the principle that clients might differ in the categories of their symptoms, with some experiencing more cognitive indices of distress, while others are more bodily oriented (Schwartz, 1978). The instrument is a short one involving 14 questions, with clients being required to "rate the degree to which you experience this symptom when you are anxious." The rating is based upon a five-point scale, with 1 meaning "not at all" and 5 meaning "very much so." Examples of the cognitive items include the questions, "I find it difficult to concentrate because of uncontrolled thoughts," and "I worry too much over some things that don't really matter." Examples of somatic items include the questions, "My heart beats faster," "I perspire," and "I get diarrhea."

Several scales do not exactly measure anxiety, but do offer some insights into stresses facing the client. Briefly, these include the Schedule of Recent Events (Holmes & Rahe, 1967), the Life Events Questionnaire (Delongis, Coyne, Dakof, Folkman, & Lazarus, 1982), and the Hassles Scale (Kanner, Coyne, Schaefer, & Lazarus, 1981). The Schedule of Recent Events (SRE) lists a series of life events which are presumed to create stress, such as marriage, death of a spouse, major illness, change of employment, etc. Clients state the number of times each event had occurred during the last 12 months (or any other prescribed time period of interest to the therapist). The life events are weighted differentially and summed to Indicate a total life stressor score.

The Life Events Questionnaire was constructed through interviews of persons involved in a community study. It is shorter than the Schedule of Recent Events, but is similar in identifying life events considered to reflect stress, such as personal injury or illness, sexual difficulties, etc. Although the administration is similar to that of the SRE, the Life Events Questionnaire also requires each respondent to rate how disturbing each event was, using a 3-point scale from "not much" to "very much." The Hassles Scale is a 117-item questionnaire which recognizes that not all sources of stress are serious life events. Instead they may be due to an accumulation of nuisances or annoying situations. Items represent the areas of family (not enough time for family), social activities (unexpected company), the environment (pollution), practical considerations (misplacing things), work (unattractive duties), finances (someone owing you money), and health (not getting enough rest). As with the Life Events Questionnaire, clients indicate the frequency of occurrence of the hassle during a specified time period, and rate the severity of the experience.

In addition to these various psychological measures of anxiety, there are also a variety of scales which assess other types of disorders, relating to anxiety states. The Fear Survey Schedule (FSS) requires clients to rate the severity of their fear response to a variety of stimuli, ranging from airplanes, to elevators, to vacuum cleaners, worms, imaginary creatures, and a "lull in the conversation." The FSS has appeared in several versions, including a shorter 50-item scale. In fact, there is a FSS-I composed by Akutagawa (1956) based upon his idea of commonly occurring fears, a FSS-II constructed by Geer (1965) based upon an empirical identification of common fears, and a FSS-III (Wolpe & Lang, 1964) based upon Wolpe and Lang's clinical observations.

Marks and Mathews (1979) have also published a phobia instrument simply called the Fear Questionnaire. This short scale invites clients to rate their level of avoidance of certain phobic circumstances, as well as rating how "troubled" they are by certain problems, such as anger, panic, depression, or upsetting thoughts. The scale offers a total phobia score, a score reflecting the client's major phobia, and subscores for anxiety/depression, agoraphobia, blood/injury, and social stimuli. Because two items are open-ended questions which permit the client to write in his or her own specific problem, the scale can assess severity of phobic conditions, even if not covered by one of the other items. The agoraphobia subscale is viewed as being especially valuable. Another measure applicable to agoraphobia is the Mobility Inventory for Agoraphobia (Chambless, Caputo, Jasin, Gracely, & Williams, 1985). This is a 27-item questionnaire aimed at assessing clients' levels of avoidance behaviors as indices of phobic severity. The clients rate the severity of their avoidance not only when alone but also under the condition of being accompanied. Further, they also rate their frequency of panic over the recent week.

Another anxiety state which has reached increasing attention by researchers and independent practitioners is Post-Traumatic Stress Disorder (PTSD). This disorder involves the reexperiencing of an unusual trauma, for instance through flashbacks, as well as persistent hyperarousal, for instance as seen in insomnia or an exaggerated startle response. The traumatic event may be war-related or from civilian catastrophic experiences, such as rape. Briefly, several standardized questionnaire approaches have been proposed. Foy, Sipprelle, Rueger, and Carroll (1984) conducted a preliminary study using the MMPI scales to discriminate between Vietnam veterans in treatment for PTSD versus those in treatment for other problems. On a small sample, they reported an 85% accuracy in separating the two groups. Fairbank, McCaffrey, and Keane (1985) have also been successful in the use of the MMPI in separating PTSD patients from a sample 'feigning' PTSD symptoms. Friedman, Schneiderman, West, and Corson (1986) expanded on Foy *et al.*'s efforts and validated the Posttraumatic Stress Disorder Scale, which involves 15 items based upon DSM-III criteria, such as questions on sleep disturbance, recurrent memories, feelings of alienation, guilt reactions, or startle reflexes. Finally, with regard to rape, Resick, Veronen, Kilpatrick, Calhoun, and Atkinson (1986) have published a factor analysis of the Veronen-Kilpatrick Fear Survey. This instrument measures both the level and the type of fear responses of sexual assault survivors.

Clinicians interested in assessing the thought processes of clients can approach this through several procedures. Cacioppo and Petty (1981) describe a general procedure for analyzing, classifying, and scoring streams of thoughts. As a general procedure, it can be adapted to specifically relate to anxiety conditions, for instance, via the instruction, "List all the thoughts that occurred when you were anxious." Glass and Merluzzi (1981) have applied the thought-listing method, but through combining role-playing and videotaping. The client is asked to role-play a problem situation which is videotaped, then the videotape is replayed and the client is asked to recall his or her thoughts during different parts of the tape. Beck and Emery (1985) provide their clients with a daily diary form, the Daily Record of Dysfunctional Thoughts. The client is to fill out the form as soon as possible after becoming anxious. In the form, the client records a description of the situation leading to the anxiety, the emotion experienced and its level of intensity, and any "automatic thoughts," as well as the client's level of belief in the thoughts. Automatic thoughts are maladaptive thoughts or mental images which repeatedly intrude and which seem plausible to the client. As cited earlier, the Cognitive and Somatic Anxiety Questionnaire developed by Schwartz provides questions related to cognitive signs of anxiety. The Agoraphobia Cognitions Questionnaire (Chambless, Caputo, Bright, & Gallagher, 1984) is also available to measure the fear of fear itself, which has been hypothesized as characterizing agoraphobics (Goldstein & Chambless, 1978). This scale is composed of 14 items covering maladaptive thoughts regarding "the potential harm that will befall the agoraphobic individual because of anxiety," for example, "I am going to go crazy" or "I am going to go blind."

Physiological Measures

It is generally believed that anxiety may appear through autonomic nervous system discharge. In fact, some somatic symptoms are actually subjective reflections of physiological events. For instance, increased heart rate and output may be expressed as "my heart pounds," heightened sweat-gland and epidermal activity is seen in sweaty palms, peripheral vasoconstriction is noticed as cold hands, and increased muscle tension as "knots" in the muscles.

By its very nature, physiological measures require complex and often bulky instrumentation (for detailed information, see Rugh & Schwitzgebel, 1977). Typically, the measuring equipment is composed of three aspects. The transducer is a unit which attaches directly to the client and which provides the input through producing an electrical signal that can be easily processed. The input signal can be varied depending upon the type of transducer; for instance, an electrode can be used to measure bioelectrical activity as indices of muscle tension or skin conductance. Or, a thermistor can instead be used to measure temperature, for example, peripheral skin temperature. There are at least four common types of transducers: mechanical, which require a movement to activate a switch; electrical, which translate bioelectric activity of the client into a signal via electrodes; thermal, which are temperature-sensitive; and optical, which convert changes in light energy via photoelectric cells. The signal from the transducer must then be amplified (or in some cases, reduced), filtered and modified to some form which can be stored; this is accomplished through a signal-processing unit.

Some transducers require special input characteristics of the signal-processing unit. For instance, transducers will differ in whether they provide analog or digital information, and therefore the signal-processing equipment must have circuitry which matches or transforms such input. Bioelectrical events, such as measured by electromyographic or electroencephalographic equipment, will require amplifiers with high input impedance, and low noise. Finally, the signal is translated into a format which can be observed and stored. If only a display is needed, then the storage/display unit might only require a display such as a voltmeter, an indicator light, or an oscilloscope. If a permanent record is desired, then the storage/display unit might rely upon paper tape cumulative event recorders, polygraph or chart recorders, tape recorders, digital printers, or computer memory.

Of the various types of physiological measurements possible, heart rate and electrodermal measures are the most frequently reported. In measuring heart rate, a baseline is obtained during a resting state against which can be compared the heart rate under the target condition. The target condition represents the circumstances under which anxiety is suspected to occur. In physiological measurement, the target condition is precipitated, while physiological changes are measured and recorded. Thus, heart rate can be measured during the interview when the client is discussing his or her anxiety experiences, or it can be assessed when the client is confronted with a laboratory-derived stressor, or measured during a naturalistic observation. Malloy, Fairbank, and Keane (1983) presented patients with videotape scenes of either a neutral shopping mall, or combat scenes of a helicopter assault. Heart rate and skin conductance were measured to discriminate differences between PTSD patients and normal controls or psychiatric patient controls.

With the improvement of technology, heart rate can now be measured in naturalistic situations. Telemetry is possible whereby the transducer emits a radio signal which is transmitted to a portable signal-processing unit. Barlow, Mavissakalian, and Schofield (1980) measured heart rate with a Holter Recorder as the agoraphobic client walked through the standardized walking course. Bellak and Lombardo (1984) have used the less expensive, portable heart rate unit known as the Exersentry Heart Rater Monitor (Leelarthaepin, Gray, & Chesworth, 1980) along with a stereo tape minirecorder. With this combination, the tape recorder can be used to record continuous heart rate on one channel and subjective reports of perceived anxiety on the other channel. With computerization advances, heart rate units have become even more miniaturized to be the size of wristwatches.

The United States Olympic Training Center's sports science research laboratories have used the Wireless Heart Rate monitor, which not only measures pulse, but has the capacity to store such information for later retrieval from a personal desk computer. Of course, even clients can obtain estimates of their own heart rate, through counting their pulse by manually pressing on the blood vessels on their wrists. This do-it-yourself, without-instrumentation approach can be surprisingly reliable (Bell & Schwartz, 1975).

In assessing electrodermal activity, such as skin conductance, a baseline is also needed during a resting state. On a polygraph with electrodes for skin conductance, the resting baseline is usually about 2–20 microns (Edelberg, 1967). As with heart rate, the actual skin conductance during a stressful situation is then obtained in order to make a diagnosis. Unlike heart rate, the data are usually transformed mathematically using a log transformation. Another alternative is to only evaluate "spontaneous fluctuations." Spontaneous fluctuations are changes in skin conductance which occur in the absence of any stimuli. There is some evidence that measures based upon spontaneous fluctuations show some relationship to anxiety (Katkin, 1975; Rappaport & Katkin, 1972). Observing spontaneous fluctuations may be the simpler procedure inasmuch as what is counted is any fluctuation reaching some minimum magnitude and no log transformations are required (Szpiler & Epstein, 1976).

One issue associated with physiological measures as diagnostic tools is the asynchrony which can sometimes be observed within clients. There is evidence that discrepancies can occur when different physiological measures are taken, such that heart rate may be reactive to stress for one client, but skin conductance show no changes in this same client. Moreover, individual differences can appear among different clients, with one client showing consistent responsivity, for example, in skin conductance under stress, but just as consistently show no heart rate reactivity. Similarly, a different client may show his or her own unique physiological response domain which is responsive while other response domains remain nonreactive (Engel, 1972; Lacey, 1967). Therefore the best recommendation is the use of multiple measures, such as cardiovascular, respiratory, electrodermal, and muscular.

Assessment of Severity

The differential diagnosis of anxiety disorders will not be discussed since there are other major sources (American Psychiatric Assocication, 1987; Cerney, Himadi, & Barlow, in press). Of some interest, however, is the assessment of the severity of the anxiety state, and identifying when to treat the anxiety.

To determine level of severity there are several guidelines that can be applied (Deffenbacher & Suinn, 1982; Suinn, 1984b). Information about both time and magnitude enable conclusions about the severity of the symptoms. Interview or other information about time would suggest a higher level of symptom severity if:

- the anxiety reactions appear more often per unit time, that is, are of high frequency;
- the anxiety reactions last for longer periods once initiated, that is the duration is longer;
- the anxiety reactions show residual effects over longer periods, that is, the recovery time is longer; or
- the period elapsing before the next anxiety reactions is shorter, that is, periods free of anxiety are less frequent.

Interview or other information relating to magnitude can also suggest a higher level of symptom severity if:

- the symptoms within any anxiety subsystem (autonomic, somatic, cognitive) are of high magnitude, for instance, extremely high heart rate (autonomic subsystem), severe speech disruption (somatic subsystem), or extreme distractibility (cognitive subsystem);
- there are numerous severe symptoms within or across several anxiety subsystems, for instance, severe diarrhea, nausea, elevated blood pressure (high magnitude autonomic symptoms), or all-

consuming ruminations, severe muscle fatigue, and continous
headaches (high magnitude cognitive and autonomic symptoms);
* the symptoms have a severe overall impact on life adjustment, for
  instance, frequent, persistent minor hassles that accumulate to
  create major disruptions or expenditures of energy.

Self-Monitoring

In addition to the details gleaned from the intake interview, AMT
clients should be required to complete a self-monitoring record. Appendix A includes a sample of the various logs which will be required
throughout AMT treatment. Stress Log 1 should be used on a daily
basis, for at least a week prior to the first actual AMT treatment session.
This log should be completed each evening prior to retiring for activities
during that day; postponing the log until the next morning would involve the risk of inaccurate recall.

The log requires the client to identify any incidents which involve
the activation of feelings which the client considers indices of anxiety.
The broader term "feelings" is used inasmuch as occasionally a client has
mislabeled their emotional reactions, for example, mixing up distress
that reflects anger or disgust or even embarrassment with distress that
truly represents anxiety. By permitting recording of any feelings which
the client associates with distress, the opportunity is available for distinc-
tions to be developed, if necessary, during review of the log.

The levels of tension or distress are also recorded on this form.
Although the concept of SUDS (Subjective Units of Distress Scale) are
frequently used in behavior therapy, this term does not appear on the
Stress Log since our major concern is to have some method for gauging
tension, and since the term SUDS may be confusing to some. Hence, the
client simply records tension levels, using the values of "0" for nonexistent tension, to "100" for maximum tension. The client is also to record
the date and hour, and a brief description of the situation associated
with the distress. Note that the client need only describe the events
associated with the tension, and is not required to describe the "events
causing" the distress. This avoids the dilemma of a client experiencing
generalized anxiety disorder being unable to report anything inasmuch
as the client cannot recognize the origins or the cues triggering the
anxiety.

This Stress Log 1, and all future logs, should be turned in to the
therapist a day before the AMT session. This provides the therapist with
the time needed to review the record, consider questions needing follow-
up, and develop a sense for the progress of the client, as well as confirm-

ing compliance. The instructions from the therapist to the client should be as follows:

> "For the next week, before our next appointment, I want you to take about fifteen minutes at the end of each day to fill in this log. There are the four columns. What you should be recording are any feelings you had during the day which might relate to feeling stressed or tense or anxious. Just put a word or two under the first column such that you can remember what that was about when we talk about it. So it might be 'butterflies,' or 'had nervous thoughts,' or 'felt my blood pressure up or my heart pounding,' or just 'felt tense, uptight, apprehensive.' Then in the second column provide a brief description of the situation. For instance, 'I was in the waiting room,' or 'I was returning something I bought to the salesclerk,' or 'I was in an argument with my spouse (friend, kids).' Then, in the third column, consider the level of the tension you were experiencing; use the scale that's at the bottom of the page, with 0 meaning no tension at all and 100 being the highest tension, really severe level. In the last column, you would put down the time of this incident. This will really help us see more clearly what is going on, and can also give us a really good sense for our progress in the training, how well we're moving along.
>
> "The best would be for you to bring it by and drop it off at my office the day before our next appointment. This will give me enough time since I want to be able to review it before we talk about it at our next session. How would this work out for you?"

Summary

The intake interview begins with the same orientation of any intake, that is, through the establishment of an atmosphere of support, respect, interest, encouragement and acceptance shown by the therapist. At the same time, the intake must aim at obtaining specific information useful towards understanding the presenting problems. One approach to conducting an intake interview has been described, covering topics one at a time through the sequence of: starting with an open-ended invitation to address a topic, followed by the identification of one topic on which to focus, followed by request for elaboration on details relating to this topic, and ending with a summary by the therapist of details to insure accuracy.

Where the intake interview is directly aimed at obtaining data on anxiety, our model of stress becomes a useful way of conceptualizing what information is needed. The nature of the anxiety symptoms may be pursued in the context of autonomic, behavioral and cognitive symptoms. The sequence of appearance of these various symptoms is also important, given the potential desynchrony of such responses. Our model also highlights the importance of obtaining information on the details of the situations under which stress is precipitated. These details include identification of the broader sources of the stressors, that is, biological, environmental, social, psychogenic, cognitive. Our particular style in conducting an intake interview emphasizes obtaining concrete details and examples in order to solidify obtaining accurate information, and minimize false assumptions or inferences. Through focusing on concrete examples from the client's life experiences, the interviewer may develop information on the nature of the anxiety experience, the similarities or differences in symptoms associated with differing settings, the cues which precipitate the anxiety reaction, the level of the anxiety experienced, the variables which influence such levels, what coping behaviors are available and their effectiveness, the actions/thoughts of the client during the stress experience, and the sequence of events ending in stress and attempts to cope.

   This chapter also covers some other examples of structured interviews, as well as other methods for doing assessment. Discussed are self-rating procedures, observer-rating methods, behavioral sampling, psychometric techniques, and physiological instruments. The chapter outlines some thoughts about criteria for evaluating the severity of anxiety, and ends with a description of the self-monitoring procedure used in AMT as a mode of obtaining information in between AMT sessions.

7

ANXIETY MANAGEMENT TRAINING— THE BASIC TECHNIQUE

The Initial Two Sessions

Anxiety Management Training Session 1

This session involves:

- Pre-interview
- Rationale
- Relaxation scene development
- Tension-Relaxation
- Post-interview
- Homework assignment

This and all subsequent individual AMT sessions will cover about one hour, with the pre- and post-interviews typically being brief (each about 5–10 minutes). If crucial issues evolve during these interviews that demand in-depth elaboration, such as major puzzling changes in symptoms or the onset of other problems which may interfere with attention to AMT skill development, then additional time might be necessary for further assessment.

Figure 7.1, entitled "Model of AMT sessions," is a convenient reference that illustrates the basic features within each AMT session (excluding the pre-/post-interviews and homework). The figure also identifies what tasks the therapist is assigned, for instance, in turning on and describing a relaxation scene, and how the signaling from the client proceeds. In Appendix B, there is a series of actual quotations which could serve as models for the exact wording which the AMT therapist uses during various AMT sessions. These quotations will provide a flavor for how a relaxation scene is initiated by the therapist, how relaxation

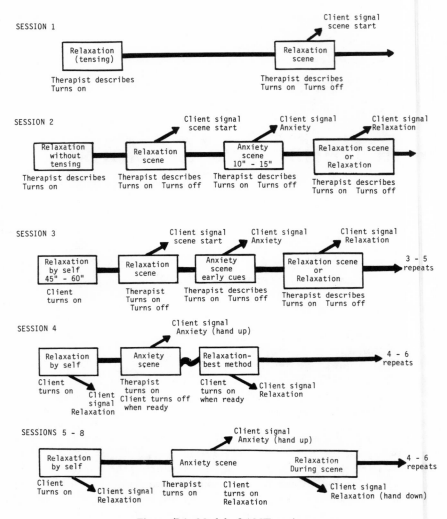

Figure 7.1. Model of AMT sessions.

exercises are introduced, and how signals are called for by the therapist. These quotations, along with quotations in this and the next chapter, are meant to provide enough details that the therapist who wishes to adopt the AMT procedure will have clear guidelines, and thereby be able either to use the same quoted statements or revise them to fit the therapist's own ways of communicating.

Pre-Interview

The pre-interview reviews the results of Stress Log 1 to determine whether anxiety does indeed seem to be the major presenting problem. The log is examined also as an initial determination of whether any patterns surface, either in terms of similarity of settings or times which precipitate the anxiety. Having the client elaborate on ambiguous descriptions can also improve communications and observational skills for clients who are unused to self-observation.

The pre-interviews prior to each session are also convenient for outlining the plans for that session. In this case, the comment might be:

> "Today I'm going to go over what Anxiety Management Training is all about as the therapy which seems best for helping you with your anxiety. I'll also be training you in the relaxation technique which will be an important basis for your learning how to control the anxiety."

Rationale

The rationale identifies the self-control orientation, and sets the stage for the client to accept that he/she will be learning a coping skill through training. The following statement can be used:

> "AMT will involve training you in recognizing the early signs of anxiety, so that you can control the anxiety before it becomes a problem. The method of control will be the use of relaxation. We'll be using a very straightforward exercise to teach you relaxation. Being able to control your anxiety will require practice. To give you this practice, we'll be having you visualize scenes of situations in which you've been anxious, in order to practice eliminating this anxiety through relaxing. That's really all there is to it. AMT is not very difficult to learn but we have good evidence that it is very successful."

The therapist can expand on this basic rationale by giving examples from the client's replies during the intake. Thus, the therapist can show how AMT is directly relevant to the client's specific symptoms or situation. The following are examples from case illustrations (cases described in more detail in Chapter 5):

The Case of Jeff. Jeff was a client originally seen for complaints of fatigue and malaise. However, during the process of psychotherapy, he began to experience increased signs of general anxiety. This was expressed in nightmares, anxiety attacks that were characterized by trembling and panic, insomnia, and an apprehension about being vulnerable to these seemingly random anxiety attacks. As an accountant he was especially upset at this loss of predictability in his life. He had been divorced after what seemed to him an idyllic marriage where his needs

220 CHAPTER 7

were cared for; now he was acquiring an ability to be self-reliant and independent. The rationale covered the following:

> "AMT is a program that would make a great deal of sense at this stage of your progress. It appears that you're now struggling with some serious waves of anxiety and you can't get a handle on what might be the cause. In the meantime, without gaining control, you're vulnerable and can't plan your life very systematically. AMT, since it involves relaxation training, should at least be helpful to you with the insomnia; many individuals actually have used the relaxation as a way of getting to sleep properly. In addition, the training is very systematic, with each step defined. The ultimate aim is for you and me to work together to give you this added way of gaining control over your life, so that the anxiety cannot overwhelm you, but you have a systematic way to control the anxiety. . . so that the anxiety would not control you."

The Case of Jennifer. Jennifer was a 16-year-old Asian-American student who had developed a severe case of test anxiety. She became anxious under a variety of situations: at the start of a school term if the teacher mentioned the exam schedule, when she overheard other students talking about preparations for an exam, if she even saw the word "test," and certainly when she was in the midst of a written examination. Her symptoms involved "butterflies" and being unable to listen attentively to the teacher because of the anxiety. The rationale added the following:

> "One of the advantages of AMT is that it provides you with a skill that will work for you in a variety of different situations. Even though we might be focusing on, let's say, anxiety from being in the exam room, the skill in relaxing will be just as useful in those situations when you hear another student talking about examinations, when you just see the word "test" somewhere, or even when you're hearing a new teacher talk about the term's testing schedule. The relaxation skill you will be using has actually been used with other individuals who sometimes have butterflies when they're under stress. I know of many Olympic athletes who describe their stress as feelings exactly like yours, the butterflies in the stomach. And the relaxation training has been for them a really useful technique."

The Case of Sandra. Sandra is a successful executive secretary and legislative aide in Washington, D.C. Her major complaint has been tension headaches. Although she does not perceive herself as a nervous person or a person under stress, she admits that all other possible causes have been ruled out, and so she is "willing to give stress management a shot." Her symptoms include grinding her teeth at night. The rationale offered the following elaboration:

> "It's possible that you are not under stress. But, the tension headaches do sound rather suspiciously like they derive from muscle tension. . . the timing seems about right, and the headache symptoms sound right for a tension headache. Sometimes a person is concentrating so hard on what they're

doing that they actually don't notice if there is muscle tension or not. One of the things about AMT is that it will teach you a relaxation method, and when you learn this muscle relaxation, it gives you a way of telling when your muscles are tense instead of being relaxed. The teeth grinding also sounds rather suspiciously like your jaws are tightening up even when you are sleeping. I think it's worth a shot as you say. Your occupation sounds really challenging and interesting, but I have to admit that it also sounds like there are elements that could be hidden stress. One of the things we'll do is have you make careful observations about what's going on so that you'll be able to do your own analysis about hidden stress, and bring it out in the open."

The Case of Chuck. Chuck is a boxer who has become so angry that he has been violent and destructive of property. The student-therapist initially seeing Chuck experienced some resistance, later identified as relating to the way in which the student addressed Chuck and failed to recognize Chuck's antagonism at being talked down to by the student. With Chuck's wish to be addressed as a peer and desire to be part of the decision making, and with his history of being responsive to learning boxing techniques, the more appropriate extension of the rationale should have included comments such as:

> "The technique we could try is rather similar to training; in fact, a number of world class athletes seem to like the approach because it is aimed at skill training rather than being like therapy. I imagine in boxing you got only as far as you were willing to put in the time in training; your manager could only guide you about what seemed to be proper technique, but you had to rely upon yourself to practice until you made it work for you. Kind of same idea with AMT. The skill involves an exercise; instead of an exercise like situps or punching the speed bag, our exercise is a muscle relaxation one. . . that we'll get to in a moment. Also, like when you're in training, some of the training will be stuff you do at home. I'm going to also need your help as we move along in putting the details to some of our steps, so I'll need to be asking you to give me feedback on how well things are going and how we can improve on tailor-making this for your characteristics."

Relaxation Scene Development

The next step involves the identification of a real life situation that is associated with being relaxed. This scene will be used at various times as a complement to the relaxation exercise itself, to cue further relaxation. The relaxation scene should be very concrete and described in such detail that an artist could sketch a picture. The usual inquiry is as follows:

> T: Describe an activity, event, or situation, that you're familiar with, a real situation in which you had felt very relaxed.

In addition to visual details, such as location, presence of others, outstanding features, activity involved, the scene should cover any other sensory aspects which can help to make the scene vivid. These might include auditory, tactile, temperature, proprioceptive, etc. To avoid confusing the choice of a relaxing event with a sexual event, it is clearer to request a scene associated with "relaxation or calmness" instead of a "pleasant scene." Furthermore, the relaxation should not be confused with tiredness or fatigue, such as might be considered by athletes— "after I've run hard and I collapse comfortably in my chair" or "that pleasantly tired feeling that comes from working out hard." Similarly, sleep should not be considered, since such an association might lead to the client actually falling asleep during the session. Finally, scenes involving artificially caused relaxation, such as "after three beers," should be avoided to prevent any impression that substance usage is approved.

The relaxation scene should be considered in terms of whether there are scene-setting elements as well as feeling-oriented elements. The scene setting elements are descriptive of the environment and circumstance, such as "on the sand, alone, with a breeze," while the feeling setting elements capture the feeling-tone, such as "I'm comfortably warm; I can feel my body completely relaxed; I have no care in the world, just peaceful." These same two types of elements are also important in later sessions for use with the anxiety scenes.

An example of a relaxation scene description that is not satisfactory would be:

> "I suppose it would be sitting on a high mesa, just simply enjoying the peace and quiet, and knowing that nothing can destroy my calm. I imagine it would be sunset."

The major issues with the example involve first the question of whether this is a fantasy ("I suppose," "I imagine") or a real event. If such a question occurs to the therapist, the interview should prompt as follows:

> T: I'm in need of knowing if this was a specific incident that actually occurred, or whether you are describing for me some common elements from a number of experiences. What would be most helpful would be for you to describe for me an actual event that occurred on one occasion. What might this have been?
>
> C: No, I was describing what might be ideal. . . my picture of an ideal, sitting on a mesa. . . watching the sunset. . . the closest that I remember is one night fishing watching the sunset.
>
> T: So this was a specific time that you recall when you were fishing? Tell me more about this, describe this incident for me in more detail so I can really picture it.
>
> C: Well, it was at a lake, I often fish there. . . about seven in the evening, this is, when the sun sets. . . very spectacular at times. . . usually quiet. . . and very peaceful.
>
> T: Now, is this a particular evening that you had gone fishing? And was this a specific lake?

C: Yes, I'm remembering late summer, last summer. . . actually, I even remember the date, it was weekend. . . Saturday night, July. . . I had been on the lake for an hour, there was someone across the lake, but otherwise I was alone. . . I was fishing with flies and had tried four patterns with three strikes, but no fish yet. . .

T: That's really helpful. Now, I'm getting a better sense of the exact situation. It would help if you could give me even more details, as though I was talking with you over the telephone, and I was an artist, a painter, and sketching out this scene on my canvas as you described all the details. . . so what else can you tell me?

C: The lake was medium size, so I could see the other side. . . it was calm, with a very slight riffle on the water. . . I was about four feet off the bank, in my fishing boots in the water. . . there are clouds reflecting the beautiful orange sunset off to my left.

(Since this still could be a description of a number of locations, and therefore a composite of an evening fishing at several lakes, the next prompt is aimed at making sure that not only was the incident at a particular date, but also a particular location and not several locations. One way of doing this is to ask about the name of the lake and how the client confirms that it was this lake in their description and not possibly another one of several lakes.)

T: So it was July, about seven in the evening. . . you were at sunset, had tried several fly patterns. . . O.K., was this a particular lake?

C: Oh, yes, I thought I had said that already. It was Lake Ramona.

T: Now as you describe this incident for me, how is it that you know it is Ramona rather than another lake that you had fished in, maybe even during that same night? What were the distinguishing features you are remembering about this particular incident at this particular time?

C: Lake Ramona has a section that I was at. . . there is a short sandy stretch at a point, and a rock about five feet out, and I am standing there just on this side of the rock. . . I did not fish any other lake that evening. . .

T: That's great, helps me to hear that extra detail. Are there other details describing this lake and the fishing and the evening that would help me really picture it clearly?

C: Every so often, there would be a splash, where a fish would be feeding. . . behind me is a cabin up on stilts; to my right are three log cabins. . . across is a big pile of rocks at the edge of the water. . .

T: O.K., I'm getting that picture. Now, how about how you were feeling. . . this was a relaxing experience, what was that like?

C: Relaxed, yes. . . peaceful, quiet. . . the sunset represents beauty, but it's also dusk, and you can see and almost feel the quietness of the dark descending. . . looking over the lake, with just the mild riffles gives a sense of calmness. . . I'm not thinking of anything except maybe how the line feels, and concentration, paying attention to the fly coming in. . . the feel of the line. . . not intense, just relaxed. . . my body feels rested and relaxed.

As illustrated in this last example, generally a scene is a real-life one when the client identifies the date of the activity, or as concrete details are added, "It's Lake Ramona, seven in the evening, July, I'm in the water, four feet out"; "It is the summer I graduated and I was. . . " or

"The room is in my apartment, I was reading the second chapter of the novel called _____, and I had my player on guitar music." Useful prompts are questions such as, "Tell me when this incident you are describing occurred, like date, time of day?", "Where was this. . . was this a specific location. . . is there a name to this particular place?", "Since this location sounds like similar other places, what are the special distinguishing characteristics about this particular place the time you are remembering?", "Now are you describing an actual incident that happened at one specific time that you were involved in or are you describing a number of times you were involved in this activity?", "I have the details now that help me identify the surroundings and the location, now tell me something about the activity, what were you involved in doing", "How about some information on what else you were aware of; were there sensory experiences, sounds, other sights, things you heard that you were aware of, that were salient for you?"

A second issue with the initial "mesa" example was the lack of sufficient details to assure that they can be relied upon to aid in retrieving the relaxation feelings. The example is more a description of the feeling state and could prove difficult to prompt at later sessions, following anxiety induction. The example of being on Lake Ramona not only has more scene setting details, but also some of the elements that seem associated with being relaxed, such as the dusk, the mild riffles, being attentive to the feel of the line instead of thoughts about daily problems, and so forth. Some questions that might help include, "Describe for me your feelings that related to your sense of relaxation," "What was the relaxation like?," "How were you experiencing the relaxation?"

A variety of other life events seem to be commonly described by individual clients. Among these are:

- being in a favorite place at home: This usually entails a favorite chair, during a quiet time of the evening, without the presence of others, and while engaging in a quiet activity such as reading a book or listening to music. The following illustration is an excellent example of this theme:

  "It was late spring, 1988, and I had finished a light dinner and settled into my favorite chair. . . it's a comfortable leather, big enough that I pull my legs up, which I had done. I was leaning on the one big arm on the left side-my left side, had one floor lamp on, so the rest of the room was dark. It was after the movie, 8 p.m. I had my soft Mozart record on, and I wasn't reading, just sitting there listening to the strings. It was nice just being alone, the peaceful feeling of isolation and quiet."

- being on a beach: This usually entails a vacation at a shore, such as lake or ocean, with sensations from the sun and the breeze and the waves being prominent, and the individual is usually suntanning. Although people may be around, there is typically no interaction. One example that clearly illustrates this is:

> "I'm at Lake Mesa, it was two years ago; I'm on a big red towel, my favorite beach towel. . . lying on my back, radio next to me, it's warm, not hot, just pleasantly warm. . . I had just come out of the water. . . I could see the blue sky and white clouds making forms, lazily drifting. . . there is a soft breeze, I can hear birds and the water lapping at the sand. . . mainly the warmth of the sun as it makes me so relaxed. . . no cares in the world."

- being at a picnic in a part of the country, the hills, the mountains, a wooded park: This usually involves a quiet break in the picnic activities, as illustrated in the following case:

> "My boyfriend and I had been on this picnic in the meadow part of the state park. . . it was just starting to be the Fall, so the air was getting cool, but not uncomfortably so since I was dressed warmly. . . Jon had left to walk to the creek to see if there were any fish. . . and I was sitting with my back to a tree. . . I was just letting my eyes gaze at this broad expanse of green, and up on the hills at a distance the beginning of some yellow and orange colors mixed with the green forest. . . it felt like one of those paintings you see with everthing peaceful. . . occasionally some birds would be singing. . . "

In these case illustrations, there are scene-setting details that identify these as real experiences that actually happened: "Spring, 1988, after the movie with the Mozart record"; "Lake Mesa, two years ago, just came out of the water"; "My boyfriend and I (at) the state park; starting to be the Fall." The scenes also identified activities and sensory experiences, "leaning on the left arm. . . listening"; "lying on my back. . . it's warm . . . pleasantly warm. . . could see the. . . lazily drifting clouds. . . (feel) soft breeze. . . (hear) water lapping. . . (feel) warmth of the sun"; "sitting with my back to the tree. . . (gazing) at the broad expanse of green. . . yellow and orange colors. . . (hearing) birds. . . singing."

Interviewing for such specificity and concreteness is worth extra time with defining and describing the relaxation scene, inasmuch as the client then is more able to understand what details are needed when the therapist requests a similar description for an anxiety incident (in a later AMT session).

Relaxation Training

The relaxation training is a revision of the version reported by Wolpe and Lazarus (1966). This exercise is outlined in full in Appendix C, and will normally take about 20–35 minutes. The exercise can be achieved on any comfortable chair, but a recliner is preferable. Low

lighting is desirable, although normal lighting will not present a problem. Contact lenses should be removed, patients suffering from angina
should not use the muscle tensing if pain develops, and clients with
dental problems should bypass the instructions involving clenching of
the teeth. The instructions should be given in a normal volume and tone,
rather than a low, hypnotic one. The exercise is an isometric type one,
with first a tensing of a muscle group, followed by relaxation. It is useful
to demonstrate prior to the instruction of having the client close his/her
eyes.

The pacing of the instructions should be such that the client is
neither asked to hold tensed muscles too long to the point of discomfort
or potential cramping, nor is the instruction to move so rapidly as to
make the client scramble to keep up. When in doubt about the pacing,
for example about how long to keep the instruction, "Now tense up your
right hand into a fist, and really pay attention to how that tension feels,"
I tend to actually flex my own fist as a way of telling how much time
seems appropriate. Since clenching the jaws can become uncomfortable
more easily, again I might use myself as a measure, by clenching my jaws
just enough so as to experience the tightening of the muscles, before
giving the instructions to release the tension. This procedure of using
your own body to establish a reasonable pace can be used for any muscle
group for which the therapist has any doubts. The length of time for the
instruction to take a deep breath and holding it is readily determined by
the therapist practicing this him/herself during the session, or prior to
the session to obtain a sense of timing. For some individuals, tensing the
leg muscles by pressing the toes downward can involve cramping; hence
I usually have a shorter period for this muscle group, about three to four
seconds instead of the more typical four to five seconds of tensing used
for the other muscles.

A cognitive component of paying attention to the muscle groups is
added to prevent distractions and to increase client awareness of muscle
relaxation. Use of deep breaths are also added to be a future cue for
enhancing the relaxation. The relaxation training begins with instructions such as the following:

"In a moment I will be giving you the instructions for the relaxation exercise.
It's actually a method that we've adopted from physical education that has
proven successful in teaching individuals how to relax their muscles. For us, it
is important because the muscle relaxation leads also to mental relaxation
and calm."

"The exercise is kind of an isometric one; by this I mean that you first
tense up a muscle group, then you just release the tension. By doing this
sequence, you use the tensing as a means of noticing just what muscle tension
feels like. Then, when you relax the muscle, you are teaching yourself how

relaxation feels. We've found that just going through each muscle group tensing them and relaxing leads to ending with a really relaxed state at the end of the exercise."

"I'll be giving you the instructions about which muscle to tense up and to relax; generally, we'll repeat each muscle group so that we've done each twice. Let me show you the general process; just watch me for a moment. So what I'll say is tense up your right hand into a fist, and you would be doing it like this (demonstrate with right hand). . . then relax that hand like this (demonstrate). . . then we'll go to the left hand, so tensing it up like this (demonstrate), holding the tension and noticing it, then releasing it (demonstrate). . . then we'll move to the right upper arm, the bicep, and you would be told to tense it up by bending your arm at the elbow, sort of flexing the bicep, the upper arm like this (demonstrate), then relaxing it and letting the arm lower back to the arm of your chair (demonstrate)."

"That's really the general idea, do you have any questions? If not, let's make sure you take out your contact lenses if you wear them. And, have you had any physical injuries so that a muscle group might give you problems if we tense them? Any medical problems, like high blood pressure, a heart condition? Let's have you settle back as comfortably as you can, close your eyes so you won't be distracted, and now we'll begin with instructions for you to follow. We'll be first having you tense up, then relax each muscle group, step by step, just as I showed you. The trick is to pay attention to the contrast between how your muscles feel when they are tensing up and how they feel when you relax them. So we'll start with the right hand, clench your right hand into a fist. . . "

(Proceed with the instructions in Appendix C.)

At various times following completion of the hands and arms, the therapist can introduce the use of the deep breath, as follows:

"All right, to further increase the level of relaxation, let's have you take a slow, deep breath, right now. . . and as you do that a couple of times, use the deep breathing to further increase your control over relaxation. . . In the future, whenever you want to quickly retrieve the relaxation, you can use this deep breath technique. . . "

By continuing to pair the deep breath cue with the muscle relaxation achieved by the exercise, the breathing can become a stimulus for relaxation.

Use of Relaxation Scene

The relaxation scene is an adjunct to further increasing the relaxation. Since the relaxation scene was selected as being already associated with relaxed feelings, then its onset in the session should further prompt relaxation. The relaxation scene can be turned on at any time following the completion of the muscle exercise, and may be repeated as often as time permits. The relaxation scene as with future anxiety scenes follow the general model of instructions for guided rehearsal scene onset and termination:

> Preliminary Signal: In a moment. . .
>
> Identification of Scene: I'm going to have you turn on the relaxation scene involving. . . (prompt for the situational cues, for example being on Lake Ramona that July evening. . . fly fishing. Really be there again, noticing all the details of this event, four feet out in the water. . . using some fly-patterns. . . the rocks across the way. . . pretty much alone. . . use any sensory experiences that also help this scene be really clear for you. . . the riffles in the water, seeing the colors of the sunset. . .)
>
> Start Signal: So right now, switch on the scene. . .
>
> Client Signal: As soon as you are into that scene, really being there and experiencing it, I want you to signal me by raising your right hand. . .
>
> Prompt for Feelings: (for example) Notice that sense of relaxation as you fish. . . the riffles bring a sense of calmness. . . the dusk descending and bringing a feeling of quiet. . . your body is rested, as you are focused on the line. . . no other disturbing thoughts. . . a relaxed attention to the fishing line. . . the beautiful sunset is capturing your attention and bringing that peaceful sense. . .
>
> End Signal: O.K., right now, I want you to turn off that scene and return to relaxing.

The use of a hand signal is arranged in order to enable the therapist to monitor the progress of the client. In this session, the major consideration is for the achievement of the relaxation scene. In later sessions, such signals will indicate the achievement of relaxation or the reattainment of relaxation following anxiety induction, or the achievement of anxiety arousal. Nearly any agreed-upon signal can be used which can readily be observed and which involves minimal effort or disruption.

Remaining Format of Session

Following the initial tension-relaxation exercise, and the onset of the relaxation scene, the remainder of the session alternates between review of the relaxed muscle groups, and the relaxation scene. The review of muscles need not repeat the tensing, but only calls for attentive review:

> "Now pay attention to the various muscle groups. Continuing to relax the right hand. . . the right forearm. . . and upper arm. . . retaining that sense of relaxation in the left hand. . . . (continue with review of other muscles). . .
>
> Take another deep breath once again to further increase the relaxation, becoming as relaxed as you wish to be. . . .
>
> O.K., in a moment, I'll have you switch on the relaxation scene again. . . so right now, switch on. . . "

The relaxation experience is ended through the following type of instructions:

> "In a moment I'm going to have you move your fingers around a little. . . so right now do that. . . and now I'll have you move your feet around. . . right now. . . O.K., when you're ready, open your eyes, retaining the relaxed feeling as long as you wish, but being alert and refreshed. . . (pause). . . (if client has not opened the eyes). . . all right, let's have you open your eyes right now, feeling refreshed and alert and relaxed. . . "

Post-Interview

The post-interview aims at determining how well the client did in achieving the relaxation, what parts of the instruction was helpful, the degree to which the deep breath was able to cue relaxation, and the vividness and control over the relaxation scene. The relaxation scene is a good measure of the readiness of the client for other types of scenes, in terms of ability to develop one that is realistic, and to maintain control over the scene.

Any indications that the client was unable to achieve relaxation would mean that extra practice in homework assignments, beyond the once-a-day/five of seven days might be needed. Or, that extra training sessions for relaxation only might need to be scheduled. Or that other adjuncts might be required, such as biofeedback or tape-recorded instructions (although decisions about such adjuncts might be held until the progress report regarding the outcome of homework practice). The norm is that it is the rare client who is unable to achieve relaxation in this session, or who is unable to improve through the week's homework. Occasionally an elderly client is slower in attaining a reasonable level.

Reports have indicated an occasional client who experiences relaxation-induced anxiety (Heide & Borkovec, 1984; Lehrer, 1982). Among the explanations are the relaxation releasing attention so the client engages in worrisome activity, a fear of anxiety to which attention is drawn during relaxation, a fear of loss of control, or a fear of events released through relaxation, such as muscle twitches or sensation of floating. Were such anxiety to be noticed, there are at least four solutions. Heide and Borkovec report that repeated exposure to relaxation can be successful. Another resolution would be to shift to alternate relaxation exercises such as heavier reliance upon relaxation imagery or biofeedback. Third, alternative treatment might be prescribed for the client's fears of loss of control. Finally, a paradoxical strategy might be utilized, such as the suggestion that learning relaxation may take time for control and that some clients experience an increase in tension during the learning period (Deffenbacher & Suinn, 1988).

Homework Assignment

Since the major skill during this session involves the learning of relaxation, the homework assigned is to practice the tension-relaxation exercise in a quiet place five of the next seven days. Hillenberg and Collins Jr. (1983) demonstrated that homework practice of relaxation helped anxious clients especially during the first week of treatment, compared to a non-homework group.

Homework involves only practicing the tension/relaxation exercise, with no relaxation scenes. This simplifies the assignment and avoids problems in the event the client finds it difficult to control the relaxation scene. The relaxation scene is basically an adjunct in expanding on the relaxation, and hence not as crucial for homework as the relaxation exercise itself.

Normally, the client is asked to set aside about an hour and a half, usually in the evening, at a place where there is quiet and privacy. The additional buffer time is to insure that there will be no rushing through the exercise. Further, the recommendation is that the time be one after which there are no appointments, tasks to be accomplished, people who need to be met by a certain time, or other such events that might distract the individual and also create a tendency to rush through the relaxation.

Generally, most clients are able to find a time, usually before going to sleep, when they can practice the exercise on their beds. However, occasionally, for a person with a family, the best quiet time may be during the midafternoon when family are all out of the house. Another solution is for the client to simply reserve a time where everyone else in the family understands that the client is "doing my exercise" and therefore should not be disturbed or interrupted, for example, by a telephone call or a member of the family or even visitors (anymore than one would be expected to come out of a shower to greet a visitor).

The exercise itself should model that accomplished during the AMT session. The client should lie or sit comfortably, remove any contact lenses or restrictive clothing, close the eyes, and begin with tensing up each muscle group, repeating each tension/relaxation cycle twice for each muscle group. The deep breath should be added at the end. Then when the exercise is complete the client can choose either to open the eyes and pick up on other activities, or to go to sleep.

The homework instruction for relaxation is a simple one, as follows:

> "For homework, I want you to practice the tensing-relaxing procedure we used today. Pick a time you can protect, reserve about one and one-half hour to yourself, where you know you won't be disturbed or interrupted. It should be a time when you won't be thinking about rushing to some other appoint-

ment afterwards, so that you can devote your entire attention just to the exercise and not be worrying or planning other things to come later.

You should also pick a place for doing the relaxation that is comfortable. Perhaps on your bed in your bedroom; or if you have a comfortable recliner. As with our sessions, you should have comfortable clothes on.

Then simply make yourself comfortable, take out contacts if you wear them, close your eyes, and go through the tensing and relaxing exercise. Use about the same pace that we did; the important point is to tense enough to notice how the tension feels, and then relax. You will not need to use the relaxation scene. But remember to take those deep, slow breaths at the end to further the relaxation. About three of these.

"I want you to practice the relaxation; it'll actually take you about 30–45 minutes each time. You should be practicing five times out of the next seven days before we meet again. I'm also going to give you some logs to fill out that I'll also explain later.

Do you have any questions? What would be a good time of the day or evening for you to set aside for the relaxation? (Wait for reply.)

And where do you think you can do the relaxation?" (Wait for reply.)

Self-monitoring continues with Stress Log 1 and adds the Relaxation Log (see Appendix A) to provide information on progress and to insure compliance. The Relaxation Log involves recording the date and hour of practice, duration, bodily areas readily relaxed, areas with tension, and tension levels before and after relaxation. These logs should be reviewed by the therapist prior to the next appointment, which should be a week later. The instructions for the Relaxation Log are as follows:

"You should fill out this log about how the relaxation went at home. The first column is about the time, the second about how long you took. . . then fill in which body areas seem easiest to relax, and those where maybe you had some leftover tension (there might not be any to report). . . then write in the level of tension before you did the exercise and the level after. . . using this scale below, with 0 meaning no tension at all, and 100 meaning you were really uptight, really quite tense."

If the Relaxation Log indicates poor compliance or poor progress, then the next true AMT session should be postponed or be a repetition of AMT Session 1 with relaxation exercises. For very poor compliance, the therapist should consider canceling the appointment, explaining, "What we do in the next session is a function of how well your homework is going, your ability to learn relaxation. Without this in hand, it'll be hard for us to see gains. I really want you to make progress. So instead of our next appointment, I'm going to give you that time instead to practice the homework, the relaxation before making another appointment. Is there something we can do to help you complete the practice this time?" For clients whose home conditions are impossible for relaxation practice, the therapist may wish to make appointments for the client to use a quiet room in the practitioner's office for practice.

Anxiety Management Training Session 2

AMT Session 2 involves:

- Pre-interview
- Anxiety scene development
- Relaxation without tensing
- Anxiety induction followed by relaxation control
- Post-interview
- Homework assignment

This session introduces three new steps: the identification of an anxiety scene, relaxation without tensing, and the use of anxiety induction and anxiety control.

Pre-Interview

The pre-interview reviews the client's progress as indicated by the Relaxation Log. Although the log can identify the bodily areas which are difficult to relax, and although some clients may not be reporting perfect relaxation, the therapist's response at this time should be reassurance rather than concern. It is somewhat early to be worried, provided that the overall report demonstrates some level of progress, about achieving relaxation and relaxing most muscle groups. In Session 2 the therapist can give the more difficult bodily areas more time. For clients suffering from tension headaches, this is likely to be the neck and shoulders.

The Stress Log is examined to determine if there is now a pattern to the anxiety condition, if new stressors or symptoms seem to have developed which might be explored, or if relaxation-induced anxiety has occurred. Following the discussion of the "feelings" reported in the last Stress Log in AMT Session 1, the client would be expected to be showing more clarity and less ambiguity in reports on distress.

As with all pre-interviews, the transition is made to the training by the therapist outlining the plans, for example:

> "You've been making really good progress in the relaxation you practiced at home. So now you're ready to move into the next step of AMT. Today we'll have you identify a scene like you did with the relaxation scene; this time we'll develop an anxiety scene—again an incident that is real from your life. Then we'll go into relaxation, but this time without tensing, since you've been doing so well. After you are relaxed, we'll have you switch on your anxiety scene, using it to experience the anxiety. When you have retrieved the anxiety, I'll give you the instructions for relaxation again, to eliminate the anxiety. We'll repeat this a number of times, and then go to the homework assignment. Any questions?"

Anxiety Scene Development

As with the development of the relaxation scene, an anxiety scene is identified. This should be a real incident, possibly one that was covered during the intake interview. The scene should be one associated with moderately high anxiety: on a scale of 0–100 where 100 is maximum intensity, this item should be about 60. As before, both scene-setting and feeling-oriented information are needed. In this case, the feeling-oriented information involves the anxiety reaction, involving the autonomic, somatic, or cognitive subsystems symptoms. A poor scene might be:

> "It's a situation in which I was anxious, about 65 level intensity. Someone was angry at me, and I always seem to become anxious in disputes. And this was one big dispute, yelling and shouting and feeling bad and panic setting in."

Although the level of anxiety associated with this scene is suitable, and there is some detail, the scene still lacks scene-setting details that enable distinguishing the specific incident itself from many other possible anger-anxiety incidents in the client's life. Further, there is a possibility that the incident is a fantasized one, or a composite of several such real incidents. The danger here is that such composites or fantasies may not be under control during the session, changing in content in the midst of the session and either leading to distraction, an inability to experience anxiety arousal, or an uncontrolled escalation of the anxiety level.

A usable anxiety scene might be as follows:

> "I'm listening to my spouse who is angrily blaming me for something that is not quite clear yet. . . I've just stepped in the front door, a week ago, after work. . . and I'm thinking 'What in the world did I step into!' Now she's boiling over and it turns out that I had forgotten to meet her for lunch and she had been waiting, alone and embarrassed. I can never handle her anger, even when she's wrong, and this time the anxiety washed over me. . . I'm thinking 'Good God, how could I do that, will she ever forgive me'. . . my stomach is knotting up and I want to leave and run away. . . I keep thinking 'She doesn't love me anymore, I'm going to have a terrible evening. . . I don't know what to say, should I apologize, but it won't matter, since I'm wrong. . . Should I turn away and ignore her. . . that'll be worse. . . this is going to last all night. . . I can't stand it. . . I have this crushed feeling inside, like bile in my stomach and inside I'm shaking. . . "

The anxiety scene should be time-limited to an event of a few moments ("We're having this argument at the door") rather than a lengthy sequence ("I'm at the door and she's yelling at me. . . and the argument moves into the dining room over dinner. . . and even after dishes, she turns to me and says snidely. . . at which point I said. . . "). Once again the reason for a time limited incident is to prevent the scene from moving out of control, or shifting from a segment that started as moderate

Table 7.1. Illustrative Anxiety Scenes

	Job	Smoking	Spouse	Tennis
What	You're being called in by your supervisor, and you don't know why.	You've been trying to stop smoking and see someone else lighting up.	You hear your spouse coming in the door; you've been having a terrible conflict all morning.	It's the club tournament; you're ahead 5–4, 30–love, your serve.
Where/who	You are sitting in front of your supervisor's desk, concentrating to see if you can tell if this is good news or bad news . . . your supervisor is (name), the most noticeable aspect of the office is (describe) . . .	This is a social gathering of people whom you don't know well . . . the kind of situation that usually makes you anxious . . . it's in (location) . . . You are standing with only two other persons, one of whom you know slightly . . . It's the cocktail party for (name) . . . A number of others are smoking.	You're in the living room, reading the evening paper . . . No one else is there so it seems especially quiet . . . and there's going to be just the two of you . . . so it seems especially intense.	You're at the service line, getting ready to serve to (name of opponent).
Symptoms				
Autonomic	You can feel the tension build . . . As your heart races, you feel a knot, and you're getting more and more tense waiting for your supervisor to say something!	—	—	You suddenly feel a little weak inside as your heart rate goes up.

	Col 1	Col 2	Col 3	Col 4
Behavioral	—	—	You find yourself talking a little too fast . . . hand trembles a litle . . . and you want to pace around . . . or even snatch a cigarette from someone.	Your muscles get shaky, your arm is no longer firm. Your timing feels off on the serve.
Cognitive	—	—	—	You keep thinking: "I can win, I'm ahead. Don't blow it . . . Am I good enough? . . . I always blow it . . ."
Triggers Responses	It's that look of superiority in your supervisor's face and that silky tone that is so condescending . . .	The other two persons seem to be waiting for you to take the lead in the conversation . . . They are looking at you expectantly . . .	Your spouse is saying, "You're always so unsure of yourself" . . . and this makes it even worse for you . . . It's the one thing that makes you even more anxious.	You're feeling really distracted . . . can't focus your thoughts as your spouse comes in the doorway . . . You keep thinking aobut how you don't want this to happen . . . Your thoughts over and over, are, "Why can't I do something aobut this?" . . .
Cues	—	—	—	Seeing your score posted and hearing the crowd around you sensing that you could win triggers being too excited . . . and you start to doubt yourself.

anxiety but moved into a very intense level. However, if the scene seems to be the one which the client considers the best example for inducing the anxiety, then care should be taken to isolate and agree upon the segment for use, identifying the beginning and ending to this segment.

The feeling-oriented elements of the scene can be elicited from the therapist's knowledge gained from the intake. Hence, if the intake revealed a heavy autonomic component, and the client's current description lacks this element, the therapist might inquire, "Were there any bodily feelings involved in this situation?" However, the feeling-oriented elements should not include avoidance or escape or defensive behaviors, since the repetition of this may strengthen their use. Hence, the following would be unsuitable:

> "I was so anxious I blocked out what she was saying. . . "
> "I had this growing trembling, and knew she was going to be angry all night, so I turned around and left, even though I knew I should stay and work it out. . . "
> "Whenever I'm anxious like this, the first thing I do is to imagine myself being somewhere else. . . "

Some types of pre-defensive behaviors are acceptable if they describe the anxiety feelings, but do not actually reflect defensive action. For instance, the following would be appropriate:

> "I was anxious and wanted to block out what she was saying, but can't do that. . . so I'm hearing all the bloody details. . . "
> "When I'm upset, I have this desire to run away, and it gets stronger and stronger, and I know this is not possible. . . meanwhile, my thoughts are awhirl, and I'm fidgeting and tied up and more and more feeling trapped."

The therapist should never change what actually has happened in the incident being described, since the anxiety scene must be used as it actually happened, in order to induce anxiety. Hence, the above examples of suitable pre-defensive anxiety scenes are acceptable because the avoidance/escape did not occur, even though the desire may have been a part of the feeling response.

Table 7.1 provides illustrations of four different anxiety scenes with different settings, anxiety subsystem responses, and identifies the stimuli triggering the anxiety (taken from Suinn, 1984). For generalized anxiety disorders, the client is unable to identify an anxiety scene if the instruction is, "Describe a circumstance which causes you to become anxious," since the client may interpret the request to mean a statement of the sources of the anxiety. Instead, the more productive request would be, "Tell me about the last time you experienced an anxiety attack, where the level of intensity was about 60." The therapist can then focus the description initially on the symptoms—"So you were feeling the anxiety through the heart rate being very high. . . "—but then move to details regarding the setting—"Now what was the setting in which you were experiencing this anxiety attack. . . ", "What was going on around you. . . ," "What was the activity you were involved in. . . "

Relaxation Exercise

Given progress in homework, this session then moves to the therapist providing the instructions for relaxation, but without the tensing (see Appendix D). This will take 15–20 minutes, and concludes with the deep breathing cue, and the switching on of the relaxation scene. A hand signal is called for to indicate the clear onset of the relaxation scene, and a similar hand signal can be used to signal the presence of relaxation:

> "Signal me by raising your right hand if you have reached a reasonably comfortable level of relaxation."

Anxiety Induction and Relaxation Control

The rest of the session involves the induction of anxiety, achievement of anxiety arousal, and control of anxiety through return to relaxation. This is repeated as many times as time allows. Thus, the client is first relaxed through the relaxation exercise and relaxation scene, then anxiety arousal is initiated through the therapist instructions to switch on the anxiety scene, to use the scene to experience the anxiety to its fullest, and to signal the onset of this anxiety. After about 10–15 seconds of exposure following the client's signaling, the anxiety scene is switched off by the therapist, who then switches on the relaxation scene and reviews relaxation across the muscle groups. The client is asked to signal when relaxation has been retrieved. In effect, the AMT procedure uses the anxiety scene to precipitate anxiety arousal, turns this scene off and along with it most of the arousal; however, by returning to relaxation, any residual anxiety arousal is being reduced through the application of relaxation. A client cannot be anxious and relaxed at the same time, hence the relaxation becomes a way of reducing, of coping with, of eliminating, of substituting for the anxiety arousal state.

This process of anxiety arousal followed by relaxation is repeated, with exposure to the anxiety induction being for a longer interval, about 20–30 seconds. Each time this cycle is repeated, the client is being provided with direct experience in anxiety and confronting this anxiety experience by first switching off the anxiety scene cueing the anxiety, then relying upon relaxation to cope with eliminating any remaining anxiety. (In later sessions, the client will gradually remain within the anxiety scene, which triggers off the anxiety arousal, and confront and cope with the anxiety through using relaxation skills for anxiety reduction.)

The process for this session involves the following therapist instructions as, for example:

> Onset of Anxiety Scene: In a moment, I'm going to have you switch on your anxiety scene, involving entering the front door and having your spouse confronting you with her anger. When I do that, put yourself right back into the situation, really be there again, and use the scene to reexperience the anxiety. As soon as you experience the anxiety, I want you to signal me. Right now, switch on that scene, you've entered the front door, your wife is angry at you about forgetting the luncheon appointment. . . (scene-setting and feeling oriented details provided). . . (therapist continues descriptions, using appropriate voice emphasis, in volume, tone to aid arousal). . .

> Anxiety Signaled; Prompting of Anxiety Feelings: O.K., I see your signal. Continue to stay in that scene, using it to feel more and more of the anxiety. Really be there, noticing how you experience anxiety. . . the feeling of stomach tension, of bile growing in the stomach, of feeling trapped. . . especially of thinking that. . . (10–15 seconds)

> Termination of Scene: All right, let me have you end that scene, switch it off, let it disappear. . .

> Relaxation Scene Onset; Call for Relaxation Signal: . . . instead I want you now to switch on the relaxation scene, involving. . . (label scene, give details). . . When you are reasonably comfortable again, signal me. So you're sitting in your favorite chair, late at night, really listening to the music and how that relaxes you. Continue to stay in this scene and using it to retrieve the relaxation. . . Use your deep breath to further increase the relaxation. . .

> (Therapist continues descriptions.)

> Relaxation Signaled: O.K., I see your signal. Switch off the relaxation scene, continue to relax. Pay attention to relaxation of the muscles, noticing the relaxation in the right hand and forearm. . . the right upper arm. . . (proceed through muscle review). . . Again use the deep breath for furthering the relaxation. (This muscle review will take about three to four minutes, thereby permitting a compete retrieval of the relaxation, which has also been enhanced by the use of the relaxation scene.)

> Repeat Onset of Anxiety Scene: Instructions are as before, with the exposure being retained for 20–30 seconds. There is no delay between the ending of the muscle review for relaxation and the next repeat of the anxiety scene and anxiety arousal.

During these early sessions, the therapist maintains maximum involvement and control over the session. The therapist gives continuous instructions for the initial relaxation exercise and relaxation scene, the onset and description of the anxiety scene, the termination of this scene, the onset and description of the relaxation scene, the termination of this scene, and the muscle review. By observing the interval between the termination of the anxiety scene and the client's signaling of return of relaxation, the therapist can gauge the client's developing skills in anxiety control. Bodily signs can also help in gauging if the anxiety is being experienced in the induction stage, for instance, through shallow and rapid breathing, frowning, change in muscle tone, movements. If necessary, hand signals can be called upon to assess such anxiety, for example, "If you are experiencing about the 60 intensity of anxiety, signal me."

Questions can be phrased to answer nearly any question about which the therapist may be puzzled and cannot be delayed until the post-interview. Such questions might entail whether the client has fallen asleep, is able to obtain clear anxiety scenes, etc. If a client has fallen asleep, then the therapist may use a two-step approach. The first is simply to say, "I'm going to have you bring yourself to a more alert level, so come up a little higher to being more alert, and signal me that you are hearing me." If this does not work, then the second level may be needed, "You're not alert enough, so I'm going to reach over and touch your wrist to bring you to a higher level of alertness."

Post-Interview

The post-interview (see Appendix E) reviews the success of the client in achieving relaxation, the ability to achieve anxiety arousal, and to accomplish later relaxation control. It is helpful to obtain information on how readily the client was able to reexperience the anxiety arousal, and what instructions helped for the anxiety induction. Also, it is helpful to have an idea of what helped the client to return quickly to relaxation control. Such information is useful for later sessions. For instance, if only naming the anxiety scene is necessary, and the therapist description of scene-setting/feeling-oriented cues are distracting, then future sessions would be revised accordingly. On the other hand, if emphasis on the feeling-oriented aspects helps to achieve the full anxiety and scene clarity, then these would be emphasized. Finally, if the relaxation scene did not seem useful and the client felt able to use the deep breath alone to recover the relaxation, then this change can be taken.

Clarity of scene is usually checked inasmuch as we assume that increased clarity produces greater relaxation (from the relaxation scene) or anxiety induction (from the anxiety scene), and this typically is the case. However, it is possible that a client may not have such clarity and still experience the necessary relaxation or anxiety induction. In this case, no problem exists. If clarity and the consequent relaxation/anxiety does become a problem, then two alternative steps may be considered. The easiest is to continue relaxation for a longer period before switching on scenes. For many clients, the clarity of scenes seems associated with level of relaxation. Failing this, the next procedure is to determine whether the client is poor in imagery skills. In this case, some training in imagery can be employed, such as having the client memorize the features of a coffee cup (color, design, shape, size, shadings, position on table, etc.) for a minute, then picture the cup in imagery with the eyes closed, opening the eyes for a brief inspection, then again visualizing it in imagery. We describe a specific imagery exercise in more detail in Chapter 9.

Finally, it should be again stated that it is not the imagery *per se* that is crucial; rather, the imagery is the tool for anxiety induction and relaxation. It is entirely possible that the client may still be able to achieve anxiety increase through simply listening to the therapist description of the incident and the anxiety feelings. Certainly the relaxation is achievable simply through attention to the muscle groups, as this is the exercise used prior to the relaxation scene.

Homework Assignment

Given the progress in relaxation, the homework involves relaxing without tensing once daily. Once again, no relaxation scene is necessary unless the client is especially capable and finds the scene especially facilitating. The deep breath cue, however, should be practiced frequently. Anxiety induction should definitely not be rehearsed, and the clients should be instructed to avoid deliberately confronting anxiety situations. Relaxation should be praticed not only in a quiet place at home, but also in places outside the home, such as when riding quietly in a car or bus, in a waiting room, while waiting for a movie to begin, etc. This assignment is a step toward generalizing the relaxation skill to settings outside of the home environment, since eventually the application of relaxation coping will be in more active settings. The Stress Log 1 and Relaxation Log are again assigned and these forms given the the client. The homework instructions are as follows:

> "The relaxation that you've practiced at home is working well; you were able to do the relaxing today quite well. So, what you'll do before we meet again is to have you practice the relaxation, again daily, but this time without tensing the muscles. Just get to your quiet location, set about an hour aside when you won't be disturbed, and go through the relaxation review. Close your eyes, and let each of the muscle groups relax themselves just as we did today when we reviewed each muscle group after the anxiety scenes. Remember to practice the deep breath technique too, using it as many times as you can so that it becomes a quick method for triggering off the relaxation for you.
>
> "If you feel it is going to be especially useful, you can use your relaxation scene, but this isn't necessary. Do not use the anxiety scene at all.
>
> "In addition to practicing the relaxation once a day in a quiet place at home, I want you also to do some quick relaxing outside the home as well. This would be when you're in a setting in your daily life when you have a minute or so. For instance, if you ride the bus, you could take a moment to do

the muscle review and relax yourself. Or if you are in a movie waiting for it to start, or waiting for your order to arrive in a restaurant. Only should take you a minute or so. Or if you're in your office, just before a coffee break. Set yourself the goal of doing this at least once daily. This will enable you in the future to rely more and more on bringing on the relaxation in settings outside your home, so that you can use the relaxation to deal with anxieties in these types of settings. So this is another important step that we're building. Keep up with filling in the daily Stress Log and the Relaxation Log. Remember to drop them off to me before we meet. Questions?"

Summary

The prior chapter introduced the intake interview, which is not considered an actual part of the formal AMT procedure. However, the intake as well as the first set of logs provides important information. This chapter focuses on the AMT method itself, specifically sessions 1 and 2. Sessions always being with a brief pre-interview to catch up on the homework or other information occurring in between sessions. Homework logs should have been submitted prior to each session to permit the therapist time to review these, and discuss them during the pre-interview. All sessions also end with a post-interview to determine the progress during the session, identify any problems, clarify any misunderstandings, determine whether revisions are needed in training, identifying what aspects of the session contributed to better progress, and assignment of the homework task.

Session 1 is basically the session to cover the rationale of AMT and to conduct relaxation training, as well as to interview for a relaxation scene. The rationale can be adapted to be congruent with the client's status, in demonstrating how AMT can be beneficial for the client's circumstances and problems. The relaxation scene development is particularly worth emphasis, since the identification of the relaxation scene will serve as the model for later identification of anxiety scenes. As the client understands what is expected through development of the relaxation scene, he/she will be much more efficient at identifying the anxiety scenes in a later session. Scenes must be reality-based, and concretely described.

Relaxation training relies upon the tension-relaxation procedure known as deep muscle relaxation, which is typically appropriate for most clients, although options are discussed in our later chapter on relaxation and imagery methods (Chapter 9). The instructions for turning on the relaxation scene to strengthen relaxation levels follow a guided rehearsal model: a preliminary signal, the identification of the scene, the start signal of the scene, a signal from the client regarding scene onset and/or clarity, a prompt to aid in focusing the feelings, and an instruction to end. The session basically repeats the cycle of relaxation of muscles followed by relaxation scene followed by review of muscle relaxation, and so forth.

The homework assignment is aimed at strengthening the client's control over the relaxation skill. Self-monitoring of stress continues, as well as monitoring of the relaxation achieved through homework practice.

Session 2 introduces three new steps: the identification of an anxiety scene, the use of relaxation instructions without tensing, and the introduction of the anxiety arousal-anxiety reduction procedure. The anxiety reduction is achieved through the use of relaxation. The anxiety scene is one that describes a real experience during which a moderately high level of anxiety had been precipitated. Scene details should include "scene-setting details" which describe location, time, activity, and so forth, and "feeling-oriented" information which describe the client's anxiety-response pattern or symptoms associated with stress. The activity portion of the session begins with relaxation instructions, but without the instruction for muscle tensing. The session then goes into the sequence of: relaxation, followed by anxiety arousal-anxiety reduction using relaxation for anxiety reduction, followed by review of muscles to maintain the relaxed state, and so forth. In these two sessions of AMT, the therapist maintains maximum control over instructions, giving the client instructions on when to start relaxation, instructions for the muscle relaxation itself, instructions for turning on the relaxation scene, instructions for turning on the anxiety scene and for when to turn it off, instructions for reviewing muscles for deepening the level of relaxation, and so forth.

Homework involves practicing relaxation without tensing in a quiet place at home. The client is also required to practice relaxing in places outside the home, such as when riding quietly in a car, in order to promote generalization of this skill. The relaxation and stress logs are continued.

8

ANXIETY MANAGEMENT TRAINING— THE BASIC TECHNIQUE

The Middle and Final Sessions

Anxiety Management Training Session 3

This session involves:

- Pre-interview
- Client-initiated relaxation
- Anxiety induction followed by relaxation control
- Attention to early cues of anxiety
- Post-interview
- Homework

AMT session 3 may be scheduled as early as three days after session 2. This session introduces two new steps. First, relaxation is self-initiated by the client. Secondly, during the anxiety induction, the client begins to attend to the ways in which he/she experiences the onset of anxiety, that is, the cues signaling anxiety. Although the interval between the intake and session 1 is recommended as one week, the span between session 1 and session 2 can be as close as three days later if the client is showing evidence of rapid progress. Typically, the previously used relaxation and anxiety scenes will be used again in this session. However, occasionally a client will recall either a better relaxation scene or anxiety scene, and these can be substituted if they achieve relaxation anxiety is induced more readily.

243

Pre-Interview

Once more the pre-interview determines whether life events have occurred that bear discussion as it relates to AMT progress. If none, the major inquiry concerns the client's progress in relaxation without tensing, and in terms of how quickly the relaxation is developing. Relaxation in this session will shift to more reliance upon the breathing technique if it is particularly successful, or to another method if the client has discovered one that works well (such as,"I just think about letting go my entire body," or "I remember my relaxation scene").

Problems in relaxing are more critical in reporting at this stage. If the client seems to still be struggling, then a search is initiated to discover how to improve, including comparing the outcomes achieved in the AMT session itself versus homework outcomes. Sometimes the environment needs to be better controlled if the home is too unpredictable and noisy, or audiotape instructions need to be offered, or appointments made to use a therapy room in the office. A judgment needs to be made based upon the client's ability to relax during the last session's relaxation training and the client's homework progress; if both looked unstable, then a clinical decision needs to be made about whether to continue with AMT session 3, or to return to the format of session 1 or 2. Such a change is typically rare.

The introduction of the client to this session might cover:

> "This session we'll have you start with initiating the relaxation yourself and without my instructions since you're making good progress here. Then we'll be doing pretty much what we did the last session, using the anxiety scene to help you experience the anxiety and then relaxation to eliminate the anxiety as a self-control procedure. The difference is that I'll have you pay attention to how you experience anxiety, your warning signals of anxiety, while you're in the anxiety scene."

Relaxation Exercise

By this session, the client should be at the point of readiness for assuming control over initial relaxation. Hence the therapist would give the following instruction:

> "Sit back comfortably, close your eyes so you won't be distracted. Now using whatever method works best for you, initiate the relaxation. And when you're reasonably relaxed, signal me by raising your right hand."

Since the responsibility is now the client's, the therapist must await the signal. It is informative as to how long it takes for the client to achieve relaxation since this is indicative of the level of self-control. The typical client will take about a minute or two.

Relaxation Scene

Upon receiving the client's signal, the following instructions will cover a brief muscle review, repeat the deep breath, and initiate the relaxation scene:

> Relaxation Signal: O.K., I see your signal. Just continue the relaxation across your body. . . flowing the relaxation in the right hand. . . right forearm. . . right upper arm. . . .etc. . .
>
> (Duration of this should be based upon a pace that enables a client to follow the muscle review without a sense of being rushed. However, since the basic relaxation should have been achieved by the client using their own skills, this muscle review simply reinforces the relaxation level. Hence the review is a "brief" review, taking about three to five minutes.)
>
> Deep Breath: Take a couple of deep breaths as your method to further increase the relaxation. (This is achieved in about 15 to 20 seconds.)
>
> Relaxation Scene: In a moment, I'll have you switch on the relaxation scene, the one (label scene). . . all right, right now, switch on your relaxation scene. . . involving (scene description). As soon as you're in this scene, signal me.
>
> (Hereafter, following the anxiety scene, relaxation retrieval and not onset of the relaxation scene will be the signal in relaxation activities. The relaxation scene is held for about 30 seconds.)
>
> Scene Signal: Muscle Review—O.K. I see your signal. . . switch off the scene, continue the relaxation, flowing it all across the body.
>
> (This brief opportunity for the client to do his/her own "flowing of the relaxation across the body" should take about one minute.)

Anxiety Induction and Relaxation Control

The anxiety scene is introduced with maximum therapist guidance as in session 2. The client signals when anxiety is experienced and the anxiety is maintained for about 30–40 seconds, again with encouragement to the client to permit the anxiety to be strongly experienced. Instructions are added to attend to the anxiety signs. These instructions can offer a general statement about what these signs may be like or can draw from the intake interview data about the special ways in which the client tends to experience anxiety. Typical instructions for this sequence are:

> Anxiety Scene Onset: In a moment I'll have you switch on the anxiety scene, the one involving (label scene). . . all right, right now switch on the anxiety scene, as soon as you experience the anxiety again, signal me. It is the scene involving (scene description). . . remember to really be there in that scene and to allow the anxiety to build. . . the scene involves (further scene description). . .
>
> Anxiety Signal: (Client signals anxiety.) O.K., I see your signal, now stay in that scene and let that anxiety really build, and notice how you experience the anxiety. . .

Cues, General Statement: It might be in your body such as your neck or
shoulders tensing, or your heart rate, or in your stomach, or in your feelings, or even in the way of various disturbing thoughts that you are
having. . .

Cues from Intake: It might be in those thoughts that your wife is right and
you feel bad, feeling trapped. . . that crushed feeling inside. . . the bile. . .
stomach knots. . . thinking "Oh, God"...shaking. However it is that you
experience anxiety. Just really notice these signs that tell you that you're
anxious. Letting the anxiety build. . .

Scene Off: All right, let's have you turn off the anxiety scene and switch on
the relaxation scene, the one (label scene). . . signal me when you're reasonably comfortable again. It's the relaxation scene involving (scene description continues until client signals relaxation)

Relaxation Signal: All right, I see your signal. Continue the relaxation, take a
deep breath to further establish relaxation control.

Relaxation Review: Switch off the relaxation scene and continue the relaxation. Focusing on the relaxation in your right hand. . . forearm. . . etc.

This sequence of anxiety arousal, maintaining the anxiety, attending
to anxiety cues, return to relaxation scene, relaxation review, is repeated
as often as time permits, usually 3–5 times. The characteristic of this step
is still the maximum control by the therapist through instructions that
guide the client in detail, the self-initiated relaxation at the beginning of
the session being the only transfer of control in this session.

Post-Interview

The signs of anxiety arousal are discussed, often leading to clients
specifying certain anxiety reactions as more important. Frequently a
client will also come up with a new sign, not previously identified that is
truly an early warning of building anxiety, for example, the mathematician client who noticed that "My hands start to clench, and I now know
this means I'm starting to feel stressed." This use of the anxiety signs as
"early warning cues" is discussed; cues that will warn the client in the
future that tension is building and that self-initiated relaxation would be
appropriate to use as coping.

The post-interview continues to gather information on how well the
self-initiated relaxation developed and the technique used by the client.
Encouragement should be offered when the therapist has observed
good progress. The interview should also cover the readiness with which
anxiety induction occurred and the return of relaxation control. There
should be a sense of further improvement and gains in this skill in this
session. As these are demonstrated, the therapist will then have the
opportunity to comment on the progress and on the way in which this

type of application will ultimately be used for coping with difficult life situations.

Homework Assignment

Homework continues with daily self-initated relaxation in settings outside the quiet home. Although the client should avoid confronting anxiety-provoking situations, the client is instructed to use self-initiated relaxation when faced with situations of minor stress. Further, anytime the client becomes aware of the beginning of stress, through noticing its early warning signs, relaxation should be immediately employed. The Relaxation Log is continued as well as Stress Log 2. Stress Log 2 involves self-monitoring situations under which stress or anxiety occurs, the level of stress, time, and the early warning cues (Appendix A). The homework instructions would be something like:

> "Until we meet for our next appointment, continue your practicing the relax-ation without tensing; you're doing so well now that you should be able to use the relaxation method to keep yourself under control if you experience anx-iety from some minor stress situations. Certainly, keep watching your early warning signals that tell you stress is building at any time. As soon as you notice this, be sure to use that relaxation.
>
> "Stress Log 2 should be filled out daily as usual. Again, you will be monitoring your daily stress just as before. The only change is to pay atten-tion to your early warning cues, and write these down. This will help you develop even more ability to recognize them early so that you can act on them and prevent your anxiety from getting out of control. Continue with the Relaxation Log as before. Be sure to get these to me before we meet again."

Anxiety Management Training Session 4

This session involves:

- Pre-interview
- Anxiety scene development
- Client-initiated relaxation
- Anxiety induction followed by relaxation control
- Post-interview
- Homework assignment

AMT session 4 may be scheduled as soon as three days after session 3, depending upon the client's observed progress in session 3. The ses-sion includes two new steps. The first involves the identification and use of a high-intensity anxiety scene, about 90 level. The second involves having the client assume one more level of responsibility during anxiety induction: determining when to end the anxiety scene and to self-initate the return of relaxation.

Pre-Interview

This interview again follows progress in the client's ability to relax, and to relax in other settings. If the client had faced a minor stress, then success in the application of relaxation control is examined. Gains in early recognition of the onset of anxiety are important to encourage. Discussion should also note the types of early warning signs identified by the client in the Stress Log.

The client can be briefly introduced to this session by the following:

> "In this session, we'll first have you develop a new anxiety scene, one that is 90 level intensity. Then we'll alternate this scene with the 60 level one to arouse the anxiety. The major difference is that I'll start the scene, and you use it to reexperience the anxiety and to pay attention to your early warning cues. But when you are ready, you make the decision, switch off the scene yourself and return to relaxation control. For signaling, I'll have you raise your hand when you have become anxious and keep it up while you're retaining the anxiety. Then lower your hand when you've regained the relaxation."
> (Demonstrate.)

Anxiety Scene Development

To promote generalization of the relaxation coping to other anxiety situations, a 90 intensity anxiety scene is now identified. The development of this scene follows the same process as for the 60 level scene in being reality based, detailed, involving scene-setting and feeling-oriented information, etc. In this session, the 60 and 90 level scenes are alternated.

Relaxation Exercise

As with the prior session, the client continues to be given responsibility for the initial relaxation induction:

> "Sit back in a comfortable position, close your eyes, and begin the relaxation, using whatever method works best for you. Signal me when you're reasonably relaxed."

It would be anticipated that the amount of time will be even further shortened to the point that some clients may be able to signal relaxation within less than a minute. The use of the relaxation scene is discontinued. By now, the client should be well in control of relaxation; hence the relaxation scene should no longer be needed as a way of enhancing the relaxation. In a future AMT session, session 5, the client will be required to remain in the anxiety scene and to retrieve relaxation. If the client is using a relaxation scene for regaining relaxation, then session 5 may be a bit confusing (since the client is in an anxiety scene, asked to remain in this scene, and may be attempting to switch on a relaxation scene to regain the relaxation). As explained earlier, the relaxation scene serves two functions early in AMT training: first, it is a concrete way of further enhancing the level of relaxation as it follows the muscle relaxation exercise; secondly, for clients in AMT session 2 who may be struggling to eliminate the anxiety arousal during their first arousal-relaxation exposure, the shift to a relaxation scene can be a beneficial way of refocusing attention from anxiety to relaxation. By session 4, the client should have progressed well enough in relaxation skills and anxiety-reduction skills that the relaxation scene should not be essential.

Anxiety Induction and Relaxation Control

The major change here is in having the client decide when to end the anxiety scene, and to retrieve relaxation control without further instructions. The instructions might be:

Signal Relaxation: "O.K. I see your signal. Just continue to relax, by flowing the relaxation throughout your body. . . using some deep breaths to further increase the relaxation (pause). . .

Anxiety Signal Instructions: In a moment, I'm going to have you switch on the anxiety scene involving (label scene) to arouse the anxiety, then whenever you wish, you will switch off the scene and reinitiate the relaxation, using whatever works best for you. When you're in the anxiety scene pay attention to how you experience anxiety, the early warning signs. For signaling, this time you will raise your hand as soon as you are experiencing the anxiety, and keep it up as long as you're anxious. Then lower it when you're reasonably relaxed again.

Anxiety Onset: All right, switch on the anxiety scene, the 60 level scene, letting the anxiety build, then reinitiate the relaxation when you are ready. Signal by raising your hand when you're anxious, keep it up while you are still anxious, and lower your hand when you're relaxed again. (Pause)

Relaxation: O.K. I see your signal. Continue the relaxation by flowing it throughout your body. Take a couple of slow deep breaths to further increase the relaxation.

Anxiety Onset: (Pause) In a moment we're going to have you switch on the anxiety scene again, this time the 90 level scene about (label scene). This is the scene involving (scene description). Once more, after you switch on the scene, let the anxiety build, paying attention to your early warning cues, and when you're ready switch the scene off, and retrieve the relaxation, using whatever works best. For signaling, hand up when you're anxious, then lower when you've retrieved the relaxation. O.K., right now, switch on that 90 level scene and really experience the intense anxiety."

This process is repeated as often as time permits, alternating between the 60 and 90 intensity scenes. This alternation simply provides some overlearning and reconfirmation to the client of his/her ability to cope with the 60 level intensity anxiety, as well as now providing practice and direct experience in using the relaxation coping for a high intensity anxiety arousal. The therapist should continue to notice how rapidly the client is able to achieve the relaxation control after the anxiety induction.

An occasional client may show some problems in regaining relaxation after the high-intensity 90 level arousal. If this is seen after the second repetition of the 90 level scene (confirmed by the client's taking a long time to signal his/her regaining of the relaxation; or if the client's bodily/facial movement signs suggest difficulty in regaining relaxation; or if the client reports still being anxious upon being asked "How's the relaxation going. . . have you retrieved the relaxed state?"), then the following would be proper steps:

First, if the client is struggling to regain the relaxation, then the therapist should go to the muscle review instructions and say:

> "Just turn off that 90 level anxiety scene. . . and focus on the relaxation, just as you did before. . . taking a few deep breaths to gain the overall relaxation. . . then letting each muscle group become relaxed. . . the right hand. . . right forearm. . . left hand. . . left forearm. . . (and so forth). . . letting the relaxation replace any signs of tension that's left. . . taking a few more deep breaths to help the relaxation process. . . and signal me when you're reasonably comfortable again. . . "

The cycle should then be repeated: 60 level arousal-relaxation by client–90 level arousal-relaxation by client. The therapist should watch and determine how well the client manages on this cycle to cope with the 90 level arousal. If the client has improved in the ability to regain the relaxation, then the session proceeds onward as usual. If the client seems to still be struggling and has not signaled the retrieval of the relaxation, then the muscle review instructions from the therapist would again be used. Secondly, if the client has been able to finally experience three repetitions of the 90 intensity arousal and regain relaxation control without the therapist's intervention, then this session could be considered as successful. However, if the client is unable to reach this criterion, then session 4 should be repeated at the next meeting.

Post-Interview

This interview adds inquiry into the improved ability to reestablish relaxation control over the 60 level scene as well as the new 90 level scene. Again information which helps includes what method the client is using to retrieve the relaxation, and new early warning signals that may be identified.

Homework Assignment

Homework continues to use the Relaxation Log and Stress Log 2. Clients are encouraged to now check routinely for "early warning signals" of building stress during the working day and evening, using the relaxation control through the deep breath cue or other method that works well for the client. The monitoring should include *time monitoring* and *situational monitoring*. In time monitoring, the client checks stress level and signs of early warning cues about every three hours (every two hours for tension headache sufferers). In situational monitoring, the client checks stress level or early warning cues before any activities or appointments which have been known to be stressors in the past. In each case, relaxation control is applied immediately if stress seems to be building. The instructions for homework might be as follows:

> "Continue the daily relaxation at home as well as at least once daily in your daily life. Remember to complete the Relaxation and Stress Logs. Now, I also want you to continue to carefully watch your stress signs, those early warning signs that tell you that you're coming under stress. There are two ways I want you to now systematically do this. About every three hours, I want you to take a quick scan of your early warning signs; just check to see if you're detecting the early signs of stress. If you notice any, then use your relaxation coping. We'll call this time-monitoring. So maybe once in the morning, once in the afternoon, once in the early evening, once in the later evening, do a quick scan, a quick check.
>
> "In addition, I want you to be attentive to whether your daily schedule has something which tended in the past to be a stressful activity. If so, just before you get to that activity, take a quick scan again of your early warning signs. . . if you detect some stress, do the relaxation and gain control before you enter that activity. We'll call this situational monitoring.
>
> "So, do the daily relaxation, complete your Relaxation and Stress Logs, and do the time monitoring and the situational monitoring. Questions?"

The early warning signs are those which were detected during AMT session 3. These are persistent patterns of bodily signs, thoughts, feelings which seem to be the early stress responses of the client. Examples could be: the mathematician who would notice his hands clenching, an executive whose shoulders would be unconsciously tightened up and raised instead of loosely lowered, the athlete who would start to have some self-doubts such as "Did I get enough warm-up?," the musician who would simply have a feeling of "logginess," or the administrator who starts the day with the feeling "I'm not up for this day's work."

Situational monitoring comes from information either from the intake interview or during AMT sessions from the Stress Logs, as the client is more and more able to identify the stressor conditions in his/her daily life. As indicated in our review of the literature, even clients suffering from generalized anxiety disorder will sometimes develop the insights during AMT of what triggers their anxieties, perhaps due to the examination of the Stress Logs, as they can see a pattern that emerged. Stress situations could range from a confrontation to come during the day, an appointment to meet with a difficult person, an undesirable task that needs to be done but has been postponed, a painful but necessary interaction, or a challenge to one's skills that will soon be tested.

In some cases, the early warning sign will be useful in pointing out that a situational stress is on the horizon. For instance, the administrator who starts off noticing his/her early warning sign of the feeling, "I'm not up to this day's work." Upon reviewing the day's schedule, and asking the question, "My early warning signal is telling me something is coming up, is there something on my schedule that I'm reacting to?," the administrator might see that he/she has been trying not to think about an employee problem or a task that needed to be confronted that day. At this point, the stress aspects can be managed through the use of the relaxation coping to reduce the anticipatory anxiety. This not only then frees the individual up to consider problem solving strategies, but also removes the person's initial inclination to engage in avoidance behaviors ("I'm not up to this day's work. . . maybe I'll take a day off" or "I'm not up to this day's work. . . I'm not even going to think about what I have to get done").

Anxiety Management Training Session 5

This session involves:

- Pre-interview
- Client-initiated relaxation
- Anxiety induction followed by relaxation control
- Post-interview

The new step added gives the client even greater self-responsibility in facing the anxiety. Instead of ending the anxiety scene prior to retrieving relaxation, the client will now remain in the anxiety scene (comparable to real life, in that a person cannot 'switch off' the life setting). Session 5 can be within 1–2 days of session 4, depending upon the progress observed in session 4.

Pre-Interview

The success in relaxation or coping for minor stresses through time or situational monitoring should be especially noted. Self-initiated relaxation should be stabilized and the client able to identify at least one consistently reliable method for achieving relaxation.

This session can be briefly introduced to the client by the following:

> "This session will be pretty much like the last. The only difference is that this time, instead of you switching off the anxiety scene before you introduce the relaxation, you will remain in the anxiety scene while you apply the relaxation control. . . comparable to what it's like in real life. The signaling is the same: hand up to indicate you're experiencing the anxiety, and hand down when you've regained the relaxation control." (demonstrate)

Relaxation Exercise

As always, the AMT sessions begin with the client achieving relaxation, to eliminate any residuals of the day's activities, to focus the client's attention on the session, to clear out any tensions, and to prepare the client for the imagery. The self-initiated relaxation process is again used, usually with clients taking no more than one minute before signaling relaxation. The instructions remain as before:

> "Get comfortable, close your eyes, and initiate the relaxation, using whatever works best for you. Signal me when you're reasonably relaxed."

Anxiety Induction and Relaxation Control

The major change is in requiring the client to remain in the anxiety scene itself while reintroducing relaxation control. Signaling remains as used in AMT session 4, with the hand up indicating anxiety, and the hand lowered indicating the return of the relaxation. The instruction can be as follows:

> Relaxation Signal: O.K., I see your signal. Just continue the relaxation for a moment. Flowing it all over your body. Use a couple of deep breaths to increase the relaxation.
>
> Anxiety Instructions: In a moment we'll have you use the 60 level scene for anxiety arousal. But this time, instead of turning off the scene, you'll stay in the scene, and while you're still in the scene, retrieve the relaxation using whatever is working best for you. So while you're still in the scene, eliminate the anxiety. . . maybe by using the deep breath technique. . . or some other method that is a fast cue for you. . . maybe reviewing your muscles and letting them lose their tenseness. . . whatever has been the method you've found most useful in gaining the relaxation control. . . After you're relaxed again, switch off the anxiety scene.

The techniques used by clients will generally involve the deep breath, since this has been practiced deliberately in prior AMT sessions and homework. However, occasionally a client will develop other equally valid methods, such as, "I just picture flowing relaxation across my muscles from my head on down, with the relaxation pushing the tension out my toes," or "I just think the words 'relax, loose'." Since the use of the relaxation scene was eliminated in the prior session, this method is not a technique for regaining relaxation during this session's anxiety arousal. As explained previously, it can become confusing for the client to be not only in an anxiety scene but to switch on a relaxation scene; it could cause the same confusion of a person watching a movie which is about a movie being watched!

> Signaling Instructions: Signal me in the same way as the last session. When you're in the anxiety scene and experiencing the anxiety, signal by raising your hand, and when you have become reasonably comfortable again, lower your hand.
>
> Onset of Anxiety: All right, let's have you switch on the 60 level scene involving (label scene). Let the anxiety build, then while you're still in the anxiety scene, return the relaxation using whatever works best for you. When you're reasonably comfortable again, signal me. (Pause)
>
> Relaxation Signal: O.K., I see your signal. Just continue the relaxing. Switch the anxiety scene off. . . (Pause). . . In a moment we'll have you switch on the 90 level anxiety scene involving (label scene). . . etc.

This process is repeated as often as time permits, about 4–6 repetitions.

Post-Interview

The client's ability to regain relaxation control should be confirmed in this session. Since the AMT sessions have been gradual in requiring more control by the client, and since the homework and the prior sessions have provided indices of progress, this session should go smoothly. The therapist should, however, be alert to any inappropriate defensive actions by the client, such as, "I remained in the anxiety scene, and eliminated the anxiety by just pretending I was elsewhere," or "I just kept telling myself this was not a real scene," or "I just occupied my mind with other thoughts."

Homework

The Relaxation Log is continued with Stress Log 3 added (Appendix A). Stress Log 3 monitors the success of the client in fully applying the relaxation control method not only to minor stresses, or as prevention, but to more difficult life situations involving anxiety. The log involves reporting whether the relaxation control was successful in controlling the anxiety, and the level of tension before and after such control. Progress on this log will form the foundation for determining how many more sessions of AMT are needed and then termination can be planned. The instructions would be as follows:

"Continue with your relaxation daily at home and outside the home. Make sure you continue with the time and situational monitoring. The time and situational monitoring should be helpful in preventing you from being faced with anxiety-provoking situations. However, even if something catches you unawares, you now have progressed well enough that you ought to be able to just employ that relaxation coping, even if you do experience some anxieties. In fact, if you do find yourself in a situation that has caused you some anxiety, make sure you use your relaxation coping technique, and use Stress Log 3 to check your success. As you can see in this log (demonstrate), the third column is for you to check your success, and the last two columns are for you to indicate your stress level before you used your relaxation coping and after. Of course, your time and situational monitoring and your responding to your early warning signals might be so good that the amount of stresses in your life might actually now be much more reduced."

Anxiety Management Training Sessions 6–8

The AMT session 5 format is repeated until self-control appears complete, typically 6–8 sessions. New anxiety scenes may be added if the prior ones seem to lose "power" in precipitating the anxiety. Termination decision is based upon the records of transfer to *in vivo* situations and the success as a preventative measure with early warning signals. Further AMT may be continued, however, to insure overlearning.

Termination

Our experience is that termination is best handled as a part of the AMT session, rather than being announced at the end of a session. Hence in the post-interview, the therapist might indicate:

"We're now at a stage where it would be helpful to obtain some progress checks. Is there a situation coming up or one you can arrange, where we can see how successful you have become in your coping?"

After collaborating with the client in identifying this "progress test," the next AMT session pre-interview would cover: what coping methods were used, on what observations does the client conclude that the coping was successful, how did the client's current reactions compare to those prior to therapy. With this approach, termination can become a mutual decision as the therapist inquires, "How do you feel about your gains?" "Does it seem to you too that we're at an ending point, that you've changed dramatically and are now in control?" This use of a real life experience to test the progress of the client was intentionally introduced as a result of my prior experiences with desensitization therapy. In spite of all the internal evidence and my own confidence that the phobia had been thoroughly eliminated in desensitization, I invariably had clients say, "Are you certain we're done? I don't feel differently; how do I know that I won't freak out again when I (see the snake, ride in the airplane, get in the elevator, and so forth)?" Therefore, we added this *in vivo* experience, labeling it as a way of "gauging progress," and use it to permit the clients an experiential way of confirming their recovery.

In Nezu's (1987) term, this step is called "verification." In problem solving as a therapeutic strategy, he requires that clients engage in implementing a solution, then comparing the real results with those outlined and anticipated during the planning stage. This is needed because, "Even though a problem may be solved 'symbolically,' the effectiveness of a solution has not yet been verified. . . If the match is satisfactory, then the problem is resolved and the individual can "exit" the problem-solving process" (p. 134). Another added advantage of this verification process is that "the positive solution outcome itself is likely to be a powerful reinforcer, (and) exiting the problem-solving process (is also) associated with self-reward. . . (which in turn) may strengthen one's perceived self-efficacy and personal control beliefs" (p. 134).

Finally, this *in vivo* experience also results in cognitive changes, according to Bandura: "Cognitive misappraisals. . . can be minimized. . . by providing opportunities for self-directed accomplishments after the desired behavior has been established. Any lingering doubts people might have, either about their capabilities or about probable response consequences under unprotected conditions, are easily dispelled. . . " (1977, p. 201).

Bandura further argues for use of self-mastery assignments by saying, "Independent performance can enhance efficacy expectations in several ways: (a) It creates additional exposure to former threats, which provides participants with further evidence that they are no longer aversively aroused by what they previously feared. Reduced emotional arousal confirms increased coping capabilities. (b) Self-directed mastery provides opportunities to perfect coping skills, which lessen personal vulnerability to stress. (c) Independent performance, if well executed, produces success experiences, which further reinforce expectations of self-competency and finally, "self-directed performance of formerly threatening activities. . . when treatments are usually terminated could also serve to reduce susceptibility to relearning of defensive patterns of behavior" (p. 202).

Where termination is agreed, the therapist should review the use of relaxation to cope with or to abort anxiety, and attention to early warning signs. The client's individual method for relaxation coping and individual early warning signs should be restated. Time and situational monitoring for prevention should be covered, along with the recommendation to take time out for relaxation periodically during the day as another preventive measure. In some cases, the therapist should be ready to provide a 'booster' session if requested or needed.

A booster session is simply a repeat of session 5, but with some defined goals. Several goals might be arranged for such booster sessions depending upon the needs of the client:

- Practice with a more recent anxiety experience which the client felt he/she handled reasonably well, but wanted to repeat through an AMT session for increased self-efficacy. This has the flavor of fully completing "unfinished business": "I did handle it pretty well. . . but I just thought it would be nice to fully prove to myself that it wasn't a fluke. . . that if I were to become that anxious again, that I really do have the skill."
- Rehearsal and reinforcement of the relaxation skill. A client might not have been practicing the relaxation as frequently, because daily stresses have been so reduced. The client therefore wishes to have a booster session with an emphasis on the self-initiation of relaxation under the therapist's supervision. This is somewhat similar to clients who have learned self-hypnosis and want a booster session.
- Preparation for an oncoming stress event. The client may have been experiencing a comfortable, stress-free life following AMT treatment, but now foresees an unusually important or stressful experience in the near future. As assurance, the individual wants to prepare by using this event as an anxiety scene in a booster session. This is typically not used in basic AMT training, since anxiety scenes must be real experiences that actually happened. However, it has been possible after training is complete to use a projected experience, along with the anticipatory anxiety as a booster session.

For some there might be a reassessment of the client's need for other training or therapy, for other problems if necessary, such as problem solving, social skills training, other emotional conflicts not amenable to AMT, etc. For instance, the client who had been referred to AMT because his anxiety was preventing further insight progress in psychotherapy, can now return to the psychotherapy content (the case of Jeff). Or the client whose high level of anxiety was blocking the ability to enter successful career or vocational planning, because the anxiety was preventing clear decision making. Or the client who suffers from interpersonal/social anxiety, but who also lacks social skills. By removing the social anxiety first, the individual is likely to be more ready to attend to social skills training through having reached a better comfort level. With the reduction of anxiety, some clients also experience an elimination of avoidance behaviors, with the result that heightened motivation appears to acquire new skills, confront problem areas, seek further insights, engage in more compliance behaviors (for instance, in medical regimes), and so forth.

Summary

This chapter concludes the detailed description of how AMT sessions are conducted, focusing on the middle and final AMT sessions, that is, sessions 3 to 5. Sessions beyond five follow the same format as used for session 5. As usual, the sessions are designed around a traditional 50- to 60-minute hour, although there is nothing that would prevent extending the time of each session, for a more extended post-session interview, or to repeat some aspects of the session.

Session 3's pre-interview is concerned about the ability of the client to achieve relaxation effectively. Also, observations from the prior session and information from the post-interview provide information on how well the client has progressed in using relaxation to eliminate the anxiety arousal in session 2. By session 3, therefore, the client should be ready for two changes: self-initiation of relaxation, and attention to bodily/cognitive cues associated with anxiety. These cues will become the foundation for future instructions involving the prevention of extreme anxiety arousal *in vivo*. Observations of progress during this session include attention to how well the client is able to initiate the relaxation by him/herself at the start of the session, and how readily the client is able to return to relaxation following the anxiety arousal during the session. Homework is based upon the client's progress in anxiety control, and involves using self-initiated relaxation when faced with situations of minor stress.

Session 4's pre-interview determines the client's success in using the relaxation for managing minor stresses, and examines the client's progress in identifying the bodily/cognitive warning signals associated with anxiety. The session introduces two new steps: the use of a high-intensity anxiety scene for arousal, that is alternated with the moderate level scene; and the client assuming responsibility for terminating the anxiety scene and reintroducing relaxation control. Observations during this session include how long it takes the client to regain relaxation following high-intensity anxiety arousal and the success of this coping; information is also gathered on what technique the client is using which aids in retrieval of the relaxation. The homework includes time-monitoring and situational monitoring. In time-monitoring, the client does a quick scan of bodily/cognitive signs about every three hours, and initiates relaxation if there are any reasons to believe that anxiety is building. In situational monitoring, the client checks stress levels prior to any activities or appointments which have been known in the past to be stressful or anxiety-provoking. These steps involve prevention of anxiety from building up and rising out of control.

Session 5's pre-interview continues to monitor progress in *in vivo* management of minor stresses, and in the prevention techniques. The client should be having excellent control at this stage of self-initiated relaxation, with at least one consistently reliable method for achieving relaxation. The client should be very clear regarding the types of bodily/cognitive cues that signal the appearance of stress. Session 5 involves one new step: during the anxiety arousal through imagery, the client now remains in the imagery and initiates the relaxation control, instead of terminating the imagery. Observations include how well the client is able to cope with the anxiety arousal, as seen in the amount of time it takes for the client to signal the return of relaxation. Following this session a decision needs to be made by the therapist regarding possible termination.

9

Management of Relaxation, Imagery, or Clients in a Group Setting

The basic steps in Chapters 6–8 will ordinarily provide the essential procedures for most clients. In fact, the research studies which have confirmed the efficacy of AMT have usually adopted these standard procedures. The current chapter is aimed at helping the practitioner or researcher in dealing with certain revisions such as in enhancing relaxation, improving on imagery, or using AMT in a group format.

Relaxation Training

The development of control over relaxation skills is an essential for AMT to be successful. Theoretically, any coping behavior which serves to eliminate the anxiety response can be used in the AMT model, and the very first procedure used included both competency scenes and relaxation. However, it was felt that chronic clients in need of help probably will also have a poor history of competency experiences. Hence the use of competency scenes has been eliminated from the standard AMT procedure. At the same time, my experience was that nearly all clients could readily respond to the deep-muscle relaxation exercise, and hence relaxation has become the coping skill of choice for AMT. In fact, during an invited presentation in Mexico, I was able to demonstrate the relaxation procedure, using an interpreter, to an audience of 200 persons, sitting on straight-back chairs, and discovered that most of the audience were able to experience the relaxation and relaxation scenes, even under these difficult conditions.

In spite of the fact that most clients are able to acquire the necessary relaxation skills to proceed in AMT, occasionally a client may experience problems. One graduate student confronted such a problem while being observed by me in supervision (from the student's perspective, not the most convenient time for a problem client to appear!). The client was a volunteer whose presenting problem was a straightforward fear of flying. She was a 68-year-old woman without any history of psychological complaints other than the single phobia. Although she was cooperative and congenial, she did have one characteristic which we had not known about, and which soon became the source of a major problem for relaxation training. This characteristic failed to show itself during the intake or during the initial part of the first session when the relaxation scene was being identified. However, within minutes of the relaxation exercise instructions, the case dramatically changed from being a routine one to a challenging one.

The client was comfortably seated on a recliner with her eyes closed, following the initial instructions to tense, then release her right hand; then to pay attention to the loosening of the muscles of her right hand and forearm; she also was progressing through the instruction to tighten the right upper arm, then to release the tension. Up to this point, the client appeared to be moving along nicely in following the instructions. But as the student-therapist introduced the instruction to tense up the left hand, the client's eyes snapped open, she sat up rigidly, looked directly at the student, and commanded, "Dearie, please speak up, I can't hear you very well!" This type of interaction was interspersed throughout the relaxation training session to such a degree that it was obvious that relaxation training was not taking place properly. Although there had been little evidence during the prior interactions with the client that she was hard of hearing, this handicap became noticeable because of the tendency of the student to soften her voice and her voice volume as she progressed through the relaxation instructions—a mistake which many novices tend to make, since they often covertly believe that relaxation training is like hypnosis, and fail to understand that the exercise alone has effects, without the addition of a soothing, calming, smooth voice quality. In addition, this elderly client had learned to compensate for her hearing loss by watching the lips of persons speaking to her. There was still another difficulty that we were yet unaware of that also explained the hearing problem, but this was discovered only at the end of the next session.

Although one solution would have been for the student to raise her voice volume and to sit closer to the client, we decided instead to use a tape recorder to make up for lost time; the audiotape training in the next session could then be assigned as part of homework. The student therefore constructed an audiotape involving the tension-relaxation instructions, and it was explained to the client as a means for resolving her hearing difficulty. Comfortable stereo earphones were used to focus the audio and as a means of also cutting down any external noises that might act as distractors. The graduate student was instructed to turn up the volume to a comfortable level for the client. With all of these preparations, we looked forward to returning to a routine procedure. Since the relaxation training was now prerecorded, the student also looked forward to a less trying session since her task was now reduced to turning on the tape recorder, and adjusting the volume control.

However, Murphy's law that "if anything at all can go wrong. . . you can bet it will," again proved itself to be correct. Soon after the tape began, the client again popped up out of her recliner and complained, "I don't know what's wrong dearie, but I can't hear. . . how can I do the right thing if I can't hear what it is!" With a calming gesture, the student-therapist settled the client back, and reached over to boost the volume, feeling confident that we had prepared for this eventuality. However, once more, the woman opened her eyes, leaned forward, and with more indignation and frustration, asserted, "I still can't hear anything that I can follow." Another boost of volume, another complaint from the client. Needless to say this pattern had us all on the brink of chaos and confusion, and the session was terminated early to "check on the problem with the audio equipment." Since I had observed this all as the supervisor behind the one-way mirror, I volunteered to help the therapist conduct a postmortem by examining the recorder to identify the problem, if we could. It only took a brief inspection to determine that the tape recorder plus another characteristic of the client had accidentally joined forces to create the mystery: the client was deaf in one ear, and the stereo recorder's volume control that was used only boosted the volume to the earphone over this deaf ear and not the good ear! Naturally we corrected this and were able to proceed thereafter without major difficulty.

However, this case brings up the broader issue of training in relaxation for older clients, given that there might be side considerations. I have conducted relaxation sessions in a variety of settings, such as with the individuals on the floor, sitting with their backs to the wall, on straight-back chairs, around the fireplace in a ski lodge, on mats in a gymnasium, and in a clinic room with occasional loud conversations coming from students walking by the room. In general, the tensing following by relaxation of muscle groups with the instruction to "really pay attention to how your muscles feel," does focus the client's concentration well enough to produce results. However, some care should be taken to determine possible sources of competition for such concentration. Among the elderly, muscles may not be as limber and flexible as in a younger person. Hence, sitting for 45 minutes, even in a comfortable recliner, might not be possible. Older clients, depending their physical condition, may become physically uncomfortable in a shorter time with muscle aches. Therefore, the relaxation and the later AMT sessions should be shortened to 20 or 25 minutes or individualized to match the particular client's endurance and comfort capabilities.

In general, all clients should be asked if they have special problems which the therapist needs to take into account. This includes a recent injury or a chronic condition that makes it impossible for tensing of a particular muscle group, for example, a person who has a stiff neck or a recent sprain. If a client has experienced a heart attack or angina pains in the chest, or arthritis in the fingers, then tensing of the hands is contraindicated. Such tensing has the capacity for increasing blood pressure, which in turn could exacerbate a heart condition. Bypassing that muscle group would be the simple solution.

Sometimes it is valuable to determine whether clients are aware of muscle groups which deserve extra attention in the relaxation training. The therapist would say, "We will be going through each of the muscle groups to help you relax them one by one. Are you aware of any particular muscle group which you think would help if we paid some extra attention in relaxing?" It is not uncommon, for example, for clients to refer to their neck or shoulders as being troublesome. In such cases, instead of doing two repetitions, the therapist should conduct three repetitions when reaching this area. Specific medical symptoms often are associated with specific muscle groups. For instance, tension headaches usually involve the neck and shoulders, while myofascial pain dysfunction syndrome (also known as temporomandibular joint syndrome) involves the jaws. Therefore, additional focus on relaxation of the neck and shoulders is especially recommended in cases of tension headaches, and practice in mild clenching and relaxing the jaws is useful for clients with myofascial pain dysfunction syndrome.

Difficulty in becoming relaxed might be attributable to a variety of circumstances. Sometimes a client has arrived after a particularly exciting experience and is unable to settle down because of continuing thoughts or an activated autonomic condition. For example, a client being seen in our clinic had a physical education class the hour before, and often needed to run across campus. For most such instances of physical activation, the pre-interview at the beginning of the session allows enough time for the client to become settled. Occasionally, the activation is due to a stressful arousal or even exhilaration from some positive news such that the client's thoughts are still either ruminating or bursting or racing. If the pre-interview coverage of what was going on does not help to control these thoughts, then the therapist may need to allow a longer relaxation exercise. A major method for removing the distracting thoughts is to replace them with another focus for their attention. Even if the AMT session has proceeded to the session whereby relaxation is accomplished without tensing, a return to tensing each muscles is a very useful method. The tensing provides the individual with a concrete experience on which to focus that can successfully compete with the distracting thoughts.

In many circumstances, the focus is the voice of the therapist. As I alluded to in the discussion of the elderly hard-of-hearing client, an hypnotic, soothing, silky voice quality is not only not needed, but should be avoided. As stated in Chapter 7, normal and natural volume and tone should be used, similar to that used when you offer any instructions or directions to someone else. A few clients will comment that "your voice really has a nice quality to it; hearing you helps me relax more quickly than anything else." The request which usually follows this statement by the client is a request for an audiotape for practicing relaxation at home. For the most part I am very reluctant to provide such tapes. The primary reason is the risk of dependency on the audiotape as the only condition that leads to achieving relaxation. Ultimately, the goal of AMT is to have the client develop self-control over initiating relaxation without being directed by the therapist or an audiotape. However, there is always the rare exception in which the client actually does not seem to be making much progress in homework levels of relaxation, as seen in the relaxation logs.

An audiotape would be reasonable to assign where this failure in relaxation appears due to inability of the client to concentrate. Such persons may be going through the motions of tensing and relaxing but not actually focusing on the muscle sensations, but instead are being distracted by their surroundings or other thoughts, such as "Am I doing this correctly?; what is the next muscle group?" Typically, this type of client is one who is anxious to please by doing everything perfectly, or who is a person who is otherwise unused to being quiet instead of continuously stimulated. This might also be a client who, in Nideffer's (1986) classification of attentional focus is more externally focused. As compared to internally focused persons, clients with an external focus of attention or concentration are more attentive to environmental as opposed to internal stimuli or events. By assigning a relaxation audiotape, such distractible clients may be more able to acquire the initial step of learning relaxation. Ultimately, the client must be weaned from the tape, a task that needs to occur by at least the start of the third AMT session, when self-initiated relaxation is required.

Sometimes the very opposite occurs, in that a client becomes too relaxed to the point of falling asleep. I have seen this happen more when giving demonstrations on relaxation to athletes, probably related to this demonstration being scheduled in the evening after a full day's work-outs. Therefore, the fatigue of the day's physical activities makes it easy for the relaxation to progress into sleep. When my first client fell asleep on me, I was rather traumatized about how to handle the situation. Since then I've learned that there are simple steps that a therapist can take to prevent sleep and to awaken the client if sleep does occur.

To prevent sleep, of course the most reasonable precaution to take is to make sure that the client does not arrive in need of sleep, for instance because of remaining up late the night before, or reporting to an appointment following extensive, exhausting physical exercise. However, even with this precautionary step, a client, especially in a group training session, might still be the type of person who is very responsive to relaxation to the degree of falling asleep when the instructions are prolonged. For such clients, the following instructions appear helpful:

> "The whole purpose of the relaxation exercise you will be going through is to reach a level of relaxation that is comfortable but not so comfortable that you fall asleep. If you discover that you have reached a level of relaxation such that by going through the rest of the exercise you will fall asleep, don't do that. Instead, stop at the point that you are comfortably relaxed and can still follow other directions. . . just hold that level of relaxation, you can do this."

Typically, this instruction will prompt some laughter from the group, but often proves effective. To prevent the laughter from escalating into a level that becomes disruptive, the comment on sleep should be given in a matter-of-fact tone, and the therapist should proceed onward with the rest of the instructions for the session.

There are times when a client still falls asleep even with the above instruction. To prepare for such an event, the following is useful to add:

> "If one of you somehow does fall asleep, what I will do is to give a general instruction to 'come to a higher level'; and if necessary I'll touch you on the wrist."

In the event that a client does in fact fall asleep, then the therapist should first give the broad instruction:

> "If any of you are into too deep a level of relaxation, just come up a little higher so you can follow my instructions. . . so come up a little higher in your level of relaxation. . . enough to hear and follow my other instructions, while still remaining comfortable."

If the client does not seem to be responding, then the therapist should reach over and touch the client on the wrist, which will usually lead to awakening. This should be followed by the general instruction:

> "All right, let's have you all continue the relaxation for a moment, staying at a level that is comfortable so that you can follow my instructions."

Alternative procedures have been used to train clients in relaxation other than the deep muscle exercise. Clients might have been exposed to procedures such as meditation, or hypnosis or biofeedback prior to AMT treatment. During the intake, this information should be obtained with a view towards determining how the client evaluated such methods. If the approach seemed successful in teaching the client relaxation and the client remains positive about the technique, then the therapist should consider relying upon the same approach. For instance, a client who has successfully mastered meditation through use of a mantra or through the Benson Relaxation Response (1975) should not need to be introduced to the deep muscle relaxation method. A person I once saw had practiced meditation daily so that she felt confident of being able to achieve a relaxed state, both mentally and physically within a short time through meditation. My procedure therefore was to have her spend a moment meditating, then to signal me when she was relaxed, at which point I used the following relaxation review and initiation of the relaxation scene:

> "That's fine. . . continue with the relaxation. . . take a deep breath to further increase your level of relaxation. . . doing that a total of three times. . . now, review the various parts of your body to also increase the relaxation. . . increased relaxation in the right hand. . . the fingers of the right hand. . . the right forearm. . . (and so forth). . . now, in a moment, I will have you switch on your relaxation scene. . . " (rest of instructions as usual for relaxation scene onset).

In another case, my client had been through hypnosis induction as preparation for childbirth, and found she was an excellent hypnosis subject. Similarly, I also have seen a client who had learned hypnosis as a method of recovering from a busy schedule as a court reporter; this client would self-induce a light trance during breaks as a type of meditative "time out." In both cases, the clients' feelings were extremely positive about the advantages of the hypnotic state, and had acquired some level of skill initially in self-hypnosis. However, both clients had also stopped using hypnosis and were no longer certain about the procedures used. One approach which seemed fruitful was modeled after a procedure I once saw Erickson use in a demonstration. My procedure is to first conduct an inquiry surrounding: recall of the setting, recall of how the hypnotist was positioned (sitting/standing, and so forth), recall of how

268 CHAPTER 9

the client was positioned (where were your hands placed, your feet, and
so forth), and recall of the procedure (did you start with your eyes open
and focused on an object; was there a count-down used). Once the specific hypnosis situation is described in full detail, then the client is asked
to reproduce each step in reality, prompted through instructions such
as:

> "Let's have you go through each step which had worked so well for you.
> Remember how you were sitting? So why don't you place yourself in the same
> position. . . putting your hands in the same place. . . and your feet. . . since
> you had your head back at that time, focusing on a spot on the ceiling, let's
> have you go through those steps too. . . and remember at some point you
> noticed your eyes were becoming tired, so when you reach that point, do what
> you did then. . . letting your eyes close. . . " (and so forth).

In Erickson's demonstration, he actually only proceeded through
having the subject in question place his hands and feet in the same
position as when he had previously been hypnotized, and the subject
immediately shifted into a trance. I have experienced similar results with
my two clients and uncovered one interesting finding. Upon terminating
the trance induction (it is also helpful to predetermine the most useful
method for achieving this too), and during my post-interview, the one
client revealed that her recall about the hypnosis technique used by the
obstetrician was somewhat inaccurate.He did not use any of the 'eyes-
open, focus-on-a-spot' method at all, but had her close her eyes and
count downward. On the other hand, the inaccuracy failed to make a
difference inasmuch as she went into a trance anyway, while noting on
one level of consciousness that she didn't need the eyes-focusing
procedure.

The use of biofeedback as an alternative method of training would
probably have relied either on a temperature feedback equipment or
electromyographic muscle feedback equipment or skin conductance via
finger measurements. Temperature feedback is dependent upon a de-
vice placed around the fingertip, which either directly senses temperature changes or measures blood flow. The feedback signal can be either
through a digital readout, or a feedback tone. With increased blood flow
comes increased temperature. Muscle feedback might involve measuring
muscle tension around the forehead or facial area, again with feedback
being provided either with a digital meter or a tone that changes in
pitch. Skin conductance can be measured through portable equipment
that involves changes in the areas around the fingers. Biofeedback relaxation does not provide subjects with a single clear instruction regarding
how to achieve the targeted changes, for example in finger temperature.
Instead the subject is told to discover the method which seems to work
best in changing the readings on the dial or the tone of the feedback

signal. For this reason, a person used to biofeedback might be able to retrieve the relaxed state without the equipment, through the instruction:

> "Recall the procedure you used when you set about making the (digital readout; tone feedback) change when you were on biofeedback. Place yourself in the same condition that (increased your peripheral temperature; relaxed your forehead muscles; produced relaxation)."

Where this approach does not retrieve the relaxation, the therapist might consider either a 'booster' session with biofeedback equipment, or shifting to the deep muscle relaxation exercise. In those cases where the client had a very concrete technique, such as visualizing a relaxing scene or being in front of a fireplace (to warm the hands), then calling upon such a technique should enhance the relaxation.

Even where the client has not reported prior successful exposure to biofeedback relaxation training, a therapist might consider whether to introduce biofeedback instead of deep muscle relaxation training. The advantage of biofeedback for research is the ability to standardize the level of relaxation achieved, if the level of temperature or of muscle tension or of skin conductance is defined. The advantage of biofeedback for a private practice or clinic or agency setting is the ability to train several clients without the continued presence of a therapist. Although clients can be trained in deep muscle relaxation through a group format, doing so still requires that the therapist be present. With biofeedback equipment, on the other hand, different clients can be assigned to individual training scheduled at their own convenience, and without the therapist present, other than in the first session for instructions on how the equipment works.

One important caution: There is some evidence that level of patient satisfaction with behavior therapy is influenced by the presence of a therapist. Thus, although the actual outcome of the therapy involved the same level of recovery, patients provided with desensitization delivered by a 'live' therapist expressed the most satisfaction with the agency services, with the least satisfaction being expressed by patients who had received completely automated desensitization (Spinelli, 1972). In between in level of expressed satisfaction were patients whose counselor appeared to turn the tape recorder on and off and answer brief questions. In other words, if an agency is concerned about client satisfaction as part of program evaluation, and if the therapy can be delivered in its entirety without therapist present, then the greatest satisfaction will be assured by having a therapist conduct the treatment in person.

For biofeedback and AMT, we are not discussing AMT treatment being delivered through a completely automated format. Instead, the biofeedback would be used for only the initial relaxation training component. We should mention that, although there are some advantages to biofeedback as a means of saving time for the overburdened therapist, there are also some disadvantages. In addition to the issue of client satisfaction with services, cost is another disadvantage. Such equipment can be expensive for an agency or a researcher who is on a limited budget, even though prices have been substantively reduced. Portability used to be a major detriment, but modern technology has now made it possible to have equipment that is very small and lightweight.

Imagery Development

The ability of clients to develop vivid and controlled imagery is a necessary part of AMT. During the initial sessions, relaxation imagery is used as an adjunct in enhancing the level of relaxation. For those clients in session 3 who find it difficult to make the transition from anxiety arousal back to relaxation, the relaxation scene is reinitiated as a means of transferring attention from anxiety to cues which are strongly associated with relaxation. The second use of imagery is in session 2 as the method for initiating anxiety arousal.

Difficulties with imagery can occur, involving poor control over scenes and in rare instances, the inability to develop imagery. Poor control over imagery might be initially a result of a poor interview during construction of the scene. As we stated in Chapter 7, the relaxation and the anxiety scenes must represent real events, concretely described. Both the relaxation and anxiety scene should be identified in such a way as to assure that the event being described actually occurred and represents a single event. What we are trying to avoid is a fantasy scene, or a scene that is a composite of several personal experiences. It is common for some persons to identify more than one event that could serve as a relaxation scene, for instance, an experience of being at the beach, as well as another experience of listening to a favorite quieting musical selection at home. What is important is that one of these scenes be *clearly* selected so that the client is focused on only this scene during the session.

I personally experienced a wonderful example of what can go wrong, which seems humorous in retrospect, but was problematical at the time. A client had two potential scenes. Scene One involved sitting in a favorite easy chair, reading a pleasant novel, with only the light from a floor lamp at 11 o'clock in the evening. Scene Two involved standing on the corner of Powell Street in San Francisco, admiring the flowers in a vendor's cart. Although the client selected the first scene for her relaxation scene, apparently this selection was only tentative. At the end of the scene, the client seemed torn between frowning and smiling, leading me to inquire as to what had happened.

She reported that the scene started off at home, with her in fact sitting in her favorite chair, but then she discovered that both her chair and the floor lamp were on the corner of Powell Street next to the flower cart! Needless to say this oddity caused her to laugh. She was instructed to reconsider which scene was associated with the greater relaxation, and we spent more time in having her describe scene details. Then, instead of going to relaxation and switching on the scene, we instead spent a moment having her close her eyes and actively picture the scene to focus her concentration, then proceeded on to muscle relaxation and to switching on the scene.

Scene control is especially important for the anxiety scene, as we mentioned earlier, since the level of arousal may be hindered if the scene is out of control. The arousal disruption could be in the direction of too low a level, because the scene has drifted to a less anxiety-provoking event. Or the scene might lead to a higher arousal than, for instance, the 60 level, because the client's scene is a fantasy that proceeds onward to more horrifying or catastrophic conclusions than did occur or could possibly occur, even in one's worst experiences. Again the major principle is to define the specific event, insuring that it is a reality experience, and identifying the actions *circumscribing* the event. By the last, I am referring to the notion that, although the anxiety scene involves reexperiencing certain sequences of thoughts, feelings, or interactions, the scene is still best viewed as a moment out of one's life akin to a still photograph of one scene, rather than as a movie or videotape that extends from one scene to another. For example, a client once selected an anxiety scene that started with a 60 level of anxiety arousal as follows:

> "I had entered my foreman's office, and was standing there waiting for him to say something about why I was called in; my thoughts were of the worst, that I had done something inadequately, that he had a complaint about me; the more these thoughts ran through my head, the more certain I felt that this was going to be a painful meeting. Meanwhile, he had not said anything or even looked up at me, but was writing something."

Although this scene does have some activity, namely thoughts, it is still a circumscribed moment in time. However, the client's first use of this scene in AMT session 2 was followed by behavioral signs of heightened anxiety, such as rapid breathing and bodily movements and a long delay before relaxation was achieved. In the inquiry, the client admitted that he had not previously described the entire circumstance to the therapist during the scene construction. The entire event actually started with the above mentioned details, but the next sequence continued:

"My supervisor finally looked up at me, and without giving me a chance to comment, started yelling at me for failing to keep an appointment with one of our customers. I was flustered because the more he yelled, the less I could remember about why I missed the meeting, yet I had the feeling it wasn't my fault. I could only think, 'He's talking so loud, everyone outside can hear that he's chewing me out.' I really felt humiliated that my friends knew I had made some kind of big mistake; but it was worse since I felt I could defend myself, that I knew it hadn't been my fault, but I was blank about why I missed the meeting. Then I became angry, but knew I couldn't do anything, and suddenly he said, 'Do you dare disagree with me? I see you clenching your hands, you think I don't know what you're thinking? I've had it with you always blaming others, making excuses, and I don't like you arguing with me.' I hadn't even said a word, and he was accusing me."

During the AMT session, the initial part of the scene continued right on to this later part of the experience, causing the initial 60 level of anxiety to escalate to 95. Such loss of control over a scene in this case is really a function of a poor scene selection and scene construction interview. The scene was better used as a 90 scene, with emphasis on the part of the scene associated with the 95 level of anxiety arousal.

I had briefly mentioned the importance of requesting a relaxation scene in Chapter 7 through the instructions, "Describe an activity or event that really happened which was associated with a sense of relaxation or calm," rather than using the phrase, "That was a pleasant situation or activity." In one revealing experience, a student of mine suffered the distracting consequences of the word "pleasant." The student I was supervising was an attractive woman working with a male client. Although he had identified a reasonable relaxation scene, we soon discovered that he substituted a fantasy, this being of engaging in sexual contact with the student therapist. . . which met the criteria of a pleasant or 'pleasurable' scene, but which proved to be a distracting interference with the progress in the session. Fortunately the student therapist was skilled enough to deal with the issue from a transference approach.

Occasionally, a client reports having had no personal experiences involving being relaxed, other than the unacceptable events of being relaxed after intake of alcohol or with fatigue associated with intense physical exercise. Therefore identifying a relaxation scene is difficult. In this circumstance, the therapist can instead rely upon the portion of the AMT session itself, involving the muscle relaxation exercise as the client's relaxation scene. Or, after the client has practiced relaxation during homework, one of these experiences can be selected.

If scene construction interviews have been correctly conducted, failures in imagery control during the first session might not represent real problems. A few clients need several repetitions with the relaxation

scene in the first session before scene vividness and control is established. If such control is not developed after 4–5 repetitions during
session 1, then session 1 should be repeated, rather than going on to the
content of session 2. One factor that seems helpful for scene control is
improved relaxation levels. The repeating of the content of session 1
during the next scheduled meeting permits the client to complete the
homework practice of relaxation for five of the next seven days. Additionally, the therapist should spend more time at the start of the session
in muscle relaxation instructions, including possibly three repetitions of
the tensing/relaxing cycle per muscle group, and more extensive review
of each muscle group at the end of the complete tension/relaxation
instructions, for example:

> "Continue to focus on relaxation of the entire body. . . again noting the
> relaxation in the right hand. . . releasing all tensions that remain. . . letting
> the relaxation increase even further up the right forearm and upper
> arm. . . " (and so forth).

In an extremely rare instance, a client might appear who seems
unable to develop imagery even after the extra relaxation and additional
repetitions with the relaxation scene. In such a circumstance, an imagery
training exercise might provide some help to achieve a breakthrough.
This exercise assumes that the client is deficient in certain skills and
provides some practice in such skills.

The exercise is as follows: Have the client focus attention on an
object that has vivid characteristics, such as a brightly wrapped object, a
simply designed vase, or a single flower. These objects should be simple
and not involve complex patterns or be surrounded by distracting features. For instance, the wrapper would preferably be of a saturated
single color, or with a simple geometric pattern. The task, then, is for the
client to focus attention for 3–4 minutes, for example, through the
following instructions:

> "I want you to pay attention to really seeing (this object) noticing its character-
> istics so that you will be able to close your eyes and picture it again. Notice the
> various characteristics. . . for instance pay attention to the color. . . what
> does it remind you of, how deep is it, is there more than one color. . . do the
> colors form some sort of pattern. . . also notice if there *is* any sort of pat-
> tern. . . ask yourself how this pattern begins at the top of the object. . . are
> there characteristics you can count (for instance, numbers of petals in a
> flower). . . what is your actual count. . . how about shape. . . what is the
> shape like, does it remind you of anything. . . and size. . . how would you
> gauge the size. . . maybe by comparing it to some other object you're familiar
> with. . . or maybe you can tell by estimating its size in inches. . . are there
> other distinguishing features that stand out. . . a sense of its weight. . .
> or bulk. . . maybe its curves or straight sides. . . think for a moment of how

you will be picturing it when you have your eyes closed later. . . color. . .
patterns. . . characteristics you counted. . . shape. . . size. . . bulk. . .
curves. . . straight sides. . . unusual characteristics. . . how about just total
impression . . . "

At this point, the therapist should now have the client close his/her
eyes and attempt to visualize the object, with the therapist giving the
instructions to:

"Just picture that object as clearly as you were seeing it a moment ago," (then
waiting about 30 seconds before providing the prompt) "recall those characteristics you were concentrating on. . . the total impression of the object. . . .color, remember the color (the therapist should now add the correct
information, for example, "remember the bright red"). . . "and the pattern,
how was the pattern. . . "(the therapist should now add a description of the
pattern, if any, for instance, "remember the wrapping was that bright red, but
with squares that were formed by green lines"... "aspects you counted. . .
"(the therapist should now add this detail). . . "the shape. . . "(add details). . . "and the size. . . "(add details). . . "and was there something relevant about bulk. . . "(add details)..curves. . . "(add details). . . "or straight
. . . "(add details) . . . "size. . . "(add details). . . "or unusual or striking characteristics. . . "(add details).

The next step would be for the client to again examine the object,
for another 3–4 minutes, then to close the eyes for a few seconds, and
reopen them to refresh the memory on relevant details. This is followed
by a prompted recall such as:

"again with your eyes closed, remember your total impression. . . get as clear
a picture as you can. . . and remember the details that help make this really
vivid again. . . it's bright red. . . this red is formed into squares by green
lines. . . " (and so forth).

The client might now be ready for the relaxation exercise under the
direction of the therapist, with the instruction to:

"Visualize that object you were paying such attention to earlier. . . letting the
image of the object develop fully and completely for you. . . letting any part
of the characteristics of this object appear, maybe the total impression. . . or
the specific color. . . or some other characteristics. . . and as this becomes
clear, let this help you have a fully developed image. . . as clearly and vividly
as possible. . . without any effort on your part. . . just now having that clear
image. . . the red color. . . the squares formed by the green lines making the
red square pattern. . . " (and so forth).

In an even rarer circumstance, a client might still be unable to
develop imagery even with the imagery-training exercise. This is truly a
rare client and it is hard to know what this implies, since no research is
available, nor sufficient clinical experiences to draw speculations. There
are a few steps that might prove useful. One is to recall that imagery does
not necessarily mean visual. Some clients are not visually inclined, al-

though I admit that the illustration of the imagery exercise described is based upon visual dominance (a substitute is to obtain a videotape of a musician, such as a soloist with a flute, for the imagery exercise).

If the client is fundamentally nonvisual in orientation, then the instructions the therapist has given should be reexamined carefully. Our instructions for AMT emphasizes giving equal attention to any or all senses, not simply the visual. If a therapist has mistakenly focused on "see yourself" or "see the details clearly" and has overlooked references to other senses, then perhaps the problem is in the instructions. If the client's inability persists, then another approach is to determine which sensory modalities are the more dominant for the client. One method for accomplishing this is to ask the client to pick some recent experience and to describe it to you, any experience that they feel they were impressed by and might have wanted to share with someone else. After the initial description, encourage the client to add more details through the prompt, "That was a good description, but continue with your description; I'd like to hear more about that event." Listen for the types of sensory words used; does the client use more adjectives describing sounds, or movements? Similarly, are there more objects that are dominant in the descriptions, or animals, or other persons? Or are there internal events that are described, rather than external ones?

From this information, the client's major orientation might be identified and the next relaxation scene described with details relying upon this dominant tendency. For instance, if movements seem more critical to the client, then the relaxation scene might (for example) focus on the swaying of the branches and leaves or the movement of the clouds. If sounds dominate, then the relaxation scene might be further analyzed for components, such as the music that is playing. If the client is more reactive to people in various events, then careful description of the mannerisms, behaviors, personalities, dress styles, and so forth, of persons in a relaxation scene would be used to start the scene. If the client is more internally focused, then internal feelings or thoughts would be emphasized as the scene is described.

Where all else fails, then it is time to remember our initial theory about AMT, and that is, that it does not really matter how the therapist precipitates anxiety arousal during the session. Our first study used imagery, recordings of Edgar Allan Poe, and synthesizer music. Any such source of stimuli that can lead to anxiety arousal should theoretically be sufficient, since AMT is fundamentally aimed at training in control over arousal through first experiencing anxiety activation, followed by the use of relaxation for control. Hence our theory is simply that anxiety arousal is needed, but through any procedure that can arouse such anxiety. Theoretically it is even possible that the very verbal description by the therapist as he/she reads the anxiety scene, along with appropriate voice emphasis, could be sufficient to accomplish anxiety arousal, even without imagery.

Finally, there may be a circumstance whereby a client is able to achieve anxiety imagery but unable to achieve relaxation imagery, even though the client has identified a real experience that had been relaxing. Such a failure to be able to switch on a relaxation scene is actually not an issue. The major function of the relaxation scene is used to help further initiate relaxation. If the client has been able to develop relaxation through the use of the muscle exercise alone, then this should suffice for AMT treatment.

Anxiety Management Training in a Group Format

We have been describing the details of AMT for individual therapy sessions. However, AMT has also been used in groups for clinical work as well as in research studies. Groups may be desirable where clients show a common anxiety complaint, or where efficient use of the therapist's time is sought. An AMT group can reasonably include up to 6–8 clients. In using AMT in a group setting, several revisions are recommended (Table 9.1 outlines the proper procedures).

Typically, the training will take a little more time. The therapist must be able to give proper attention to insure that all clients understand the training and homework procedures, have successfully developed relaxation and anxiety scenes, have acquired relaxation skills and the ability to switch on the scenes, and are able to demonstrate anxiety coping. A client who is more skilled in sessions than others represents no issues in contrast with a client who is lagging behind. Therefore, the pace of the sessions should be geared to that of the slowest client to insure that no one is being pushed beyond their ability to profit from AMT. In general, session 1 and certain later sessions should be repeated (see Table 9.1 for the sessions that are repeated). By repeating session 1, all clients are assured of having control over the relaxation method and will have extra experiences with imagery (of the relaxation scene); by repeating later anxiety-coping sessions, all clients will have additional practice in self-control over anxiety arousal. Of course, the feedback information from the various logs serves an even more crucial role in aiding the therapist in gauging the progress of each client, and his/her readiness for the next session's activities.

Another revision in group AMT involves the method for development of the relaxation scene. The relaxation scene is developed in ses-

Table 9.1. Group AMT Format

(In general, except for repetitions of some sessions, the overall content and the homework assignments are similar to those of the individual AMT format.)

I. Session 1 (60–75 minutes)
  a. Structure AMT if not accomplished in intake meeting
  b. Develop Relaxation scene
  c. Instruct in tension-release relaxation
  d. Use Relaxation scene visualization
  e. Homework: Practice relaxation in quiet protected surroundings
    Write Relaxation scene on index card for next session
    Stress Log 1
    Relaxation Log

II. Session 2 (60 minutes) (repetition of Session 1)
  a. Refine Relaxation scene if needed
  b. Instruct in tension-release relaxation
  c. Use Relaxation scene visualization
  d. Homework: Practice relaxation in quiet protected surroundings
    Stress Log 1
    Relaxation Log
    Write two 60-level Anxiety scenes for next session

III. Session 3 (60–75 minutes)
  a. Review and refine two 60-level Anxiety scenes as needed
  b. Relaxation instruction, T control, no tensing
  c. Anxiety arousal with first Anxiety scene, followed by anxiety control
  d. Alternate Anxiety scenes for anxiety arousal/anxiety control
  e. Homework: Practice relaxation in nonactive "real-life" surroundings
    Stress Log 1
    Relaxation Log

IV. Session 4 (60 minutes)
  a. Relaxation instructions, C control
  b. Anxiety arousal with awarenss of bodily/cognitive signs of anxiety
  c. Homework: Practice relaxation in a variety of real-life surroundings
    Stress Log 2
    Relaxation Log
    Apply relaxation if needed during minor stress

V. Session 5 (60 minutes) (repetition of Session 4)
  a. Relaxation instructions, C control
  b. Anxiety arousal with awareness of bodily/cognitive signs of anxiety
  c. Homework: Practice relaxation in a variety of real-life surroundings
    Stress Log 2
    Relaxation Log
    Apply relaxation if needed during minor stress
    Write one 90-level Anxiety scene for next session

(continued)

Table 9.1. (*Continued*)

VI. Session 6 (60 minutes)
    a. Review and refine 90-level scene as needed
    b. Relaxation instructions, C control
    c. Anxiety arousal, followed by anxiety control through C terminating A-scene and using best relaxation method (hand signal format changes); alternate 90 and best (most impactful) 60-level scenes
    d. Homework: Stress Log 2
                Relaxation Log
                Time monitoring
                Situational monitoring

VII. Session 7 (60 minutes) (repetition of Session 6)
    a. Relaxation instructions, C control
    b. Anxiety arousal, followed by anxiety control through C terminating A-scene and using best relaxation method; alternate 90 and 60-level scenes
    c. Homework: Stress Log 2
       Relaxation Log
       Time monitoring
       Situational monitoring

VIII. Sessions 8–10 (60 minutes)
    a. Relaxation instructions, C control
    b. Anxiety arousal, followed by anxiety control with C *remaining* in A-scene; alternate 90 and 60-level scenes
    c. Homework: Stress Log 3
       Relaxation Log

IX. Termination interview (follows assignment of *in vivo* test)
    a. Review behavioral evidence of *in vivo* test
    b. Contrast characteristics prior to therapy and current
    c. Review coping skills learned, use of time, and situational monitoring for prevention
    d. Agree on termination

sion 1 as usual, although the session might be extended from 60 to 75 minutes. The therapist should use the standard inquiry addressed to the group in general, then accept a description from the first client to volunteer (this client is usually the most comfortable within the group). By careful use of open-ended queries, the therapist can guide this client to a detailed scene description that can serve as a model for the others. The therapist can then comment on the salient characteristics of this scene, and encourage another client to identify and describe a relaxation scene for him/herself. The therapist should obtain a relaxation scene from each client, although the amount of interviewing time involved will be greatly shortened as a function of the success of the first one modeled. Clients are asked to write their scenes on an index card, to be used as reminders at the next AMT session (homework relaxation practice involves muscle relaxation only, and not scene visualization). All clients should be told that their own personal relaxation scene, as described, will be the scene to visualize whenever they are asked to switch on "*the relaxation scene*" by the therapist.

There are also similar revisions in the method for anxiety scene development. Between the second and third group sessions, clients should be asked to write down two separate anxiety scenes of moderate level anxiety, and to turn these in on an index card to the therapist prior to the next AMT meeting. The therapist uses the standard instruction of what is included in an anxiety scene, emphasizing that the scene should be concrete, a reality situation, and as detailed as the relaxation scene had been. The level of anxiety of each of the scenes should be "moderate," that is, about 60 on a scale from 0–100, where 100 is maximum anxiety.

Session 3 in the group AMT format is the first session in which the anxiety scenes are used. Part of the session is allocated to further refinement of the clients' anxiety scenes, and to insuring that all clients have identified and developed useful descriptions of two anxiety scenes arousing moderate levels of anxiety. This session might therefore be extended from 60 to 75 minutes. The therapist assigns the labels "*your first moderate anxiety scene*" and "*your second moderate anxiety scene*" as the method for the clients to know which anxiety scene to visualize during the session. During session 3, the therapist alternates switching on the first anxiety scene (followed by return of relaxation) with the second anxiety scene (followed by relaxation), etc. This alternating procedure insures that all clients will experience anxiety arousal through at least one of the scenes.

The procedure of writing out and turning in an anxiety scene is also used between sessions 5 and 6. As homework between sessions 5 and 6, the clients are to identify and write out one high level anxiety scene, associated with a 90 level intensity. During session 6, this scene is further refined where necessary through further discussion and interviewing. Each client's anxiety scene is then given the label of "your high anxiety scene." Session 6 follows the same format as session 4 under individual treatment format.

Specifically, the session begins with client-initiated relaxation, followed by anxiety arousal through the 90 level scene, followed by termination of this scene, followed by relaxation retrieval. The termination of the anxiety scene is initiated by the client when he/she is ready to do so. Once this cycle is completed with the 90 level scene, then the client is instructed to use the 60 level scene that had the most impact in the prior sessions. The remainder of this session simply repeats this procedure of alternation between the high-intensity and the low-intensity scenes. As with the individual AMT format, each client relies upon whatever self-control method (relaxation scene, deep breath cue, muscle review, etc.) has been most useful in elimination of the anxiety response.

Another revision in using the AMT group format involves the method for obtaining signals within sessions, e.g., during scene development. With individual treatment, a hand signal is used to signal the initiation of a scene, or to initiate the achievement of relaxation, etc. This same method is also used in the group format; however, the signal should involve a movement that is clearly visible to the therapist, such as raising the hand rather than simply one finger. Furthermore, the therapist must remember to verbally acknowledge each time one of the clients in the group signals, e.g., by saying, "O.K., I see your signal." In some instances, a client will continue to hold his/her hand up even after such acknowledgment. When the last client has signaled, the therapist should handle this by the instruction, "All right, you can put your hands down now."

In the group AMT format, signals provide a useful method for determining the progress of each client. If the therapist needs to determine what is occurring with a client, a general instruction can be given to all clients, and attention paid to the reply of the client in question, for instance, "If you were able to experience about a 60 level of anxiety in your last scene, signal me by raising your right hand, now."

Managing the AMT group is similar in some ways to managing psychotherapy groups. Clients should be removed if their characteristics are such as to interfere with their own progress or that of others. Such characteristics include dominating the use of the group's time, being disruptive or antagonistic, or habitually failing to complete homework or log assignments. Since AMT relies upon a skill training model, the successful completion of each level of skill before the next session is essential. Without such progress, the training provided at the next session will not have much constructive impact. If a client's characteristics are an obstacle to progress in skill development, then the entire group may be kept from showing gains.

One behavior which sometimes occurs involves falling asleep during the session. To avoid this, AMT sessions should be scheduled at times during which clients are not expected to be especially tired physically. Since falling asleep does occasionally happen, the therapist should routinely inform the group that a touch to the wrist will be used by the therapist to quietly awaken any client who needs to be more alert. As with other client characteristics, if falling asleep appears to be a habitual response by a client, then this client might be transferred to another group with a better time schedule, or seen on an individual basis.

The group AMT format requires the therapist to be particularly attentive during the early sessions, to gauge the understanding and progress of each client, to use feedback and signals to determine the responsiveness of each client, and to manage the logistics of the scene interviews, homework assignments, and post-session interviews. As the sessions progress, the group setting can be a source of encouragement and reinforcement as group members share their progress with one another. Such mutual support can be used as a positive influence in maintaining attention to homework and record-keeping with logs.

Summary

This chapter has focused on the practicalities of conducting AMT. Relaxation training and the development of imagery are two of the mainstays of successful AMT treatment. Although most clients move readily through the standard AMT procedures, occasionally a difficulty arises that needs attention.

Successful achievement of relaxation training must take into account physical as well as environmental factors which could hinder the process. Among the physical factors are hearing loss, especially among the elderly, or physical aches and pains which might affect comfort. The level of relaxation achieved might prove to be an issue in either direction: an inadequate level of relaxation, or too deep a level, so that sleep takes over. We have covered the various ways of avoiding or resolving these types of relaxation issues, as through revising the instructions or shortening the time. In addition, since there are alternative methods for relaxation training, this chapter devoted some attention to how an AMT therapist can take advantage of these. There is an especial advantage if a client has already learned relaxation skills, such as through hypnosis training, meditation, or biofeedback. By relying upon these as foundation skills, the therapist can substitute these for the muscle relaxation procedure and thereby save some time, while making the client more comfortable in relying upon a skill they already possess. One major caution that we cited with biofeedback equipment, however, are the data that suggest that a completely automated system, where the therapist never spends time with the client, tends to create client dissatisfaction.

Imagery can be an issue in terms of either failure to gain control or complete failure of imagery development. The greatest concern regarding the control of imagery or the use of fantasy in imagery is the possible uncontrolled escalation of anxiety, or the inability to achieve relaxation because of an improper relaxation scene. A major element of imagery instructions, therefore, is the absolute insistence on the scenes being descriptions of actual, reality experiences. This prevents loss of scene control, and also enables clients to provide specific, detailed descriptions of the events. In those rare cases where imagery development seems impossible for the client, one solution may be found in the interview process used by the therapist. Since a few clients are less visualizers in the sense of being sight oriented, and more attuned to other sensory experiences (such as sounds), the interview to identify scenes might require broadening to: "What sensory experiences are you aware of that help to describe that scene for you more fully?"

The description of how to conduct AMT in groups has been added to this chapter since it is another practical issue. I have preferred to conduct group sessions where possible inasmuch as it is a more efficient use of time. A group format also had the potential advantage of providing some increased motivation as members become supportive of one another, as well as opening up insights as members suggest ideas to one another, for instance regarding ways of scheduling days so as to gain the needed time for homework practice of relaxation. In addition to these values, the research report of Deffenbacher, which we cited in Chapter 2, demonstrated that it is even possible to conduct groups of clients with mixed symptoms or complaints.

However, most AMT groups would be made up of clients with the same type of psychological difficulty, such as those with the same phobias, or those experiencing generalized anxiety disorder, or those with tension headaches or hypertension, or all Type A persons, and so forth. The group sessions tend to take a greater number of sessions, and would be helped by being longer than the 45–50 minutes of individual sessions. Group dynamics are as important for AMT groups as they are for other psychotherapy groups, with the interpersonal and group dynamics being met through the same procedures for AMT groups as for psychotherapy groups. The optimal size of an AMT group is really a function of the size which the therapist is capable of giving his/her fullest attention, but probably will seldom range beyond 10 clients.

IV

APPLICATIONS OF ANXIETY MANAGEMENT TRAINING

10

Behavioral Medicine

Since the early 1970s, the vast talents of behavioral science researchers and practitioners have devoted their attention to the issues of medicine, leading to major contributions to behavioral medicine (Agras, 1982). One review of such contributions can be found in a special issue of the *Journal of Consulting and Clinical Psychology* edited by Blanchard (1982). This chapter will review some of the ways in which Anxiety Management Training has proven relevant to a variety of such medical issues, including Type A behaviors, hypertension, dysmenorrhea, and tension headaches.

Type A Behaviors

Since the seminal writing of Friedman and Rosenman (1974) and the classic research of the Western Collaborative Group Study (Rosenman, 1975), the Type A behavioral pattern has been recognized as a major risk factor in cardiovascular disease, along with obesity, smoking, lack of exercise, cholesterol levels, etc. The Type A pattern is viewed as an extremely important one for professional services, since it is most prevalent among upwardly mobile, achievement-oriented managers and professionals (Matthews, Helmreich, Beane, & Lucker, 1980). In addition, it is estimated that the prevalence rate is as high as 50–75% of middle-class managers (Howard, Cunningham, & Rechnitzer, 1977). Suinn (1976) and Dembroski, MacDougall, Eliot, and Buell (1983) suggest that physiological mediators of heart disease among Type A persons involve the high level of stress associated with being Type A. Type A persons, through their behaviors, expose themselves to stressors and challenges, such as self-imposed deadlines, but are also in danger of heart attacks if they are also psychophysiologically reactive to such events ("hot reactors"). The relationship between Type A behaviors, stress, psy-

chophysiological reactivity, and cardiovascular disease has been speculated as connnected with sympathetic nervous system hormones, the
catecholamines (Krantz & Manuck, 1984; Wright, Contrada, & Glass,
1985).

Anxiety Management Training

The possible value of AMT becomes clear from these theories of
stress and Type A behaviors. In fact, the very first published behavioral
intervention study was on the effects of AMT with Type A patients
recovering from a heart attack. Suinn, Brock, and Edie (1975) compared
AMT combined with imagery rehearsal in a cardiac rehabilitation program to results from the cardiac rehabilitation program alone, and reported changes in patients' Type A life-styles for the AMT group, but no
changes for the non-AMT group. This was replicated by a number of
other studies as we summarized in Chapter 3, including a study by Suinn
and Bloom (1978). The application of AMT for Type A persons can be
illustrated from this study's approach which is described next.

Announcements through the newspaper identified Type A persons
from a variety of occupations, including a mathematics professor, a high
level manager, a dentist, a sales manager, a farmer, and an executive
secretary. As might be expected, since men tend to outnumber women
among Type A persons, the sample was predominately male. AMT was
adapted for Type A training in the following ways:

Rationale. Acknowledging the self-reliant and competitive charac-
ter of Type A's, AMT:

- was described as training, not as therapy. The Type A persons
  were in high level positions and were persons who viewed themselves as successful. Hence any implication of being engaged in
  psychotherapy would have been incongruent with their self-
  perceptions, and would likely have led to resistance and a high
  dropout rate. Hence, Anxiety Management Training was introduced by its title, with the emphasis on "training." In fact, my
  involvement with the psychological training of Olympic athletes
  and the application of AMT in their training made the concept of
  skill training even more accepted.
- was presented as training to enhance efficiency through eliminating the obstructive features of being Type A. The issue as to why
  one should even want to alter Type A behaviors needed to be
  addressed. Type A individuals tend to attribute their success to
  their hard-driving nature, their tendency to rush toward deadlines, and their aggressiveness. It was explained that such char-

acteristics also bring certain disadvantages, namely of loss of efficiency. The example of research on workers who work energetically but continuously versus those who have rest breaks was cited. The Type A style would encourage this hard-working pattern of "staying with it once you start, and seeing it through to the finish." However, the research has in fact dramatically demonstrated that even a brief coffee break permits a breather to regain concentration, avoid exhaustion, achieve a sort of "second wind," so that the work productivity actually increases. Thus, by giving up a little time, the end product is a significant gain in efficiency and output that more than makes up for the time. In a similar sense, the Type A characteristics might actually not be the most efficient style.

- was described as enabling them to to retain the beneficial elements of being Type A, would not change them into B's nor eliminate their success or drive levels. Type A individuals tend to perceive their Type A characteristic as the source of their major drive or motivation. Their fear is that altering their Type A characteristics occurs in an all-or-none fashion: either a person is completely a Type A and being Type A insures success and drive, or a person is stripped of all the Type A characteristics with the consequence of losing all drive and becoming a failure. It is clarified that a person can reduce some of the intensity of the Type A characteristics without losing all of the characteristics; that it is possible also to retain one's drive to succeed but in more efficient ways other than Type A ways, that one's high drive and high achievement motivations are likely to continue, and that altering one's Type A characteristics might involve knowing how to rely appropriately upon Type A characteristics, and when such characteristics are not essential.
- was presented as increasing their self-control. Type A persons typically also pride themselves on high levels of self-control. They drive themselves, set their own deadlines, are likely to discipline themselves in engaging in multiple activities, and see themselves as being self-motivated. Because of this valuing of self-control, the AMT program is explained as an appropriate form of training, since AMT emphasizes a method for increasing self-control.

Motivation. Accepting the fact that Type A's are high-drive and competitive, but also time impatient, we turned these traits around to work for us, by:

- announcing that by their very nature, they will want to speed up the pace of reaching the training goals, but

- that the challenge of the AMT training program was in achieving the skills through the "productive" way, which was to proceed at a steady pace. The comment was made: "I just know that some of you are going to want to try to get through this training as fast as you can, to see if you can beat the record. . . you wouldn't be Type A if you didn't have this impatient quality. (There is typically laughter as the participants recognize the accuracy of this insight.) However, the individuals who do the best job of acquiring the skill we'll be covering are those who make it a point to practice every step fully and completely, and who can develop the skill of doing this systematically and without rushing. In other words, there is a "Type A way" which will urge you to rush through and perhaps be a little sloppy, and there is a "productive way" which means being systematic and complete."

Homework. The pre-interview review at the start of each session which examines the progress made in the homework assignments (the format of this interview is described both in Chapter 7 and in Chapter 8) turned out to be a form of competition that was useful in maintaining motivation. Those who had shown compliance in homework practice were publicly praised by the therapist, leading noncompliant participants to work harder the next time. However, such competitiveness needs to be carefully monitored to insure that the striving does not become all-important and lead to misrepresenting actual progress at pre-interview review of homework, or post-interview of how well the session went.

Anxiety Scene. This is the major area in which AMT is adapted, with the anxiety scene referred to as the "stress" scene, and with the content derived from the characteristics common to Type A persons. Therefore scenes centered around stressors such as time impatience and anger/hostility elements. Examples from our clients are:

"I'm in my car, going home from work. . . this happens every day, but it was yesterday. . . warm in the car. . . I am at a traffic light that I just missed getting through, so I'm sitting and getting impatient. . . I'd like to get home and hate delays. . . I start to drum my fingers, turn to another radio station, can't find one I'm satisfied with. . . it's this waiting for no good reason that gets me. . . reminds me of waiting lines we have everywhere these days, a nuisance. . . I grip the steering wheel, I guess that's how I can tell I'm under stress, my hands start to clench. . . I'm thinking 'C'mon, c'mon light, turn, turn. . . "

"I'm having this meeting with some of my colleagues, one is reporting on his part of our project. He's one of these slow talkers, never gets to the point quickly. I'm thinking this meeting could be more efficient if I just did everything, I'm quicker and can get things done if only I didn't have to wait for others on the team. . . so he's reporting on the students he's interviewed. . . we're in the conference room in the Georgia building, and I'm sitting on this swivel chair at the head of the table. . . I'm thinking that I want to break in and shout, 'Get on with it, stop all this drivel' but I don't want to insult him. . . yet I'm getting angry inside, have to hold it in and not show it. . . I find myself interrupting and finishing his statments several times, so he is saying '_____' and before he finishes, I complete the statement with '_____'. . . all the time, I'm kind of moving fast in my thoughts, planning ahead, wishing this thing were over. . . knowing I have others I have to listen to. . . I want out!"

Homework assignments for transfer of the relaxation coping were readily identified in real life settings, since such stress experiences occurred almost daily. Applications thus involved using relaxation coping at traffic lights, in cashier lines, and in place of being stimulated to rush to complete a deadline ahead of time. As we will elaborate upon later, the use of AMT for the anger/hostility component of Type A persons, or other persons with difficulty in anger control, is also a very relevant part of the Type A training.

This AMT study and those of others, such as Hart, focused solely on the stress management approach in order to provide research confirmation of the importance of stress and the value of AMT. Although significant results were achieved, in practice other elements would be important to combine with AMT. Friedman *et al.* (1981) combined stress management with homework assignments, cognitive and values intervention, into a broad spectrum program. However, AMT should continue to have a core role in service delivery for Type A persons. Behavioral therapies appear to be particularly helpful in promoting Type A change with those Type A persons shown to be more reactive to stress (Jacob & Chesney, 1986). We know that anxiety induction procedures have proven their value with stress reduction. We also know that imagery induction is an important element in AMT. We also now know that Type A persons have been found particularly able to develop arousal with Type A-relevant stress imagery. Hence, it seems sensible again to conclude that AMT should be a major part of a therapist's armament for Type A treatment (Baker, Hastings, & Hart, 1984).

Essential Hypertension

Essential hypertension involves the presence of chronic elevated blood pressure with no known organic cause. It is estimated to account for 90% of the approximately 25 million cases of hypertension. Hypertension contributes heavily to the risk of heart disease, and heart disease is among the leading causes of death in the United States. Hypertension is clearly linked to stress (Shapiro, Benson, Chobanian, Herd, Julius, Kaplan, Lazarus, Ostfeld, & Syme, 1979) and is associated with sympathetic nervous system arousal, possibly involving norepinephrine and cortisol (Lawler, Cox, Sanders, & Mitchell, 1988; McGrady, Woerner, Bernal, & Higgins Jr., 1987). Humans exposed to repeated stressors are subject to hypertension: air traffic controllers annually develop hypertension at a pace nearly six times greater than pilots, and workers under constant noise stress tend to suffer from high blood pressure (Cobb & Rose, 1973; Jonsson & Hansson, 1978).

Anxiety Management Training

Given the role of stress in essential hypertension, AMT seems ideally suited as a treatment of choice, particularly since hypertensive stress involves chronic stress. This very chronicity implies that clients may need to develop stress management methods which not only cope with existing transient stressors, but also stressors which have persisted in the past and new stressors that may evolve in the future. AMT provides for generalization of the coping skill as well as enabling clients to show continued gains in the future, after therapy terminates.

An especially good example of the added advantage of AMT was the case reported by Bloom and Cantrell (1978). The client was actually the spouse of one author, who was found to be hypertensive in the initial trimester of her pregnancy. Both the obstetrician and the authors were reluctant to rely upon medication, for fear of the possible consequences for the fetus. Therefore, AMT was tried. The basic AMT method was used covering six treatment sessions over six weeks. Sample anxiety scenes were:

> "You're trying to get to your class on time, because it's important. . . but it's quite clear that you're going to be late. . . and this bothers you as you try to rush. . . "
>
> "You're sitting in the waiting room of your doctor's office. . . the waiting is giving you time to worry about how the baby is doing. . . you're apprehensive enough about the pregnancy, much less about the hypertension. . . your feelings are. . . "

Figure 10.1 illustrates the progress of blood pressure during baseline, treatment, and for an eight-week follow-up. The first trimester of the pregnancy had been just prior to the baseline period. The second trimester included the baseline period and the first two weeks of treatment. The third trimester of the pregnancy began with the four last weeks of treatment. As Figure 10.1 illustrates, blood pressure during baseline was declining already. This trend for blood pressure to decline

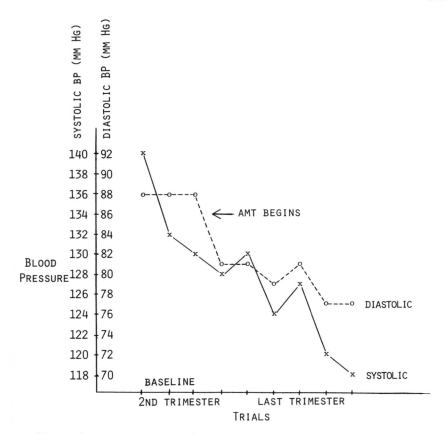

Figure 10.1. AMT results with hypertension. (From Bloom & Cantrell, 1978.)

during the baseline turned out to be consistent with known findings that blood pressure tends to rise in the first trimester, fall during the second, and rise again in the last trimester of pregnancy. Baseline for this client was taken during her second trimester, a period which is normally associated with blood pressure declines. The important results are in the third trimester, which corresponded to the last four weeks of AMT and the entire follow-up. What is seen in the results is the decline of blood pressure during treatment, that is, during the third trimester, a period in which blood pressure would be normally expected to be climbing. Hence, the effect of AMT appeared to be even greater than the measures actually showed. Also, the systolic and diastolic blood pressures during treatment reached normal levels, although the client had been hypertensive prior to treatment. During follow-up of eight more weeks, there was found some increases in blood pressure, although the mean systolic and diastolic blood pressure levels over this follow-up were still equivalent to that achieved during treatment (systolic mean at baseline = 133.14 mm Hg, at treatment = 124.50, at follow-up = 123.63; diastolic mean at baseline = 88.00 mm Hg., at treatment = 79.30, at follow-up = 81.25).

The application of AMT for hypertension does not require any changes in the basic AMT procedure. Perhaps the more important initial step is to assess the client's understanding that the hypertensive condition is associated with stress in the client's life. Without this appreciation, AMT may appear to be an irrelevant treatment plan and the client might drop out from therapy. The following intake procedure can be adopted to aid such clients:

- Exploration of other factors relating to hypertension in the client's life, such as amount of salt intake, use of stimulants such as caffeine, etc. While obtaining data through daily diaries on these factors, the therapist should include self-monitoring of stress levels and blood pressure as well. By imbedding the stress monitoring with monitoring of other factors more acceptable to the client, the therapist avoids conflict over the patient's beliefs.
- These diaries/logs can now be reviewed to determine whether there is a relationship between the reporting of stress and the client's level of reported blood pressure. Pennebaker (1982) reported that patients' systolic blood pressures were highly correlated with physical symptoms. This led others to speculate whether hypertensives could therefore monitor their blood pressures through their observations of their physical symptoms. Data has been quite inconclusive in replicating Pennebaker's results (Baumann & Leventhal, 1985; Stewart & Olbrisch, 1986). But even if clients are poor at estimating their blood pressure, the stress log alone can offer a source for intake discussions with the client at hand about the relevance of stress in the client's current life.

As with other medical disorders being reviewed for possible AMT treatment, hypertensive patients should have complete medical evaluations. This is meant to rule out any possible non-anxiety origins which are the primary determinant of the hypertension, with the therapist's own intake being aimed at ruling in the role of anxiety as a differential diagnosis. Such medical consultation can be extremely valuable, since medications or unique medical conditions can imitate anxiety reactions. I recall being stunned to discover that potassium was being prescribed to a case of mine involving symptoms of general anxiety and loss of emotional control. Even though I had required a full medical and laboratory workup before proceeding with the case based upon the intensity of the symptoms, the physician's course of action still came as a shock. Furthermore, the patient's laboratory report confirmed that her level of potassium was actually normal; the prescription was based on the internist's "intuition based upon nine years' experience." The client did regain more control over her emotionality with the potassium, however, she still was able to profit from AMT.

Given the availability of inexpensive home sphygnomamometers with some accuracy, the AMT therapist might include self-monitoring of blood pressure before and after events which are suspected to be stressors. This then can be used to strengthen the situational monitoring assignment following AMT session 4. Situations proven to raise blood pressure and which are experienced as stressors by the client would then be especially targeted for preventive use of relaxation coping. Naturally, such home equipment can also be used to obtain daily blood pressure records as indices of progress in AMT therapy.

Dysmenorrhea

Primary dysmenorrhea involves menstrual pain which occurs in the absence of known organic pelvic disease and composes one of the most common gynecological disorders. Primary spasmodic dysmenorrhea involves acute pain which begins with the onset of menstruation. Primary congestive dysmenorrhea involves more diffuse or dull aches occurring several days before the onset of menstruation. It is estimated that about one-third of women will suffer severe enough symptoms as to alter their daily routines, such as being absent from work, remaining in bed, or seeing a physician (Sommer, 1978). Spasmodic dysmenorrhea is considered to be the result of increased muscle tension and hence pain management might profitably focus on the region of this tension, the subabdominal area.

Anxiety Management Training

Quillen and Denney (1982) adapted AMT for particular application for women suffering from either spasmodic or congestive dysmenorrhea. The following shows the use of their AMT model for these types of clients:

Rationale. Clients are informed that the goal is the management of pain, and that they will learn a self-control approach to achieve this goal.

The role of muscle tension in pain can be explained and tied to the relaxation coping. One sample rationale would be as follows:

> "The pain you experience with your menstrual cycle is partly a function of your normal physiology, but might be made worse by the fact that your muscles are tensing up perhaps more than is typical. We know that a mild ache can become much more painful if we are also experiencing muscle tension in that same area. In addition, if your menstural period also happens to include a time of stress for you, a time during which you are particularly vulnerable to being tired and vulnerable to irritable moods, then these also tend to tighten up your muscles. Muscle tension is a common reflection of stress and tension and emotional conditions. All of which serve to increase your painful sensations. What we will be teaching you is a method for relaxing the muscles. In addition, we have learned that this muscle relaxation procedure also seems to be associated with helping a person be more resistant to stresses, to pressures, to things which cause further irritability. So by applying the relaxation skills which you will be learning, you will also be developing a method for controlling your menstrual pain."

Relaxation. The initial AMT session remains identical, with tension-relaxing as the procedure. Since the dysmenorrheic tension tends to be maximum in the subabdominal region, the relaxation is focused in this area. Session 2 also includes the briefer relaxation without the tensing. However, in addition the following is added:

- Turning off (distracting) sensations of pain through visualizing a warm, soothing liquid flowing from the abdominal region slowly downward to the knees,
- Clients use their hands to press their abdomen to simulate the pressure of menstrual pain, then they initiate relaxation of this area to neutralize the pressure,
- Similar simulation using the hands is used with the pelvic area and the thighs.

Pain (Menstrual Discomfort) Scenes and Relaxation Coping. Session 3 involves self-initiated relaxation, followed by menstrual discomfort scenes. Clients use these scenes to increase menstrual discomfort arousal, then apply the relaxation coping. Five scenes were identified in the study involving situations in which menstrual distress might appear, such as:

> "It's the middle of the night, you've been comfortable but suddenly awaken because you feel the menstrual pain beginning. . . there is that (acute, diffuse) pain. . . "
> "You have been menstruating but doing what you normally do to retain some comfort. . . you're sitting in a class on sociology with there being about five minutes before the end. . . you begin to feel the pain and your muscles are starting to cramp, you hope that this won't be happening. . . "

"You're out on a dinner date with your boyfriend, you've dressed up nicely and used your favorite body powder and perfume. . . you're at the table in _____ restaurant, your meal includes chicken Kiev. You've been having a nice conversation, and your boyfriend is looking at you as you are talking. . . you start to experience the bloated sensations, the discomfort that's inside you but not specifically in one place. . . and you start to lose that good feeling. . . "

Session 3 also introduces the typical instruction to pay attention to the cues asssociated with discomfort. The rest of the AMT for dysmenorrhea is similar to AMT for anxiety conditions, including the reliance upon prevention through early use of relaxation before the onset of dymenorrhea.

The results obtained from this AMT approach were successful for both spasmodic and congestive clients. Significant reductions were found for pain levels, discomfort, interference behaviors (i.e., staying in bed, loss of concentration), and time loss. The gains were maintained over the 18 month follow-up. An interesting unexpected outcome was the delay of menstruation following AMT, an outcome that is not necessarily recurrent among all AMT clients, but which the authors called attention to because it did occur several times. They recommend therefore that future clients be alerted to the possibility that such a delay can occur.

Tension Headaches

Tension or muscle contraction headaches involve recurring dull pressure and a band-like tightness at the forehead, the back of the head, and/or the neck. Tension headaches compose about 80% of headaches experienced, with headache complaints being the 14th most common symptom in medical general practices. The muscle contraction headache tends to last four hours and occurs in excess of five times monthly. Additional symptoms include fatigue, anxiety, tension, dizziness, and spots before the eyes. Nausea and vomiting are not common. Onset is gradual (Feuerstein & Gainer, 1982). Migraine headaches are different, and involve an aura that is a sensory precursor of the headache, nausea, vomiting, and pulsing pain.

Anxiety Management Training

Muscle contraction headache sufferers appear to be characterized by skeletal muscular tension of the shoulders (Williamson, 1981) and higher resting autonomic arousal (Cohen, Williamson, Monguillot, Hutchinson, Gottlieve, & Waters, 1983). Also, as might be expected, stress plays a major role as a precursor to the headache pain (Gannon, Haynes, Cuevas, & Chavez, 1987). Given the role of stress, AMT should be a perfect match for tension headache patients. However, only one report has indirectly evaluated the efficacy of AMT for this problem. Suinn and Vattano (1979), using the AMT model, treated severe headache patients and reported a reduction in the frequency of tension headaches, but not in the intensity of headaches. In effect, once a tension headache appeared, it was full-blown.

Where AMT is used with a client with muscle-contraction headaches, the major revisions involve the relaxation training and the use of time monitoring. Since the muscle contraction is likely to involve the neck and shoulder regions, relaxation training should emphasize gaining control over these areas. Teaching relaxation of the neck can be achieved by having the client first bend the head to the left to tense the muscles, then to the right side. For the shoulders, shrugging will accomplish the necessary tensing. An example of the instructions for relaxation would be as follows:

> (Instructions for the hands, arms, head are as usual: see Appendix C). . . (for the neck and shoulders the instruction would be:) ". . . All right, now we'll pay a little more attention to your neck and shoulders since these are the areas that typically cause the tension headaches. . . first let me have you bend your head to the left side. . . now really stretch the neck muscle as you do this. . . notice the tenseness this creates in the neck. . . this is muscle tension. . . (hold this for about five to ten seconds). . . really tense and tight. . . now relax the muscles by straightening your head, and notice the relaxation taking over, much more relaxed (about ten seconds). . . now once more tense up the neck by bending your head to the left and really stretch that muscle. . . noticing the tension, the tightness. . . O.K., now relax by straightening up your head and just enjoy the relaxation taking over. . . next, we'll have you do the same thing but by bending your head to the right side. . . O.K., right now, let's have you bend your head to the right side, so that you're really stretching, tensing the neck muscle. . . (and so forth for three repetitions for tension headache clients; more repetitions can be added if the therapist feels such extra attention is appropriate for better training). . .
>
> Now, we'll move to the shoulders. . . in order to tense up the shoulders I'm going to have you shrug them. . . like you're going to have them reach to your ears. . . so right now shrug your shoulders, really high. . . like they're trying to reach your ears . . . very tense, very tight. . . notice that tenseness and how it feels. . . now relax them. . . " (and so forth for three repetitions).

In time monitoring, the best guess is that tension headaches are the consequences of the gradual building of skeletal muscle tightness over a course of about 2–3 hours. In order to abort this chronic tension and therefore the headache, the client is taught to do time monitoring every two hours.

Again, as with all medical conditions, accurate diagnosis is important. Certainly the separate diagnosis of muscle contraction from migraine headaches is crucial. Also, other types of headache-like syndromes should be assessed, such as myofascial pain-dysfunction syndrome also known as temporomandibular joint pain syndrome (Scott, 1981).

Diabetes

Insulin-dependent diabetes is the result of inadequate insulin production by the pancreas. It is a chronic disease and the most common endocrine disorder of childhood. Symptoms involve fatigue, excessive thirst and urination, and weight loss despite eating. Although blood sugar may be abnormally high, the lack of insulin prevents utilization of this sugar and the individual may lapse into a coma. Approximately 150,00 children and adolescents are diagnosed as suffering from this disorder. Stress has been examined since insulin production is further decreased, blood glucose is affected, and urine volume increased, all of which influence the patient's diabetes metabolic stability (Hanson & Pichert, 1986; Johnson, 1980).

Anxiety Management Training

Rose, Firestone, Heick, and Faught (1983) have the only published research on AMT. They relied upon AMT on the supposition that control over emotional stress would be the outcome, which in turn would lead to more stable metabolic control over glucose. Patients were provided with seven hours of AMT over a two-week period, a very short treatment time. However, follow-up training involved assigning each patient an audiotape for future relaxation practice, to be used three times per week at minimum. Furthermore, they were reminded to use the relaxation control for stress management over the next 2–5 months. On a multiple baseline design, diabetes control was considered positively improved through the AMT training. Given the lack of further replication at this time, and given the complexity of diabetes, we can only comment that this use of AMT is a promising one, but one which needs further cautious investigation by clinical researchers and practitioners.

Summary

AMT has its best applications in behavioral medicine where there is a stress component or arousal level involved. For instance, the result with regard to essential hypertension seems to be a strong application as AMT permits the client to cope with the stress conditions which influence the blood pressure. Certainly, tension headaches should be amenable to AMT intervention, with the special emphasis in training on relaxation of the neck and shoulder muscles, and on time monitoring to prevent muscle tension from building throughout the day. The results on the Type A behavioral pattern were initially stimulated by my theorizing that anxiety is a crucial part of the daily experiences of Type A persons, brought about by their own characteristics. For instance, the self-imposed deadlines and tendency to engage in multiple tasks simultaneously would be expected to be associated with stress. Further, we speculated that Type A persons were unwilling or unable to change their behaviors because of anxiety reduction. Each time the Type A person meets his/her deadline or completes a task, this reinforces the sense of achievement and satisfies the sense of competitiveness. But it also reduces the anxiety or stress associated with this activity; and anxiety reduction has been proven to be a form of reinforcement that prevents a behavior from extinction. Finally, the evidence of AMT's application to anger management, and the attention to anger and hostility as part of the link of Type A behaviors and cardiovascular disease, complete the rationale for using AMT with Type A individuals. The use of AMT with dysmenorrhea and with certain forms of diabetes raises interesting possibilities, although research is still sorely needed. With dysmenorrhea the AMT procedure is revised to focus on pain, although stress reduction in and of itself can have pain reducing benefits. For diabetes, the hypothesis is that stress may be a contributor to diabetic disregulation symptoms.

This chapter sought not only to highlight the possible behavioral medicine applications of AMT, but also to provide illustrations of the revisions needed in the AMT procedure. Where necessary, we have provided some exact quotes regarding revisions in the rationale or method for obtaining anxiety scenes. Further illustration is also found in Chapter 5, for example, regarding tension headaches. Finally, we should note that AMT might well be appropriate for the patients seeing family practice physicians or in similar medical settings where broad somatic symptoms are presented. As we noted in Chapter 3 on the Scientific Evidence for AMT, research has discovered that many medical patients appear to have symptoms which may be more due to stress than to a physical disease process.

11

Human Performance Enhancement

Thus far, we have been demonstrating the applications of Anxiety Management Training to different types of human disorders. In each case maladaptive behaviors are implicitly assumed to be characteristic of the help-seeker. In this chapter, no such assumption is made. Instead we are working with persons who have proven themselves to be extremely talented but whose life setting confronts them with stresses not usually faced by others with less talent. We are referring to athletes, musicians, theatre and dance performers.

The Elite Athlete

The Olympic athlete epitomizes the normal person confronting abnormal stressors. At the same time, even the varsity athlete playing for his/her own high school shares such stress in common with the elite world class competitor. Unlike the nonparticipant in organized sport, these competitive athletes are involved in seeking success simultaneously on two levels: their own routine daily lives, and their athletic lives. These persons are committed to traditional activities such as those at work or school, but also to activities preparing for competition such as training and practice. With the modern development of sport psychology (Mahoney & Suinn, 1986), stress management for these healthy individuals has become an essential factor in performance enhancement (Suinn, 1986b).

By performance enhancement, we refer to the means for reaching one's potential rather than remediation of deficits, or the removal of unique obstacles to free up skills instrumental for reaching such potential. At all times, the individual involved is accepted as possessing the normal level of adaptive skills for the more normative life issues. On the other hand, the athlete, for instance, must additionally confront the stress of competition, the need to be at maximum efficiency for the right amount of time and at the right time, and the ability to weather internal or external stressors that may interfere with the learning or display of higher level performance skills.

Anxiety Management Training

AMT's special contribution to athletic performance can be seen in three types of benefits: its use for multiple or extraordinary events, its use for endurance enhancement, and it use for recovery from injury.

Multiple or Extraordinary Events. Regarding multiple or extraordinary events, we are calling upon the unique ability of individuals trained in AMT to be able to transfer the stress management skill to diverse settings and events. Remember that AMT proved superior in its being applied by clients to situations different from the anxiety scenes used within AMT sessions. For competitive situations that have multiple or changing conditions, AMT is ideally suited. One clear example of a multiple condition is the high-glamor Olympic track and field event, the decathlon. Here the athlete must be prepared for 10 different types of distinctive challenges, each with a different type of psychological stressor. I have had the opportunity to use AMT for the military version of the decathlon, the Modern Pentathlon, which is more stressful in some ways, even though having less events. The pentathlon demands outstanding skills in pistol shooting, horseback riding, fencing, running, and swimming. The first three, when combined, probably represent the most intense stressors for even the best Olympians. For the U.S. team, the policy has been to identify those persons who appear naturally gifted in running and/or swimming, and to make these persons into decent marksmen, riders, and fencers. The reason is the belief that speed is innate and therefore there are limits to how much faster a person can move through even the best training. There is in fact scientific proof that sprinters have innate "fast twitch" muscles associated with bursts of speed, different from the "slow twitch" muscles associated more with endurance over long distances.

CASE HISTORY:
    Allen, who had missed earning a place on the prior Olympic Team, was a hopeful for the next Olympics in the Modern Pentathlon event. As with the majority of elite U.S. competitors in the pentathlon, Allen was in the military, spending most of his tour of

duty stationed at the training center for pentathlon. Allen was actually a youngster, 19 years old, who had been an outstanding runner in high school and on the swimming team. In the military, he found a home in this multiple event sport despite his inexperience with shooting and his total lack of exposure to either horses or to fencing.

When we met, Allen was already a likely candidate for the Olympic Team, with his strengths in running and swimming. However, these were the last events in the coming meet, and he felt he simply had to do well in shooting, and hold his own in horsemanship and fencing. There are unusual stresses in each of these events. In his view: "Shooting is rapid-fire, you have a time limit and must squeeze off all your rounds when the target turns to face you. . . since it's automatically controlled there's the psychological pressure. Then you have to sit down and wait while the judges inspect your target. The longer they take, and the more they discuss, the more you think you didn't do well. And then there's the pressure of knowing that when they finish, they post your score for everyone to know. So you sit and try to keep occupied, to keep your mind off what's going on.

"Now, for me, riding is the most chancy. We don't get to bring our own horse, they have a stable of new horses, and you get a random draw. If you're lucky, it'll be a good horse, an easy one to ride. If you're not, then you could be in with one that's nasty. I never rode before, I was never near a horse growing up. So these animals can be scary for some of us. Do you realize how big a horse is, and how dangerous the riding can be. . . I mean you can fall and really get hurt, and there goes all your hard work."

Given the mutiple events of the pentathlon and time constraints for training, AMT was the clear treatment of choice. For the 90 intensity scene, Allen selected the pistol shooting event:

"It was my very first international competition, and I was on the very first position. . . I couldn't believe I was actually competing. I had just fired my last round, and we were all seated as the judges were at my target inspecting it. The longer they take, the more you wonder about your score. . . did you actually miss the target completely. . . this can happen. . . I'm waiting, trying to not think about anything, but I'm fooling myself. . . I keep looking at the judges. . . I think how terrible if I missed. . . I was O.K. before, but I'm starting to get tight inside, feeling my neck get sore. . . my heart is pounding now, like I've swallowed something huge that's beating away. . . feeling real hot, sweaty. . . can I calm down for the next event. . . they're going to post my score, I know it. . . everyone will see if I did badly. . . am I good enough to really be in this competition. . . ?"

Allen had been exceptionally responsive to relaxation training, since he had tried his own version before fencing events, and highly motivated to use sport psychology training such as AMT for his events. Because of his progress in relaxation and imagery control, and his ability to regain relaxation after arousal, and because I was scheduled to leave the next day, AMT was speeded up by reliance only on the 90 intensity scene (actually AMT had been originally designed to use only one intense scene; the second was later added to the procedure to promote more generalization). The meet the coming day was an international one, and included a former bronze medalist. I was able to watch the shooting, horsemanship, and fencing events, but did not know of the final outcome since my plane left before the final two events. Allen telephoned the next day to report that he felt particularly good about AMT with the shooting, had found himself comfortable and in control in riding, and was just trying keep it all together in fencing. Most important, he actually had his best performance in his career, leading to winning the meet!

Allen applied the relaxation coping at several times during the competition:

- On the evenings in between the events, he used only the relaxation as a procedure for getting to sleep. As indicated earlier, he was particularly good at accomplishing a relaxed state.
- Since he had selected a pistol shooting experience as his 90 intensity scene for AMT training, it turned out that he found himself almost automatically relaxing when he actually encountered this event during the meet. I noticed his taking a few deep breaths, and his closing his eyes as he was waiting for the judges to declare that everything was in order. He later told me that he had closed his eyes to concentrate further on relaxing his arms and shoulders, since this would help his steadiness in shooting, and would also keep him calm.
- For the horsemanship, he prepared himself as he was walking to his horse, focusing on keeping his entire body loose, comfortable, and relaxed. Since he was somewhat uncomfortable about the strange horse he had drawn, he kept his attention on his shoulders, keeping them relaxed. This tended to accomplish not only retaining the relaxation and preventing anxiety from building up, but also kept him from staring at the horse and thereby becoming anxious at seeing the beast.
- For the fencing, which involved intense periods of battling followed by long periods of no activity, he used the rest periods to sit with a towel over his head. Under this towel, he reviewed his muscle groups, looking for any signs of tenseness from the prior bout. If there were any signs, he practiced relaxing those muscles involved.

The appropriateness of AMT for multiple events entails not only the multiple events of a pentathlon, but also multiple in the sense of changing competitive situations. For instance, changing conditions would include facing the challenge of a different opponent each round, or being in a stadium with totally different characteristics, or with an audience that is sometimes demanding, sometimes outright rude. The ability of AMT results to generalize is especially useful.

AMT is also valid for extraordinary events, again for the transferability of the skill. It is difficult enough to transfer from the practice court or field to the real competition; as much as an athlete pretends that practice is like the real thing, everyone knows it is not fully comparable in terms of the emotions generated. Consider how much more critical it is to be preparing for the extraordinary event of the Olympic Games or the World Championships or the National Championships. . . or, for a young athlete, even the city school championships. Preparing for the worst upon entering the Moscow Stadium, with an audience of intense patriotism and loyalty, and in a country viewed as anti-American, is in fact an extraordinary circumstance. For such settings, AMT should be the first type of stress management program considered; since AMT does not rely heavily upon the specific stimulus conditions, but emphasizes coping in the presence of anxiety arousal. Then the conditions creating the anxiety arousal are really secondary. Hence, once the athlete learns AMT coping, it does not matter if the stress derives from jitters prior to a local meet, or the major tensions from the Olympic Games.

Endurance Enhancement. The presence of tension may actually not be as major a concern for short-distance performance, but can become magnified for the longer distances. Being somewhat tense may have little influence on a 100-yard sprinter, but could lead to cramps, loss of time, or even failure to finish for a marathoner. The basic premise is that stress leads to muscle tension, and this tension uses up precious energy. For the endurance sport, such energy can drastically interfere with peak performance.

Ziegler, Klinzing, and Williamson (1982) trained well-conditioned members of a men's cross-country track team with either AMT or SIT. In exercise physiology, the efficiency of the athlete is readily measured through the analysis of oxygen consumption, under a workload controlled by a treadmill test. On a 20-minute treadmill run, both AMT and SIT athletes showed increased efficiency as shown by their lower oxygen consumption and lower heart rate, while a control group did not show such improvements (Figures 11.1 and 11.2). Sample anxiety scenes for AMT include:

> "You're in the meet against Ohio State. . . you were running pretty smoothly to the beginning of the hill. . . now you're noticing that your breathing is harsher and you start to feel some tightness in your left leg. . . you begin to worry about cramping up. . . you just came off a really poor race. . . and

you're starting to feel like the heat is going to get to you. . . you're feeling discouraged, because you really want to do well, but you're breathing is now in spurts and you start to make sounds with each exertion. . . you're really mad at yourself. . . "

"It's the day of the regionals, and you're on the field warming up and stretching. . . you haven't felt good since arriving. . . didn't sleep well. . . you notice the other competitors and start to feel anxious. . . your whole body feels like a violin, all strung up, tight like a bow. . . stiff. . . you can't bend your body into loosening up. . . you're feeling nauseous with the butterflies that won't go away, feel like throwing up. . . "

A very interesting part of this study was the researchers' interest in knowing more about what was going on in the "inner athlete" following training, hence they interviewed the competitors. The SIT trained athletes reported feeling more confidence, ability to control stress over "those little things that get in your way," and an increased appreciation for how positive thoughts can be helpful. The AMT trained competitors felt they had a new mental set for preparation, an increased confidence in handling "emergency stress" during competition, and an awareness that stress could be handled rather than being "something you just had to live with."

Based upon similar premises about muscle tension and endurance, Suinn, Morton, and Dickinson (1980) also tested varsity team cross-country runners. An AMT-like approach showed improvements in oxygen consumption, with greater gains for the women athletes than for the men. The instructions are described in more detail in Chapter 5 as part of that chapter's case illustrations.

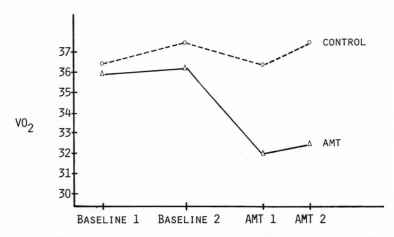

Figure 11.1. VO$_2$ consumption on treadmill test. (From Ziegler, Klinzing, & Williamson, 1982.)

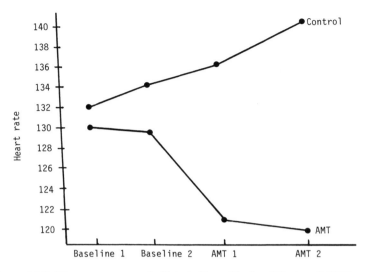

Figure 11.2. Heart rate on treadmill test. (From Ziegler, Klinzing, & Williamson.)

Recovery from Injury. AMT can be applied for the problems of sports injury. A major accident or injury can prove not only physically debilitating, but can also entail exteroceptive learning similar to a minor situational anxiety state. A football player who pulls a hamstring on a wet field, cutting away from a defensive back, can become conditioned to fear a similar injury when on a similar field. Even given assurances from the surgeon that the tendon has been repaired to be stronger than before, there can still be the unconscious tendency to hold back. In keeping with our discussion of social learning principles, the more intense and hurtful the pain during the initial injury, the greater the avoidance conditioning.

AMT can be used along the same guidelines as for treatment of situational anxieties, except that the anxiety scene used is the single incident of the injury. One revision, however, that makes this retraining with AMT complete is the addition of other imagery involving positive outcomes, for instance, having the running back now envision making the cut strongly and firmly, and completing the run successfully (Suinn, 1984). This approach leads to the AMT working more like desensitization but in a brief application. The anxiety scene should also avoid retrieving the total intensity of the pain, but instead should be used to prompt the early stages of the injury event, with the relaxation being used to abort the pain arousal. Hence, the anxiety scene guided rehearsal would actually be in two stages:

Stage One, Controlling the Pain: "In a moment I'll have you switch on the injury scene, the one (label scene). . . just at the moment when you began to feel the tendons under pressure, signal me and we'll immediately go to relaxation. . . O.K. switch on the injury scene right now. . . (signal). . . All right, switch off that scene and focus on relaxation. . . releasing the pressure. . . "

Stage Two, Completion of Recovery: "In a moment I'll have you switch on the scene of the linebacker charging at you, and you sidestepping by him. . . the grass was wet, but you were running full speed, and then cutting by the linebacker to slip away. . . this time, I want you to complete this move, and to successfully escape the tackle, and then turning it on down the field. . . feeling strong in this move. . . All right, right now, switch on. . . "

The use of AMT for injury recovery requires this type of revision. In contrast, AMT for preparation for coping with stress for multiple or extraordinary events, or for endurance enhancement, do not require such revisions, but is conducted in the standard manner. The primary difference is that recovery from injury involves a real situation when an actual injury has occurred. Hence, it is to be expected, possibly through classical conditioning principles, that the athlete might have been conditioned to react with self-protecting behaviors to the situational cues, for instance, when running again on wet grass. By having the athlete rehearse the successful scene, this replaces the conditioned negative reaction. On the other hand, for other competition events where failure, damage, or injury has not occurred, the usual AMT procedure has proven sufficient to eliminate or control the anxiety. I should remark that I have sometimes used guided rehearsal involving the "Stage Two" recovery or success type of scenes for clients who are phobic, anxious, under stress, even though I have just argued that this is not essential for their recovery. Adding this approach can be a helpful adjunct to build efficacy, or to provide the client with practice in success behaviors beyond the anxiety-management behaviors of applied relaxation.

Enhancing Musical Performance

In working with the first musician to raise the question of improvement on music performance, my first thought was to wonder just how vivid would be the auditory aspects of the guided rehearsal. This was of concern in spite of earlier experiences with athletes that confirmed that the anxiety imagery following relaxation training was multisensory. Nevertheless, for athletes a primarily visual and proprioceptive vividness would be satisfactory, but the musician is reliant upon auditory cues on the darkened stage. On the other hand, the musician is also superbly trained to process and be aware dominantly via sound. As it turns out, the imagery for a musician can be vivid in all dimensions, sight and sound and all the others. Any difficulties are not caused by the fact that the sensory domain is auditory, but are rather general problems of imagery control. As we said in Chapter 9, the usual solution to such problems is to do a little more training in relaxation. It seems to me that always preceding imagery rehearsal with good relaxation is what provides for the type of realistic imagery and control that is needed. Without the relaxation, the imagery can slip into being the more artificial mental practice or role playing (Suinn, 1982).

The consequences of anxiety for the musician with a wind instrument includes interference with breath control. The anxiety can produce shallow breathing and hence weakened "power" of the musical note, or erratic breathing rhythm such that wind reserves are not available at the proper moments. For the instrumental musician where wind is not a factor, the interference may be in other ways. If the somatic subsystem is the dominant area of symptoms, then even minor motor trembling can mean lack of "cleanness" in a musical phrase or improper timing. If the cognitive subsystem is affected, then the musician's concentration could be lost, perhaps leading to as blatant an outcome as losing one's place or even forgetting the memorized score. An example of an anxiety scene would be the following:

> "You're having the trumpet solo during the concert performance. . . this is for the commencement exercise, it is spring, May. . . you are sitting in the brass section. . . the crowd has settled down, a large, interested crowd. . . you notice many looking at the orchestra players, feel many are actually looking at you. . . you have this brief rest period when you are not playing. . . fiddling with your fingers. . . wondering if you can handle that passage smoothly. . . feel a little tight in the chest. . . leading to you catching your breath, your breathing doesn't feel right. . . little catch in your throat too. . . thinking, 'gotta be smooth, mellow' . . . everyone will know if you aren't right on. . . thinking 'can't rush it, that's your common error when you're nervous, to rush'. . . "

For musicians preparing for improved performance for their major solo, the AMT training will approximate that of using AMT for athletic injury. For the injury, the AMT arousal avoided the full exposure to the pain of the injury incident. Furthermore, there is a "Step Two" in the guided rehearsal which includes a scene of correctly completing the task; for the musician it would be performing the musical passage fluently and smoothly. AMT also aims at achieving prevention of anxiety arousal, so that the musician is not faced with anxiety arousal during the critical stages of performing. For the musician who must perform perfectly there is simply no time for time-out moments for reinstating coping. Contrast the demands for test anxiety, for instance. During the test, any recurrence of anxiety is dealt with by the client returning to relaxation for coping. Meanwhile, the client need not be answering the question on the test paper. Even in public speaking, the client can afford a brief pause that will seem natural, take a calm breath and trigger off the coping. The musician in the midst of a musical phrase does not have the same opportunity. Therefore, the identifying of early warning signals prior to entering the performance hall or going on stage becomes even more important. The musician should be especially attentive to monitoring these early warning signals, and to initiate preventive relaxation so that the anxiety is prevented from having any effects.

Regarding this prevention phase of AMT, the application of AMT for musical performance enhancement is similar to the prevention procedures for all groups. With time and situational monitoring and with the awareness of early warning signals, all clients eventually learn to deal with anxiety "before it starts." The test anxious student can initiate controlled relaxation prior to entering the examination room, and the public speaker can relax while walking to the front of the room. In the same way, the musician can use the relaxation to remain in control prior to being on stage. And the previously injured athlete can keep his stress subsystems under control prior to running onto the field.

Except for this ultimate emphasis on emphasizing the prevention stage of AMT, the training for musicians would follow the usual model. Where the solo represents the crucial part of the performance, the scene setting cues would involve not only the environment, but also the bars in the musical score leading up to the solo.

Enhancing Theater and Dance Performance

Here the application of AMT is identical to that for traditional referral problems. As with Olympic athletes, it sometimes amazes me that even professional stage performers experience anxiety, until I again remember that these are normal persons often facing abnormal stress. Also, it is not simply the experience of anxiety that connotes maladjustment, since everyone is subject to such experiences. Anxiety is no more than a built-in human mechanism that cautions that some threat exists, an innate early warning signal to prevent real harm. The stressors facing professional performers may be specific to their circumstances. The following case provides a sense for such situations:

CASE HISTORY:
    A professional dancer from a popular off-Broadway show had many first-night openings, since the show was now on the road.

Although interpersonal conflicts, home and family issues, and career difficulties were routinely handled by a New York psychological consultant, Jennifer visited the Lake Placid Olympic Training Center. She had heard of the use of sport psychologists for performance enhancement and was interested in similar training. I was available to see her, and we worked together on identifying the stressor cues related to a stress scene for AMT:

"Even though we are all supportive of one another, still dancers cannot help but watch one another to see who's doing best, even for that night's peformance, since the best performer may change from night to night. So you know that it's your friends on the stage who may be your most intense critics, and not the audience in the theater. . . unless you know that the theater critics from the media are in attendance. Still you play *to* the audience, but you're always aware inside you that the other dancers are watching, watching, watching. Opening night, of course, is special. No matter how many times, it never gets old. You're excited, and that's usually good, it gives you fire and motivation. The trick is to not let it get into nervous tension to such a level as to ruin your fluidity or grace or timing or getting into the dance itself."

The stress scene we used involved:

"It's opening night in New York. . . you're in the wings just before your entrance. . . your entrance is slow and dramatic and you are in a pose. You feel the excitement, and it builds inside your body. . . on the verge of being too strong and like a force that could take you over, instead of you being in control. . . you don't want this to happen, you must control your body. . . you are aware of the other dancers. 'Are you going to be good enough? They can tell. They demand perfection. Are you better than they are tonight?'. . . The excitement builds as you make your entrance, it's starting to wash over you, too excited, too many thoughts, must be more relaxed. . . " (scene switched off, relaxation on)

The stress scene obviously did not have extreme intensity anxiety for this performer, although it could for other performers. Jennifer really only needed to sharpen her self-control skills a bit, since the stress reactions were nowhere near being severely disruptive. Training was for one day, similar to that for Allen, since Jennifer also turned out to be quite responsive to relaxation and guided rehearsal imagery. She was well received in her next opening, especially by the critics who singled her out in their columns. Both Allen and Jennifer illustrate the potential for AMT sessions to be speeded up. AMT aims at skill development, and the pace of the learning experience can be adjusted to how readily the client is capable of acquiring the relaxation, the imagery arousal, and the relaxation coping skills. In traditional use of AMT, with clients for whom relaxation is new and unique in their lives, the first two AMT sessions are spaced a week apart in order to insure proper relaxation competencies. Also, the anxiety scenes for clients or patients tend to be intense and disruptive. Further, such individuals have few coping or adaptive skills. Hence, the pace of AMT is more conservative, with homework reports and pre- and post-interviews providing more direct information on whether the pace can be escalated. For this athlete and dancer, it was possible to mass training into 1–2 days, with some breaks for interviewing to identify progress in the various skills.

Summary

The application of AMT to performance enhancement is actually a logical extension of stress management as a program. In fact, my first initiation in the area of sport psychology was because my interests in stress matched the needs of a ski team, which needed stress-reduction training. The advantage of working with elite athletes or dance performers is the fact that many have already been exposed to the value of and the technique of relaxation training. In fact, it is not uncommon to discover a person who had learned the tension-relaxation method as part of a physical education course. Approaching some athletes involves issues similar to work with Type A persons. Both groups of individuals tends to be self-assured and initially less willing to admit to either stress or the need for help. The more successful the individual has become in his/her endeavor, the more delicate is the issue of whether outside help is needed, or for that matter, any help. However, as with the Type A person, athletes generally become responsive upon recognizing that stress management is a skill routinely adopted by elite and Olympic athletes across the world, and can provide the individual with an 'edge' to achieve one's potential during competition. For the theater arts performer, the role of stress is often recognized in the opening night jitters which disrupts motor coordination or voice or breath control.

Thus far, the various applications of AMT have developed more from direct clinical experiences than from controlled research studies, although there are a smattering of research reports. AMT is especially useful where there are multiple stressors from changing events or from changing settings. The case of Allen in the Modern Pentathlon is a prime illustration of a multiple-event stress, and an excellent example of the usefulness of AMT. Theater performers who are in traveling shows so that there are many "opening nights," or who must audition for different producers under diverse conditions would represent an example of stress that is triggered by differing settings.

The few studies of the value of stress reduction through AMT for endurance events is an interesting one. The improvement in efficiency of consumption of energy demonstrates a purely physiological benefit of stress management. Ordinarily, we tend to think of AMT as improving one's psychological or emotional status, but here is an example of an actual physiological gain. On the other hand, the application of AMT to recover from the psychological residuals of injury is a sensible extension of AMT. Accomplishing this application involves a modification of the AMT approach, but this is readily accomplished.

Perhaps the most intriguing aspect of my clinical experience is the short-term possibilities of AMT. In a number of circumstances, I had very little time with the athlete or performer, sometimes as brief as one day. Hence a full AMT set of sessions had to be truncated to: one hour of relaxation training, with many repetitions of the relaxation scene and muscle review; and one to two hours of anxiety arousal followed by relaxation modeled after AMT session 2. To avoid fatigue, there is usually a rest period introduced between the first and second anxiety-arousal periods. This also permits an interview to determine progress. These short-term AMT sessions have usually been conducted under necessity, because of the travel schedule of either the performer/athlete or myself. Two factors are important for me to monitor: first, the ability of the individual to acquire the relaxation skill; and secondly, the ability of the individual to experience the arousal and the return to relaxation. In the few cases of short-term training which I have accepted, both of these were present and probably the key to the success.

12

Intense Emotions

Thus far, we have limited the discussion to details regarding AMT for traditional applications, such as anxiety conditions, or for performers. We did discuss, however, the new appropriateness of AMT as a more general impulse control procedure. Anxiety and phobias involve a state of arousal, an impulse of sorts. The restlessness of generalized anxiety disorder may be the behavioral aspect of the impulse seeking an outlet. For the phobic disorder, the impulse is escape or avoidance. With the conceptualization of AMT as an arousal, impulse control procedure, then other forms of emotional arousal would be subject to AMT management. These include anger along with the impulse to strike out, and frustration along with the impulse to break free. It would make sense for AMT to be examined for hyperactivity control, although we actually have only theory and no research nor case experiences. We do have research for anger control, and some case experience for frustration. Finally, this chapter will provide illustrative case material for another type of disorder with severe emotional loss of control, post-traumatic stress disorder (PTSD).

Anger Management

The importance of general anger states, akin to general anxiety, has reached a new level of prominence. This tendency to become easily and frequently angered and to be out of control over the arousal, contributes to verbal or physical aggressiveness, personal injury and property damage, ineffective problem solving or maladaptive withdrawal, child or spouse abuse, and health problems such as essential hypertension or cardiovascular disease (Deffenbacher, Demm, & Brandon, 1986; Gentry, Chesney, Gary, Hall, & Harburg, 1982; Krantz, Contrada, Hill, & Friedler, 1988; Novaco, 1979). Anger and hostility have been highlighted as perhaps the most critical features of Type A behaviors that link to heart disease, with one study reporting that hostility is predictive of the incidence of heart attacks and cardiac deaths at a 10-year follow-up of 1800 patients (Barefoot, Williams, Dahlstrom, & Dodge, 1987; Hearn, Murray, & Luepker, 1989; MacDougall, Dembroski, Dimsdale, & Hackett, 1985; Shekelle, Gale, Mostfeld, & Paul, 1983). Finally, anger expression was found to be significantly correlated with health problems in a national survey of 1277 black adults (Hohnson & Broman, 1987).

Anxiety Management Training

The application of AMT to anger control is a straightforward one, with simple substitution of "anger" for "anxiety." The following format is recommended:

Rationale. "AMT is a procedure which will help you develop control over those strong angry impulses. Instead of being overwhelmed by them, we'll be teaching you a method to eliminate the strong feelings. . . etc."

Anger Scene. Similar to anxiety scenes, 60 and 90 intensity scenes are identified, from real life incidents. The scene setting details are in the way of those cues that basically are the provocations for the anger.

The feeling-oriented components of the scene are similar to anxiety scenes in identifying the autonomic, somatic, or cognitive elements associated with the anger response.

As with anxiety scenes, the anger scenes avoid content that is maladaptive. For instance, it is unacceptable to have the scene, "You are raging inside and you can't stop yourself, so you cuss out your supervisor" or "In order to stop his words from getting to you and making you more angry, you shut him out of your mind." Acceptable scenes, however, would be: "You are raging inside and you want to cuss out your supervisor," or "You keep getting mad because he is calling you names, and you want to shut him out, but you continue to hear his outburst. . . " (these are acceptable scenes provided that these events actually characterize the client's real reactions).

The therapist should exercise great caution about using a scene with unacceptable elements. If such unacceptable events are described, the therapist has two options. As a first and preferred option, the therapist should search for a different scene with acceptable elements. If such a reality scene is impossible to identify, then the only available option is to use the early portions of the scene leading up to the moments involving the unacceptable behaviors, and then ending the scene at that point. By this time, it is likely that the anger arousal will have been accomplished using the situational scene-setting cues.

For instance, consider the scene:

> "I was in the bar. . . and the fella in the next booth had just insulted me by saying, 'I think you drink just like a woman. . . and you smell like one too'. . . and I was humiliated. . . my friends were with me, egging me on, saying 'Are you going to stand for that?'. . . and I knew I was really angry, fuming, burning up. . . I was reaching that point of no return. . . my fists were bunching up, I was seeing red. . . and I couldn't stop myself, I just rushed over, arms flailing, letting it all bust out. . . "

If there are no other options available, then this scene could be used but truncated as follows:

> "You are in the bar. . . the fella in the next booth had just insulted you by saying, 'I think you drink just like a woman. . . and you smell like one too'. . . and you are feeling humiliated. . . your friends are egging you on, saying 'Are you going to stand for that?'. . . and you're really angry, fuming, burning up. . . hands bunching, seeing red. . . just let that anger build to that level. . . noticing how that anger feels again at this high level. . . concentrating on the experience of the anger. . . now switch off the scene and return to the relaxation. . . "

AMT Sessions. The AMT sessions for anger management duplicate the sessions for anxiety management, such as the use of guided rehearsal for anger arousal followed by relaxation coping, the fading of therapist guidance, the use of homework, including time and situational monitoring, the identification of early warning signals, and practice in prevention. Anger logs are substituted for Stress logs, but have the same elements.

The following is a case illustration of anger management with AMT:

> David is currently unemployed as a result of his temper. He is an exceptionally good automobile mechanic, and was actually managing the Phillips service station. However, he continued to feel put upon by his employer and often perceived customers as demanding too much for too little. He did what was necessary, but found it hard to hide his impatience when customers did not have the right change or couldn't make up their minds about whether to purchase cigarettes or a lottery ticket. Others describe Dave as a "seething volcano," a person who never smiled, and always seemed on the verge of erupting into violence. After being rude to several customers, and breaking expensive electronic equipment in the shop when he threw a wrench, David was fired. In seeking help, he recognized that he has a history of losing his temper that is pervasive. He has yelled and screamed at the Little League coach of the team for which his child

plays and even literally grabbed an umpire after a game. He remembers being afraid when his boy was an infant that he would bash its head during crying spells.

Relaxation training proceeded slower inasmuch as David was restless and distractible during the training session. He kept opening his eyes, and moving on the chair to "find a more comfortable position." Judging that David was reacting to the length of the session that required reduced activity, the next AMT session was solely devoted to relaxation training, and held for 20 minutes' duration. Further, he was left alone in the treatment room, using an audio relaxation tape for the relaxation exercise. Once beyond this issue, David acquired the relaxation skill with one more training session, and his other AMT sessions proceeded unabated.

His 90 intensity scene was as follows:

> "You are in the shop of the service station trying to meet a deadline for a tune-up. All day the bell has been constantly ringing as customers come in for gas. . . it seems as though the bell has rung nonstop. At this moment, your employer was using the telephone next to your tool chest. You hear another customer driving up, your boss is in your way, you asked him politely to move, but he says, 'Keep your pants on dummy.' You want to jam on his foot, he makes you so angry. . . it's that tone of voice he has. . . and it's just been nonstop work today. . . too many problems to deal with. . . you feel tense and angry all over. Your stomach is churning, in a fiery knot. You feel the cords of tension up your neck and shoulders. . . You grind your teeth and clench your jaws. You're thinking, 'What the heck now. Do I need this? He needs me more than I need this stinking job.' Your thoughts start to get jumbled, and your vision starts to blur, you are sweating and you see this haze of red. . . You feel this rush of blood to your face, you're heating up, you want to punch out your employer. . . "

The AMT sessions for David were slower as a result of his initial distractibility during the relaxation training. Three relaxation sessions, one reduced to 20 minutes with an audiotape, were required before the therapist was able to return to the usual AMT format. After eight more sessions, David appeared to be making significant progress, first noticeable in his feeling of "being more patient" with his child. "I think I'm a better parent now, and a better spectator. I can enjoy the game a little more, more mellow about seeing it as a game, see, not a life-or-death situation. I even sometimes laugh at how the other parents seem to make such a big deal, yelling and all that." He has moved to another part of the city for employment, and spends extra attention in time monitoring. Specifically, he engages in brief relaxation about every two hours on his service station job. Before waiting on a customer, he also reminds himself, "Keep loose." He still occasionally finds himself getting impatient during busy periods, but has recognized that the busy times are during the time in the morning when everyone is driving to work and stopping for gas, about 10 in the morning when shoppers are heading for stores and stopping at the station for service, about the lunch hour, and again at quitting time. In preparation for these busy periods, he takes special pains to monitor his early warning signals, and to abort any building feelings of impatience or irritation. He has bought himself an oil rag that has printed the words, "Loose and easy."

The recent research on AMT with anger management has confirmed that AMT is clearly suitable as an arousal control method with applications to anger arousal. In addition, these studies suggest that, at least for a student population, the control of anger enables these subjects to rely upon more constructive coping methods. As with the theoretical analysis of delinquents, the likelihood of such constructive coping being released will depend upon whether the client's anxiety was suppressing such skills. If the client never possessed such coping methods, then AMT treatment would need to be followed with other social skills training (Nally, 1975).

Frustration and Impulse Control

Frustration and impulse problems are actually very similar to anger problems. The difference may be that the provocation for frustration is the clear blocking of the client's goal-directed actions. Also, the impulse to strike out is not necessarily the major impulse. The frustrated adolescent might instead experience the impulse to just finish the task, even poorly or to give it all up and quit.

Hsi offered a stress management workshop for underprivileged and minority youths, as a summer program. She introduced AMT for anxiety and anger management, but also suggested that feelings of frustration would be acceptable for discussion by these adolescents. As with AMT for anger, AMT for frustration involves the same type of training steps, with the exception that a frustration scene is substituted for anxiety scenes. The following are two case illustrations:

> "You're trying to fix the brake shoes, getting the springs back in, but they keep slipping. It's happened twice already, and your girlfriend is watching, expecting you to be good at fixing her car. You're hot and sweaty, losing your patience. You're getting close this time. . . and it slips again. . . you feel frustrated, you have this impulse to just jam it all together, just eliminate the one piece, and everything will fit. . . won't work real well, but it would get it done. . . finished. . . no more messing around. . . "
>
> "It's lunchtime, Tuesday afternoon, and you've been sitting with your boyfriend. . . or a boy you want to be your boyfriend. . . you have been talking politely, trying to show him you're interested, but he seems so dense. . .

like he doesn't see you the way you are. . . he's talking about this weekend movie he saw. . . and you're trying to steer his conversation around to talking about you. . . or at least to pay attention to you. . . it's so frustrating, like he's like a brick wall, more a blank wall. . . and you can't move him. . . you start to clench your teeth, you want to throw up your hands in exasperation. . . you know you'll say or do something stupid. . . "

As with other maladaptive arousal problems, the details for frustration and impulse scenes must avoid including maladaptive actions. On the other hand, the distinction between anger management and frustration management may not be as important. The understanding by the therapist of the nature of the client's presenting difficulty is more important in the design of the AMT therapy than whether the anger elements make the scene an anger management scene or a frustration scene.

Post-Traumatic Stress Disorder

Post-traumatic stress disorder (PTSD) is defined in part by the precipitating event, a catastrophic circumstance such as war or an airplane disaster, that go beyond common stressors. Examples of such catastrophes range from natural disasters such as Mount St. Helens (Shore, Tatum, & Vollmer, 1986), technological disasters such as the Buffalo Creek Disaster and Three Mile Island (Baum, Gatchel, & Schaeffer, 1983; Bromet, 1980; Gleser, Green, & Winget, 1981); and man-made disasters such as war and sexual assault (Bard & Sangery, 1986; Kilpatrick, Veronen, & Resick, 1979; Kulka, Schlenger, Fairbank, Hough, Jordan, Marmar, & Weiss, 1988). The associations from this trauma form the basic fear structure, with symptoms persisting long beyond the termination of the trauma (Fairbank, Langley, Jarvie, & Keane, 1981). Epidemiological research estimates the prevalence of post-traumatic stress disorder from all sources to be between one and two percent of the adult population, close to the prevalence of schizophrenia in the United States (Helzer, Robins, & McEvoy, 1987; Kulka et al., 1988). Hence it is believed that there are some 2.4 to 4.8 million cases of post-traumatic stress disorder just in the United States. For combat veterans symptoms include recurrent, intrusive memories of battle events, either as a flashback in a waking state, or as nightmares during sleep. About 500,000 veterans are in need of help as a result of their battle experiences (Pensk & Robinowitz, 1987; Yager, Laufer, & Gallops, 1984). The following illustrates the memories of one veteran:

"Things happen so fast up front, you never knew what was on your left or even behind you. I used to get turned around and think I was surrounded. I was scared all the time.

"The constant feeling of being all alone. . . unreal. . . sounds, explosions, vague crying, then dark, and light again, flashes. . . everything goes on and on.

"I used to be sick all the time or afraid of being sick, from the blood. . . and the smell of blood. . . I remember over and over again the arm falling in front of me. . . you couldn't afford to make friends, it rips you up too much if they bleed on you, or if you see them crippled for no good reason. . . or worse, if they die next to you." (Suinn, 1988, p. 144)

Anxiety Management Training

Drs. Richard Borrego (personal communication, 1988) and Ricardo Rivas (personal communication, 1988) have been using AMT successfully with post-traumatic stress disorder patients either through the veterans' center or private practice. They have reported that AMT appears to directly confront the very arousal that is unpredictable and uncontrolled in flashbacks or nightmares, and brings these under control. Ultimately, the trauma attacks themselves are eliminated. Although, theoretically, one would feel initially cautious, given the intensity of these patients' anxiety symptoms, the work with generalized anxiety disorder patients and with anxious schizophrenics should have been reassuring. As it turns out, Borrego and Rivas have found the standard AMT procedures quite suited to post-traumatic stress disorder. Naturally, the identification of the anxiety scene is very straightforward, inasmuch as the veterans are keenly aware of their flashbacks. On the other hand, the relaxation scene may be more difficult to identify, if the patient has been experiencing chronic, unresolved tensions on a daily basis. Since relaxation activity resulting from medication is not appropriate, some other solution needs to be found. Doing away with the relaxation scene is not a very good option. The major use of this scene is as one method to remove the anxiety scene's residuals, through substituting the cognitive imagery of the relaxation scene for the cognitive imagery of the anxiety scene. In addition, having the concreteness of the relaxation scene along with its strong associations with relaxation enables a firm systematic method for relaxation retrieval. One solution to a patient lacking any relaxation scene from real life is to conduct several relaxation sessions, and to use the best of these sessions as the relaxation scene to be recalled. The following case is an example of AMT with post-traumatic stress disorder:

Harold had been raised in a pleasant, middle-class, rural town. After seeing some movies and television commercials about the military, he enlisted and asked to be sent to "where the fighting was." He pictured himself as aggressively masculine, and believed the battlefield would prove his mettle and harden his fighting skills.

He was completely unprepared for Vietnam. There were no battle lines, and no courageous testing of face-to-face combat. Instead the jungle hid the enemy, and the heat and bugs were wearing, and everything smelled. Boredom alternated with fear. Rocket attacks, nighttime forays, persistent suspicions about which friendlies were really Vietcong made for chronic anxiety. Nerves were on edge, and an animal existence the way of life.

Harold was discharged an older and more somber person, with anger, depression, and a loss of any ideals whatsoever. He would jump to sudden small sounds, be unable to fall asleep unless he used alcohol, and would awaken suddenly in the evening. He remembers some but not all nightmares, which were so realistic that he would thrash around and shout incoherently. During the day, unpredictable flashbacks would occur, leaving him depressed, empty and shaking. He avoided all movies, TV programs, or magazines that even mentioned war. Still, this did not prevent his trauma from reappearing.

Harold's anxiety scene involved: "You're on patrol, it's very dark. . . you know your buddies are in a line, but you can't see them because of the thick undergrowths. . . you feel isolated, alone, like it's a nightmare movie and you're suddenly in a different world. . . someone makes contact.. there's firing all around, flashes. . . you instinctively fire yourself. . . you're so scared, you're yelling at the top of your lungs, and you're even crying. . . suddenly a Vietcong jumps up out of nowhere, his face is large in your face. . . you know you're going to die. . . somehow, his face explodes. . . and you have his blood all over you, and you see his eye hanging out. . . you're yelling and crying and sobbing and running. . . "

In the event that the patient not only lacks a relaxation scene, but does not seem to be able to use the AMT relaxation training as his/her scene, then the alternative to regaining relaxation is to return directly to the muscle review. With this method, on the first exposure of the anxiety scene, the muscle review should return to tensing followed by relaxing. The purpose is to focus attention on a concrete sensation as a means of countering any residual anxiety stimuli. If the patient is showing reasonable ability to return to relaxation, the tensing is eliminated and only review of relaxation across each muscle group is needed. However, the patient should be reminded to: "Pay attention to each muscle group, again noticing how the relaxation feels. . . so letting go the right hand and arm. . . pay attention to the right hand and arm, and just let the relaxation flow there. . . " This type of detailed instruction focuses the attention, and avoids drifting back into anxiety. Such continuing descriptions by the therapist in the early sessions is the method for maximum therapist control and assurance that the client is returning to the relaxation. It is a common format for any client during AMT session 2 or for any client who seems to need this type of concrete instructions to regain a focus on relaxation.

A revision of AMT for post-traumatic stress disorder recommended by Dr. Riccardo Rivas (personal communication, 1988) involves extending both the intake session time and the addition of personal interviewing sessions interspersed between AMT sessions. This "down time" he defines as a "needed break from training/therapy" to consolidate gains, retrace historical events associated with the trauma, deal with efficacy or analysis of potential gains in the therapy, etc. Rivas reports a total course of treatment of approximately 16 sessions, with the AMT components covering about 10 sessions.

Dr. Richard Borrego has extensive experiences with Vietnam veterans and has provided treatment services to them through the Vet Center in Boulder, Colorado. His experience is that AMT has particular value for four common symptom areas associated with combat post-traumatic stress disorder: generalized anxiety and panic attacks; hypervigilance; anger control and fear of loss of control over anger; and dissociative, flashback episodes and nightmares. In evaluating these symptoms, he observes:

Anxiety and Panic. ". . . panic attacks. . . often. . . occur in supermarkets or department stores, and large crowds. . . (originating from) suppressed feelings. . . that. . . are beginning to surface. . . The overwhelming anxiety experienced, particularly rapid heart rate and shallow breathing, can trigger fear of death which was experienced and suppressed many times on the battlefield. . . The physiological symptoms of the anxiety attack trigger fears of death or physical harm which have been suppressed, and these symptoms trigger more anxiety. Thus the anxiety stimulates more anxiety and fear. Anxiety Management Training has been particularly useful in breaking the chain of physiological symptoms which result in the panic attack."

"That these panic attacks occur in supermarkets or large crowds indicates that they may be related to social phobia. Certainly, a large number of veterans suffering from PTSD have isolated themselves from society. The result of this isolation has been social anxiety and a need for resocialization. Also, in Vietnam, the combat soldier learned that being in a group on a patrol or even in town could be hazardous to your health. Resocialization groups and individual therapy are helpful; however, AMT. . . as an adjunct to deal with the anxiety can be helpful."

Hypervigilance. Borrego associates this with the state of being constantly tense and anxious. "I have found that roughly 10%–15% suffer from a conditioned fear/anxiety response which has not relaxed since the war. . . Extreme hypervigilance is a common trait. . . With those that do fall in this category (of hypervigilance), individual talk therapy and group therapy are not sufficient to reduce what I believe to be a conditioned physiological response which requires a treatment regime of specific physiological deconditioning. . . The procedure involved in AMT, when traumatic incidents are (used) for the anxiety scene, has been reported by (my) PTSD clients to free up their feeling of being tense all the time."

Anger Control; Fear of Losing Control. Borrego calls attention to the DSM III-R recognition that the post-traumatic stress disorder patient may experience a fear of losing control. Furthermore, if the patient is a combat veteran who has committed acts of violence during the war, the fear may center on the fear of losing control over these aggressive and violent impulses. Borrego adds his own view that another experience relates to the "rage toward the enemy which was never released. It was not uncommon to be attacked by rockets, mortars, or small arms fire and never see the enemy or have a chance to fire back. Thus, the soldier was left with a desire to retaliate which was not discharged." In addition, a variety of other factors contribute to the heightened feelings of anger: "(1) return from the war to a society that was often hostile toward the veteran, and the resulting isolation/alienation; (2) frustration in finding and maintaining employment; (3) anti-authority issues stemming from the political/controversial nature of the war; and (4) lack of proper rest due to disturbed sleep." Regarding treatment with AMT, he indicates that he ". . . found that AMT used in conjunction with other anger control techniques, e.g., assertive training, time outs, etc., can be helpful in controlling impulsive aggressive behavior and domestic violence. . . "

The fear of losing control, the anxiety, and the anger may all be intertwined for the veteran: ". . . there is a circular process whereby the fear of losing control of rage triggers anxiety, which in turn may be cognitively associated with the rage response previously experienced in Vietnam, thus, validating the possibility that the veteran may lose control." The fact that AMT emphasizes the development of self-control, therefore, becomes an extremely important contribution toward aiding the veteran in acquiring a greater self-confidence regarding maintaining control.

Flashbacks and Nightmares. Borrego confirms that "Nightmares are fairly common amongst Vietnam veterans with PTSD," as well as

similar reexperiencing of prior traumatic events through daytime flashbacks. As we stated earlier, these nightmares and/or the flashbacks can
serve as the content for the anxiety arousal scenes for AMT, and has
been so used by Borrego.

As with Dr. Rivas, Dr. Borrego has also shared with me some of his
recommendations regarding therapeutic strategies to improve on AMT
applications for post-traumatic stress disorder. Borrego offers the following advice:

> "Due to the intensity of feelings which can be aroused in employing AMT
> with PTSD clients, I highly recommend that (AMT) not be implemented
> until the therapist has developed rapport and trust with the client. I think it is
> crucial that the client feels a sense of safety and confidence in the therapist's
> ability to deal with what is presented. Many Vietnam veterans with PTSD
> have suppressed feelings and memories about Vietnam for years, indicating
> some preconceived notion about what might happen if they opened 'Pan-
> dora's box.' It is often necessary to spend a session or more just talking about
> their fears about getting in touch with traumatic memories and the feeling
> associated with those memories. I have gotten responses such as, 'If I allow
> myself to feel the pain I may never stop crying,' or 'If I really start remem-
> bering and feel the anger I'll lose control and go into a rage'. Another
> response has been, 'I'm afraid if I started getting in touch with what's inside
> me I'll explode or go crazy.' By exploring the fears and reassuring the vet-
> eran, the AMT can proceed more effectively."

Finally, Borrego offers two methodological suggestions that appear
to reflect success in his practice. He estimates that "For the high intensity,
chronic anxiety type of PTSD client. . . 15 sessions may be enough to
reduce symptoms." However, he indicates that he has "also used a shortened version. . . with clients. . . (for whom) recurring nightmares (are)
the key to the most pressing issue which needs resolution. . . when
nightmares persist, I will employ an AMT model of one session relaxation and two to three sessions of relax—nightmare scene—relax."

Summary

AMT was initially developed as an intervention method for anxiety
states. However, partly stimulated by the early work of Hart with Type A
persons and anger, I have become sensitive to the fact that AMT is
actually an arousal-control technique. Stress responses and anxiety happen to be one form of arousal. But other arousal states include anger, as
well as the arousal associated with frustration. In some regards, AMT
therefore has the qualities of an impulse control procedure. With anxiety or phobic conditions, there is a situation that triggers a state of
arousal, with an attending impulse for action. For the phobic person, the

impulse is a desire to leave, to run away from the phobic stimulant. With generalized anxiety, the impulse shows up in agitated motor behaviors or in persisting thoughts of gloom and doom. Similarly, anger must be conceived as involving an anger stimulus, the precipitation of anger arousal, and an impulse to aggress. Problems of impulse control, such as hyperactivity, might follow the same model, with a precipitant to the impulse, the arousal, and the desire to act in some way. The precipitant might be a new task that the person is starting, or possibly even time, that is, the person has been sitting quietly for a certain length of time and has now reached his/her limit for patience. The impulse is for some form of action, and in some cases the action is to charge into the task without planning. In other cases, the action is the uncontrolled, unfocused hyperactivity.

We now have a number of studies on anger management with the AMT model. These have confirmed that AMT can indeed be applied to anger, by simply substituting the use of anger scenes for anxiety scenes. Furthermore, the research has involved subjects whose aggressive actions have been of a serious nature. Further details of the application of AMT for anger management can be found in Chapter 5 through a case illustration. The application of AMT to frustration is a sensible one, with the evidence coming from a workshop for adolescents, rather than a research report. On the other hand, impulse control and hyperactivity are applications which seem logical extensions of AMT, but for which we lack either clinical or research confirmation.

Another way of conceptualizing AMT is reflected in this chapter's title, as a procedure for working with "intense emotional states." Certainly anxiety and anger fit this category. But it also represents the application to post-traumatic stress disorder. This condition, especially with regard to combat stress, appropriately deals with the high level of residual stress. The recurring nightmares or the flashbacks present a direct access to the content for the AMT anxiety scenes. The systematic, guided steps of AMT also offer the combat veteran with assurance that he/she will not be faced with an experience in therapy which is out of control. Finally, as Borrego noted, the focus on the development of self-control through AMT offers the veteran a crucial achievement to bring closure and self-assurance to the prior persisting and distressing symptoms. Finally, Borrego calls attention to the anger-management application of AMT for post-traumatic stress disorder.

APPENDIXES

A

Logs for Client Self-Monitoring of Stress and of Relaxation

Stress Log 1

Feelings	Situation	Tension level*	Date and hour

*0 = Nonexistent tension.
 100 = Maximum tension.

Stress Log 2

Feelings	Physical/ cognitive cues	Situation	Level of stress (0–100)	Day/hour

Stress Log 3

Situation	Physical/ cognitive cues	Anxiety control success Yes	No	Tension level before control (0–100)	Tension level after control (0–100)

Log for Relaxation Practice

Date and hour of practice	Duration of practice	Body areas easily relaxed	Body areas with tension	Tension level (0–100)*	
				Before	After

*0–100 scale: 0 = Nonexistent tension.
              100 = Maximum tension.

B

Model for Therapist Instructions to Clients for AMT Segments

Session 1

The instructions for the tension-relaxation exercise are straightforward. During session 1, the therapist also asks for a signal to indicate the relaxation scene. The instructions may follow the model:

> "In a moment, I'll have you switch on the relaxing scene about (label). The scene involves. . . (give details). So right now, switch your relaxing scene on, letting the details come as realistically as possible, using whatever senses which help this scene to develop realistically for you. As soon as you get any part of the scene, signal me. . . Be there and use the scene to help you further increase your relaxation. . . , etc. . . ."

Session 2

Relaxation without tension is used for clients who have sufficiently practiced the exercise in homework meetings. The instruction for relaxation without tension follows the usual model (Appendix D), such as:

> "Let's have you sit back in a comfortable position, close your eyes, and now start focusing on relaxing the various muscle groups, starting with loosening up the fingers of the right hand. . . increasing a sense of relaxation in the right forearm. . . and the right upper arm. . . etc. Now, use the deep breath to further increase the relaxation. . . ."

The instructions for session 2 will also call for switching on the relaxation scene, and the instructions for asking for a scene onset signal are along the model indicated under session 1 previously.

333

The session also calls for the use of an anxiety scene. During this first exposure to an anxiety scene, the duration is kept brief, i.e., 10–15 seconds. The model for instructing the client may be as follows:

> "In a moment I will have you switch on the anxiety scene you originally identified about _____. It's the scene about. . . (give details). All right, let's have you switch on that scene right now. As soon as you begin to experience the anxiety, signal me. . . (pause). Really be there, let the scene develop as realistically as possible; allow yourself to experience the anxiety again." (When client signals, then proceed with the next instruction after about 10–15 seconds.) "That's fine. Let that scene disappear, let it go, and switch on the relaxing scene. . . switch on the relaxation scene as clearly and completely as possible, really be there. . . Signal me when you're reasonably comfortable again. . . The relaxing scene in which you are (insert description). . . etc."

After the client has shown the ability to obtain anxiety arousal through the establishment of the anxiety scene, then from this point onward the anxiety scenes are initiated and held for 20–30 seconds; this time interval is the time interval from the client signaling the onset of the scene to the period that the therapist turns off the scene.

Session 3

This session involves relaxation initiated by the client after the client has demonstrated the acquisition of this skill. The instructions may follow the model of:

> "Let's have you sit back in a comfortable position on the chair, close your eyes, and begin the relaxation technique using whatever procedure seems to be working best for you. Signal me when you're reasonably relaxed." (Pause—until a signal of relaxation, then the therapist continues with the instructions as follows.) "Continue relaxing, focusing on flowing the relaxation through the right hand, forearm, and upper arm. . . , the left hand. . . , etc."

The client also is given the relaxation scene, with scene onset signal, followed by the anxiety scene. For the anxiety scene, the following instruction is used:

> "In a moment, I'm going to have you switch on the anxiety scene about _____. As you experience this anxiety, I want you to signal me. . . All right, let's have you switch on that scene right now, really be there, let the scene develop as realistically as possible; allow yourself to experience the anxiety again higher and higher, just let the anxiety build. As you experience the anxiety, now pay attention to how it is that you experience anxiety. . . , perhaps it's in your neck or shoulder muscles tensing, body signs such as your heart rate, or in your stomach, or in your feelings or in the various disturbing thoughts that you're having.* Let the anxiety continue to build, all the while noticing your signs, how you experience anxiety. . . (hold the scene for a total of 20–30 seconds after client signals). Now switch that scene off, and switch

on the relaxation scene. . . , that scene involving _____ (insert appropriate description) and signal me when you're reasonably comfortable again,. . . etc."

*Where a client has identified specific anxiety cues, cite these instead.

Session 4

In session 4 the client once again is given instructions to self-initiate relaxation, signaling when a reasonably relaxed level is achieved. The client is then instructed by the therapist to turn on the anxiety scene and to self-initiate terminating that scene and initiate the relaxation scene, using the following model for instructions:

> "In a moment, I'll have you switch on the anxiety scene about _____ to arouse anxiety again; then whenever you wish, terminate that scene and reinitiate the relaxation, using whatever works best for you. For signaling, this time I'll ask you to raise your hand when you experience the anxiety, and keep it up as long as you're still anxious; then lower it when you've retrieved the relaxation. All right, switch on the anxiety scene now, let the anxiety build, then reinitiate the relaxation when you are ready. Signal by raising your hand when you experience the anxiety, and lower your hand when you're relaxed again. (Silence until client signals reachievement of relaxation.). . . All right, continue that relaxation for a moment. . . etc."

Session 5

Session 5 again begins with the client using self-initiated relaxation, signaling the therapist when a comfortable level of relaxation is attained. The therapist then initiates the anxiety scene, following the instructional model of:

> "In a moment, I will have you switch on the anxiety scene about _____ to raise the anxiety again; then *while you're still in the anxiety scene*, reinitiate the relaxation. For signaling, raise your hand when you experience the anxiety, keep it up while you're still anxious, then lower it when you have retrieved relaxation. All right, switch on the anxiety scene now, let the anxiety build, then while you're still in the anxiety scene, return the controlled relaxation. (Silence until client signals reachievement of relaxation). . . That's fine, now continue that relaxation. . . etc."

C

Relaxation Training Instructions*

Pre-Instructions

If on recliner, have person push back to a comfortable incline, saying "I think you'll be more comfortable if you have your hands on the arms (of the recliner) and your feet straight." Describe the steps of the muscle exercise and demonstrate, e.g., making your hand into a fist, etc. Have client remove any contact lenses.

Relaxation of Hands and Arms

Settle back as comfortably as you can. Close your eyes so you won't be distracted. . . . Now, as you relax like that, clench your right fist, just clench your fist tighter and tighter, and study the tension as you do so. Keep it clenched and feel the tension in your right fist, hand, forearm. . . and now relax. Let the fingers of your right hand become loose, and observe the contrast in your feelings between the tension that was there a moment ago and the greater sense of relaxation now. . . Now, once more, clench your right fist really tight. . . hold it, and notice the tension again. . . Now let go, relax; let your fingers straighten out, . . . and notice the difference once more. . . O.K. we'll leave the right hand and attend to the left hand. . . Clench your left hand into a fist. . . very tense, very tight. . . Clench that fist tighter and notice the tension. . . and now relax. Again notice the contrast. . . Repeat that once more,

*Adapted from Wolpe, J., and Lazarus, A., 1966.

clench the left fist, tight and tense. . . Now relax your hand. Continue relaxing like that for a while, both hands and fingers becoming much more loose and relaxed.

Now, we'll leave both hands comfortably relaxed and move to the right bicep. Bend your right arm at the elbow to tense your right bicep, the right upper arm. . . Tense them harder and study the tension. . . All right, straighten out your arm, let it relax and feel that difference again between tension and relaxation—the absence of tension. . . Let the re- laxation develop. . . Once more, tense your right bicep, hold the tension and observe it carefully. . . Now, straighten the arm and relax; let your arm move to a comfortable position. Let the relaxation proceed on its own.

All right, now we'll move to the left upper arm, the left bi- cep. . . Tense up the upper arm by bending your left arm at the elbow, very tight, very tense. . . feel the tension in the bicep and the upper arm. . . this is muscle tension. . . All right, now release the tension; let your arm return to a comfortable supported position, and notice the relaxation. . . a greater sense of relaxation in the entire left upper arm. . . Now once more, tense up the left upper arm right now, very tense, very tight. . . and notice the tension. This is how tenseness feels. . . Now, relax the arm, letting the tension be replaced by relaxa- tion, and let your arm move to a comfortably supported position.

So, right now, you can notice the increased sense of relaxation in the right hand. . . and the fingers of the right hand. . . and the right fore- arm, and also the right upper arm. . . Similarly, relaxation in the left hand. . . the fingers of the left hand. . . the left forearm, and the left upper arm. . . very relaxed in both hands and both arms. . . Now we'll leave both hands and arms comfortably supported and shift our atten- tion to the area around the head.

Relaxation of Forehead, Eyes, Facial Area, Neck, and Shoulders

We'll start with the forehead. In order to tense up the forehead, I'll have you wrinkle up your forehead right now; wrinkle it tighter. . . like you're frowning. . . tense, and tight. . . Now, relax the forehead and smooth it out. Picture the entire forehead becoming smoother as the relaxation increases. . . Now, frown once more and wrinkle your brows and study the tension. . . very tight. . . Now, let go of the tension and smooth out the forehead once more. . . Now, we'll move to the eyes. . . Close your eyes tighter and tighter. . . feel the tension. . . Now, relax your eyes; keeping your eyes closed, but comfortably relaxed and notice the sense of relaxation. . . All right, once more, close your eyes really tight, and notice the tension. . . tight and tense. . . and now relax, let the tension disappear and be replaced by a greater sense of relaxation, while your eyes are comfortably closed. . . much more relaxed. . . O.K., we'll now move to the rest of the facial areas by having you clench your jaws. . . bite your teeth together; study the tension throughout the jaws. . . All right now, relax your jaws. . . notice the relaxation all over your face. . . your forehead. . . your eyes, lips, and jaws. . . Now once more, bite your teeth, clench your jaws and notice the tension that creates. . . O.K., now relax the jaws and the entire facial area. . . Let the relaxation proceed on its own to cover the forehead, the eyes, the jaws, the entire facial areas. . . Now attend to your neck muscles. Press your head back as far as it can go and feel the tension in the neck. . . tense and tight. . . Now let your head return forward to a comfortable position, and notice the relaxation. Let the relaxation develop further. . . Once more, press your head back and notice the tension. . . All right, now relax the neck and let your head return to a comfortable position. . . Now, we'll move to the shoulders. . . Shrug your shoulders, right up. Hold the tension. . . Drop your shoulders and feel the relaxation. . . let the relaxation increase in the neck and shoulders. . . Shrug your shoulders again. Feel the tension in your shoulders and upper back. . . Now drop your shoulders once more and relax. Let the relaxation spread deep into the shoulders, right into your back muscles; relax your neck and shoulders. . . and your forehead and eyes and the entire facial area. Now we'll move from the head and shoulders to your upper body.

Relaxation of Chest and Stomach

Breathe easily and freely in and out. Notice how the relaxation has increased across your body. . . As you breathe comfortably, just feel that relaxation. . . Now inhale deeply and hold your breath. Study the tension. . . Now exhale, let the walls of your chest grow loose and push the air out automatically. Continue relaxing and breathe freely and easily. Feel the relaxation and enjoy it. . . Now breathe in deeply and hold it again. . . That's fine, breathe out and appreciate the relief. Just breathe normally. . . Continue relaxing your chest and let the relaxation spread to your shoulders, your neck, your facial area, and your arms. Merely let go. . . and enjoy the relaxation. Now let's pay attention to your abdominal muscles, your stomach area. Tighten your stomach muscles, make your abdomen hard. Notice the tension. . . and relax. Let the muscles loosen and notice the contrast. . . Once more, press and tighten your stomach muscles. Hold the tension and study it. . . and relax. All right, we'll now move to your legs and feet.

Relaxation of Feet and Legs

To tense up your legs and feet, press your feet and toes downwards, away from your body, so that your calf muscles become tense. (To avoid cramps, make this brief). . . All right, now relax, allow the relaxation to proceed on its own. . . Now, once more, press your feet and toes downwards, away from your face, so that your calf muscles become tense. Study that tension. . . O.K., now relax your feet and legs. . .

Now you can become twice as relaxed as you are merely by taking in a really deep breath and slowly exhaling. Take in a long deep breath and let it out very slowly, using that method to become as relaxed as you would like to be. In the future, we'll use this deep breath as a quick signal to achieve relaxation. . . Once more, take a deep breath and flow the relaxation across your body. . . relaxing your hands and arms. . . your facial area. . . the muscles of your neck and shoulders. . . your stomach. . . and both legs and both feet.

Relaxation Scene Instruction

In a moment, I'm going to have you switch on the relaxation scene about (label). So right now, switch your relaxation scene on, letting the details come as realistically as possible, using whatever senses which help this scene to develop realistically for you. (See also "Model for Therapist Instructions, Session 1.")

Termination of Relaxation

In a moment, I'll count backwards from 3 to 1. When I get to 1, you'll be alert and refreshed, without aches or pains. O.K., "3," much more alert; "2" without aches or pains, and "1" quite refreshed and alert. (Pause while client refocuses attention.) (If in a group format, and not all clients are alert, then add, "Let's have you all open your eyes now.") All right, let's have you sit up.

D

Relaxation without Tensing

Settle back comfortably. Close your eyes so you won't be distracted. . . now start focusing on relaxing the various muscle groups, starting with loosening up the fingers of the right hand. . . increasing the relaxation there and throughout the entire right hand. . . and flowing that relaxation to include the right forearm. . . .and now, the right upper arm. . .

And now also attending to relaxing the fingers of the left arm. . . the entire hand. . . and increasing the relaxation to include the left forearm. . . and now the left upper arm. . . so much more relaxed and tension-free in both hands. . . both forearms. . . both upper arms. . .

Take a slow deep breath and slowly exhale, using this method to further the relaxation process. . . then returning to breathing normally. . .

Now, while the hands and arms are relaxed, we'll have you focus on loosening up the forehead. . . letting any tensions remove themselves, to become wrinkle free. . . smoothening out the forehead area. . . and flowing that relaxation across the eyes. . . and the entire facial area, including the lips and the jaws. . . much more relaxed, and tension-free in the whole head and facial area. . .

Spreading that relaxation across the neck and shoulders. . . letting the muscle tension be replaced by a greater sense of relaxation. . .

And continuing the relaxation across the chest. . . the stomach. . . and both legs and both feet. . . much more relaxed. . .

Take another slow deep breath, and use this to again remove any last tensions. . . slowly exhaling and feeling that tension just leave your body. . . then returning to breathing normally again. . . so much more loose, relaxed in your entire body. . .

341

Take three more of those deep breaths, with the slow exhaling each time to increase the relaxation even further. . . as relaxed and comfortable as you would like to be. . . then continuing to breathe normally. . . retaining the sense of relaxation.

E

Samples of AMT Post-Session Interviews

The following is a transcript from an AMT session. There are too many missing details in this interview.

T–1: "3 - 2 - 1, open your eyes when you're ready. (client does) How did the scene go?"

C–1: "That anxiety scene was better, really made me anxious this time."

T–2: "That's important, we need to have the anxiety for you to learn control. Now, how was the relaxation?"

C–2: "Went fine. This really works. I've been noticing it in my everyday problems."

T–3: "Tell me about the relaxing today."

C–3: "Was really good. Had some trouble in leaving it though when you'd tell me to go to the anxiety scene, it's too comfortable. But I got better as we went along, seems to depend."

T–4: "So you had some trouble, but could shift?"

C–4: "Yes, I would want to stay with the relaxing and it would take some time before leaving it."

T–5: "Tell me about this, you would stay relaxing and not leave it for the anxiety scene?"

C–5: "That's really because your instructions are so good; you have a good voice. The signaling helped because I could tell you I was anxious and you knew it and we could go to something else."

T–6: "It is really important that you understand AMT—it's meant to help you eventually in everyday problems. However, I don't want you to try it yet, but do practice the relaxing. I'll see you at

10 again; is that a good time? You've had some trouble with that time before, missed sometimes."

C–6:   "Yes, it's a good time, it's just that I had a dental exam once, a meeting with my prof the other time, and I was on the phone and couldn't get off the last time."

T–7:   "OK, I'll see you again. Meantime, keep on with the practice."
END

This interview does a good job of obtaining useful data:

T–1:   "3 - 2 - 1, open your eyes when you're ready. (client does) How did session go?"

C–1:   "That anxiety scene was better, really made me anxious this time."

T–2:   "That's important, we need to have the anxiety for you to learn control. Tell me about it."

C–2:   "I think I had more time to get into the scene; you weren't saying as much and I could concentrate on the scene; I knew that scene since we used it before; earlier it helped for you to describe the scene to me, but now I can get into it myself. . . and actually, your descriptions are a little distracting because I want to get ahead of you to the next part of the scene."

T–3:   "So it helps the scene for me to be more quiet. . . tell me something about the anxiety."

C–3:   "I could really get into it; at the very start of the scene, I could feel my stomach tighten and my heart start to pound, and I think I felt it hard to breathe. . . really started to feel panic."

T–4:   "That's really good - that you could get into the scene and feel the anxiety. Describe the scene you were using - did it differ from how I described it?"

C–4:   "No, it was the same, it's just that I guess I don't need you to help talk me through it; it's clear without you helping. I was there, could see the people talking; I was walking to them, felt reluctant, then anxious; there were two men wearing ties and a woman leading the conversation."

T–5:   "So the scene was very clear. And how was the relaxation control?"

C–5:   "You mean the first relaxation, or the relaxation to get rid of the anxiety?"

T–6:   "First tell me about relaxation to control the anxiety."

C–6:   "Went good, real good."

T–7:   "How do you mean?"

C–7:   "I was able to take a deep breath and flow away the anxiety. I also can now sense the situations that make me anxious more clearly now."

T–8: "So the deep breath helps. What else seems useful to gain control?"

C–8: "The deep breath. . . the "relax" word doesn't seem to add much. . . and I practice the deep breath during the day too, like you said, when I'm not under stress, just to practice. . . don't know of other methods which help."

T–9: "That's really good, you're practicing and apparently having gains. Now, go back apiece, you were going to say something about relaxation before anxiety scenes?"

C–9: "Yes, the relaxing went real good today. You have a good voice. . . I was so comfortable, in fact I had some trouble in leaving it though when you'd tell me to go to the anxiety scene, too comfortable. But I got better as we went along, seems to depend."

T–10: "So if anything you were too relaxed, and had some difficulty shifting to the anxiety scene?"

C–10: "Yes, I like the relaxing, it feels good to me. . . better than the anxiety."

T–11: "Yes, the relaxation experience is really positive. . . but somehow your transition to the anxiety was difficult. . . yet for you to be gaining even more in self-control, it's important to get to the anxiety scene. You described getting into it well once you shift, so maybe we need to get a feel for what helps you to shift more easily from relaxation to anxiety scene. . . what's your thought?"

C–11: "After the first time, it usually goes all right. But the first time we do the anxiety scene in the session, I'm slow, I guess I'm reluctant to give up the relaxation and get to work. . . "

T–12: "What do you suppose is going on?"

C–12: "Maybe I feel that the anxiety won't go away. . . I won't be able to control it away. . . "

T–13: "I understand that. That's the reason we go at it carefully and systematically. I first want to be sure you have the ability to use the relaxation, so I have you practice relaxing at home, and we look at your logs. We start the anxiety control process only when you're at the stage of readiness, and I think you see yourself from how the session went, the gains in self-control you've achieved. Is there something we can do for that first scene to help you?"

C–13: "Maybe if you can start with some neutral parts of the scene, like the things leading up to the anxiety part and gradually move to

it, like entering the room, hanging my coat, talking to the hostess, and then going to where the strangers are."

T–14: "Sure, sounds like a useful approach we should use in our next
meeting. How do you feel now about your comment a moment
ago. . . about whether you will have control?"

C–14: "I feel better, I did really do well today didn't I. . . and I forgot
what you had said about what the home practicing does."

T–15: "That's fine, and we should make sure to always leave time for
you to go over any feelings you might have about the program,
or your concerns. Are there others?"

C–15: "No, that was the main one."

T–16: "I am interested in your homework practice. We were talking
earlier about your log (what progress, what's helping, how much
practice, etc.), is there anything more you want to add?"

C–16: "No."

T–17: "On another topic, you had also talked today about sensing the
anxiety sources more clearly?"

C–17: "Yes, it's not just strangers. It's if they're already talking among
themselves as if they know one another, and if no one turns to
say hello to me, or if the speaker doesn't glance at me to include
me by looking at me, and particularly if it's women. . . but not
really if there are more men than women, or only men in the
group."

T–18: "Does that seem to be a common distinction, men versus women
in other situations that make you anxious?"

C–18: "Maybe, I hadn't seen that before, just recently. But I think it's
an important thing in a variety of circumstances."

T–19: "What would be an example?"

(Interview continues)

References

Aberle, D. F. (1952). "Artic hysteria" and latah in Mongolia. *Trans. New York Academy of Sciences, 14,* 291.

Abey-Wickrama, I., A'Brook, M. F., Gattoni, F. G., & Herridge, C. F. (1969). Mental hospital admissions and aircraft noise. *Lancet, 2,* 1275–1277.

Adler, J. (1982, January 4). Looking back at '81. *Newsweek,* 26–52.

Agras, W. (1982). Behavioral medicine in the 1980's: Nonrandom connections. *Journal of Consulting and Clinical Psychology, 50,* 797–803.

Agras, W. S., Sylvester, D., & Oliveau, D. (1969). The epidemiology of common fears and phobia. *Comprehensive Psychiatry, 10,* 151–156.

Aiello, J. R., Epstein, Y. M., & Karlin, R. A. (1975). Effects of crowding on electrodermal activity. *Sociological Symposium, 14,* 43–57.

Akutagawa, D. (1956). *A study in construct validity of the psychoanalytic concept of latent anxiety and a test of projection distance hypothesis.* Unpublished doctoral dissertation, University of Pittsburgh.

Albee, G. (1980). A competency model to replace the deficit mode. In M. Gibbs, J. Lachenmayer, & J. Sigal (Eds.), *Community psychology: Theoretical and empirical approaches.* New York: Gardner Press.

Alpert, R., & Haber, R. N. (1960). Anxiety in academic achievement situations. *Journal of Abnormal and Social Psychology, 61,* 207–215.

Altmaier, E., Ross, S., Leary, M., & Thornbrough, M. (1982). Matching stress inoculation treatment components to client's anxiety mode. *Journal of Counseling Psychology, 29,* 331–334.

Amies, P., Gelder, M., & Shaw, P. (1983). Social phobia: A comparative clinical study. *British Journal of Psychiatry, 142,* 174–179.

Baker, L., Hastings, J., & Hart, J. (1984). Enhanced psychophysiological responses of Type A coronary patients during Type A-relevant imagery. *Journal of Behavioral Medicine, 7,* 287–306.

Bandura, A. (1977a). Self-efficacy: Toward a unifying theory of behavioral change. *Psychological Review, 84,* 191–215.2 Bandura, A. (1977b). *Social learning theory.* Englewood Cliffs, New Jersey: Prentice-Hall.

Bandura, A. (1978). The self-system in reciprocal determinism. *American Psychologist, 33,* 344–358.

Bandura, A. (1982). Self-efficacy mechanism in human agency. *American Psychologist, 37,* 122–147.

Bard, M., & Sangrey, D. (1986). *The crime victim's book* (2nd ed.). New York: Basic Books.

Barefoot, J. C., Williams, R. B., Dahlstrom, W. G., & Dodge, K. A. (1987). Predicting mortality from scores on the Cook-Medley scale: A follow-up study of 118 lawyers. *Psychosomatic Medicine, 49,* 210.

Barlow, D. H. (1988). *Anxiety and its disorders: The nature and treatment of anxiety and panic.* New York: Guilford Press.

Barlow, D. H., Mavissakalian, M. R., & Schofield, L. D. (1980). Patterns of desynchrony in agoraphobia: A preliminary report. *Behaviour Research and Therapy, 18,* 441–448.

Barlow, D. H., O'Brien, G. T., & Last, C. G. (1984). Couples treatment of agoraphobia. *Behavior Therapy, 15,* 41–58.

Barlow, D. H., Vermilyea, P. B., Vermilyea, J. A., & Di Nardo, P. A. (1984). Co-morbidity in anxiety disorders. Manuscript submitted for publication.

Bash, K. W., & Bash-Liechti, J. (1969). Studies on the epidemiology of neuropsychiatric disorders among the rural population of the province of Khuzestan, Iran. *Social Psychiatry, 4,* 137–143.

Bash, K. W., & Bash-Liechti, J. (1974). Studies on the epidemiology of neuropsychiatric disorders among the population of the city of Shiraz, Iran. *Social Psychiatry, 9,* 163–171.

Baskin, S. (1980). Anxiety management training for the reduction of Type A coronary-prone behavior. *Dissertation Abstracts International, 35,* (12-B, Pt. 1), 6102–6103.

Bates, H. D., & Zimmerman, S. F. (1971). Toward the development of a screening scale for assertive training. *Psychological Reports, 28,* 99–107.

Baum, A., Gatchel, R., & Schaeffer, M. (1983). Emotional, behavioral, and physiological effects of chronic stress at Three Mile Island. *Journal of Consulting and Clinical Psychology, 51,* 565–572.

Baum, A., & Koman, S. (1976). Differential response to anticipated crowding: Psychological effects of social and spatial density. *Journal of Personality and Social Psychology, 34,* 351–360.

Baumann, L., & Leventhal, H. (1985). "I can tell when my blood pressure is up, can't I?" *Health Psychology, 4,* 203–218.

Beck, A. T. (1967). *Depression: Clinical, experimental, and theoretical aspects.* New York: Harper & Row. Republished as *Depression: Causes and treatment.* Philadelphia: University of Pennsylvania Press, 1972.

Beck, A. T. (1978). *PDR checklist.* Philadelphia: University of Pennsylvania, Center for Cognitive Therapy.

Beck, A. T. (1982). *Situational Anxiety Checklist (SAC).* Philadelphia: University of Pennsylvania, Center for Cognitive Therapy.

Beck, A. (1983). Negative cognitions. In E. Levitt, B. Lubin, & J. Brooks (Eds.), *Depression: Concepts, controversies, and some new facts* (2nd ed.). Hillsdale, New Jersey: Erlbaum.

Beck, A. T. (1985). Theoretical perspectives on clinical anxiety. In A. H. Tuma & J. D. Maser (Eds.), *Anxiety and the anxiety disorders,* pp. 183–196. Hillsdale, New Jersey: Lawrence Erlbaum.

Beck, A. T., & Emery, G. (1985). *Anxiety disorders and phobias: A cognitive perspective.* New York: Basic Books.

Beck, A. T., Steer, R. A., & Brown, G. (1985). *Beck Anxiety Checklist.* Unpublished manuscript, University of Pennsylvania.

Beitman, B. D., DeRosear, L., Basha, I., Flaker, G., & Corcoran, C. (1987). Panic disorder in cardiology patients with atypical or non-anginal chest pain: A pilot study. *Journal of Anxiety Disorders, 1,* 277–282.

Bell, I. R., & Schwartz, G. E. (1975). Voluntary control and reactivity of human heart rate. *Psychophysiology, 12,* 339–348.

Bellack, A. S., & Lombardo, T. W. (1984). Measurement of anxiety. In S. M. Turner (Ed.), *Behavioral theories and treatment of anxiety.* New York: Plenum Press.

Benson, H. (1975). *The relaxation response*. New York: Avon.

Berghausen, P. (1977). *Anxiety management training: Need for arousal-cued relaxation*. Unpublished doctoral dissertation, Colorado State University, Fort Collins, CO.

Bernstein, D. A., & Beatty, W. E. (1971). The use of in vivo desensitization as part of a total therapeutic intervention. *Journal of Behavior Therapy and Experimental Psychiatry, 2*, 259–266.

Blanchard, E. (Ed.) (1982). Special issue: Behavioral medicine. *Journal of Consulting and Clinical Psychology, 50*, 795–1053.

Bliss, E. L., Migeon, C. J., Branch, C. H. H., & Samuels, L. T. (1956). Reaction of the andrenocortex to emotional stress. *Psychosomatic Medicine, 18*, 56–76.

Bloom, L., & Cantrell, D. (1978). Anxiety management training for essential hypertension in pregnancy. *Behavior Therapy, 9*, 377–382.

Bourne, P. G., Rose, R. M., & Mason, J. W. (1967). Urinary 17-OCHS levels. Data on seven helicopter ambulance medics in combat. *Archives of General Psychiatry, 17*, 104–110.

Bourne, P. G., Rose, R. M., & Mason, J. W. (1968). 17-OCHS levels in combat. Special forces "A" team under threat of attack. *Archives of General Psychiatry, 19*, 135–140.

Boyd, J. H. (1986). Use of mental health services for the treatment of panic disorder. *American Journal of Psychiatry, 143*, 1569–1574.

Braestrup, C., Nielsen, M., Honore, J., Jensen, L. M., & Petersen, E. N. (1983). Benzodiazepine receptor ligands with positive and negative efficacy. *Neuropharmacologyy, 22*, 1451–1457.

Breggin, P. R. (1964). The psychophysiology of anxiety with a review of the literature concerning adrenaline. *Journal of Nervous and Mental Disease, 139*, 558–568.

Bremer, J. (1951). A social psychiatric investigation of a small community in Northern Norway. *Acta Psychiatrica Scandinavica Supplementum, 62*, 1–62.

Breznitz, S. (1971). A study of worrying. *British Journal of Social and Clinical Psychology, 10*, 271–279.

Bromet, E. (1980). *Three Mile Island: Mental health findings*. Final Report. Rockville, MD: National Institute of Mental Health.

Brooks, G., & Richardson, F. (1980). Emotional skills training: A treatment program for duodenal ulcer. *Behavior Therapy, 11*, 198–207.

Brown, J. (1980). Coping skills training: An evaluation of a psychoeducational program in a community mental health setting. *Journal of Counseling Psychology, 27*, 340–345.

Burns, L. E., & Thorpe, G. L. (1977). Fears and clinical phobias: Epidemiological aspects and the national survey of agoraphobia. *Journal of International Medical Research, 5*, 132–139.

Butler, G., Cullington, A., Mumby, M., Amies, P., & Gelder, M. (1984). Exposure and anxiety management in the treatment of social phobia. *Journal of Consulting and Clinical Psychology, 52*, 641–650.

Cacioppo, J. T., & Petty, R. E. (1981). Social psychological procedures for cognitive response assessment: The thought-listing technique. In T. V. Merluzzi, C. R. Glass, & M. Genest (Eds.), *Cognitive assessment*, pp. 309–337. New York: Guilford Press.

Cannon, W. (1929). *Bodily changes in pain, hunger, fear and rage*. Boston, MA: Branford Press.

Carey, G., & Gottesman, I. I. (1981). Twin and family studies of anxiety, phobic, and obsessive disorders. In D. K. Klein & J. Rabkin (Eds.), *Anxiety: New research and changing concepts*. New York: Raven Press.

Carr, D. B., & Sheehan, D. V. (1984). Evidence that panic disorder has a metabolic cause. In J. C. Ballenger (Ed.), *Biology of agoraphobia*. Washington, D.C.: American Psychiatric Press.

Cattell, R. B., & Scheier, I. H. (1963). *Handbook for the IPAT Anxiety Scale Questionnaire (Self Analysis Form)*. Champaign, IL: IPAT.

Cawte, J. (1972). *Poor, cruel and brutal nations*. Honolulu, HI: University of Hawaii Press.

Cerney, J., Himadi, W., & Barlow, D. (in press). Issues in diagnosing anxiety disorders. *Journal of Behavioral Assessment*.

Chambless, D. L., Caputo, G. C., Bright, P., & Gallagher, R. (1984). Assessment of fear in agoraphobics: The Body Sensations Questionnaire and the Agoraphobic Cognitions Questionnaire. *Journal of Consulting and Clinical Psychology, 52*, 1090–1097.

Chambless, D. L., Caputo, G. C., Jasin, S. E., Gracely, E. J., & Williams, C. (1985). The mobility inventory for agoraphobia. *Behaviour Research and Therapy, 23*, 35–44.

Chambless, D. L., Cherney, J., Caputo, G. C., & Rheinstein, B. J. G. (1987). Anxiety disorders and alcoholism: A study with inpatient alcoholics. *Journal of Anxiety Disorders, 1*, 29–40.

Charlesworth, E. A., & Nathan, R. G. (1981). *Stress management: A comprehensive guide to wellness*. Houston, TX: Biobehavioral Publishers.

Charney, D. S., Heninger, G. R., & Breier, A. (1984). Noradrenergic function in pain attacks. *Archives of General Psychiatry, 41*, 751–763.

Charney, D. S., Heninger, G. R., & Jatlow, P. I. (1985). Increased anxiogenic effects of caffeine in panic disorders. *Archives of General Psychiatry, 42*, 223–243.

Charney, D. S., Heninger, G. R., & Redmond, D. E., Jr. (1983). Yohimbine induced anxiety and increased noradrenergic function in humans: Effects of diazepam and clonidine. *Life Science, 33*, 19–29.

Charney, D. S., & Redmond, D. E., Jr. (1983). Neurobiological mechanisms in human anxiety. *Neuropharmacology, 22*, 1531–1536.

Chesney, M., & Tasto, D. (1975a). The development of the Menstrual Symptoms Question-naire. *Behaviour Research and Therapy, 13*, 237–244.

Chesney, M., & Tasto, D. (1975b). The effectiveness of behavior modification with spas-modic and congestive dysmenorrhea. *Behaviour Research and Therapy, 13*, 245–253.

Clark, D., Salkovskis, P., & Chalkey, A. (1985). Respiratory control as a treatment for panic attacks. *Journal of Behavior Therapy and Experimental Psychiatry, 16*, 23–30.

Cobb, S., & Rose, R. (1973). Hypertension, peptic ulcer, and diabetes in air traffic control-lers. *Journal of the American Medical Association, 224*, 489–492.

Cohen, M. E., & White P. D. (1950). Life situations, emotions and neurocirculatory as-thenia (anxiety neurosis, neurasthenia, effort syndrome). In H. G. Wolff (Ed.), *Life stress and bodily disease* (Nervous and Mental Disease, Research Publication No. 29). Baltimore, MD: Williams & Wilkins.

Cohen, R., Williamson, D., Monguillot, J., Hutchinson, P., Gottlieve, J., & Waters, W. (1983). Psychophysiological response patterns in vascular and muscle-contraction headaches. *Journal of Behavioral Medicine, 10*, 411–423.

Cole, C. W., & Oetting, E. R. (1972). *Concept specific anxiety scale (CAS): Informational brief*. Fort Collins, CO: Rocky Mountain Behavioral Sciences Institute, Inc.

Comas-Diaz, L., & Griffith, E. E. H. (Eds.) (1988). *Clinical guidelines in cross-cultural mental health*. New York: Wiley.

Cooper, B. (1978). Epidemiology. In J. Wing (Ed.), *Schizophrenia: Towards a new synthesis*. London: Academic Press.

Costello, C. G. (1982). Fears and phobias in women: A community study. *Journal of Abnor-mal Psychology, 91*, 280–286.

Cowden, R. C., & Ford, L. I. (1962). Systematic desensitization with phobic schizophrenics. *American Journal of Psychiatry, 119*, 241–245.

Cox, B. J., Norton, G. R., Dorward, J., & Fergusson, P. A. (in press). The relationship between panic attacks and chemical dependencies. *Addictive Behaviors*.

Cragan, M., & Deffenbacher, J. (1984). Anxiety management training and relaxation as self-control in the treatment of generalized anxiety in medical outpatients. *Journal of Counseling Psychology, 31,* 123–131.

Crocker, P., Alderman, R., & Smith, F. (1988). Cognitive-affective stress management training with high performance youth volleyball players: Effects on affect, cognition, and performance. *Journal of Sport and Exercise Psychology, 10,* 448–460.

Curtis, G. C., Nesse, R. M., Buxton, M., & Lippman, D. (1979). Plasma growth hormone: Effect of anxiety during flooding in vivo. *American Journal of Psychiatry, 136,* 410–414.

Daley, P., Bloom, L., Deffenbacher, J., & Stewart, R. (1983). Treatment effectiveness of anxiety management training in small and large group formats. *Journal of Counseling Psychology, 30,* 104–107.

Darwin, C. (1872). *The expression of the emotions in man and animals.* Chicago: University of Chicago Press, 1965.

Deffenbacher, J., (1988). Cognitive-relaxation and social skills treatments of anger: A year later. *Journal of Counseling Psychology, 35,* 234–236.

Deffenbacher, J., & Craun, A. (1985). Anxiety management training with stressed student gynecology patients: A collaborative approach. *Journal of College Student Personnel, 26,* 513–518.

Deffenbacher, J., Demm, P., & Brandon, A. (1986). High general anger: Correlates and treatment. *Behaviour Research and Therapy, 24,* 481–489.

Deffenbacher, J., & Hahnloser, R. (1981). Cognitive and relaxation coping skills in stress inoculation. *Cognitive Therapy and Research, 5,* 211–215.

Deffenbacher, J., McNamara, K., Stark, R., & Sabadell, P. (in press a). A comparison of cognitive-behavioral and process oriented group counseling for general anger reduction. *Journal of Counseling and Development.*

Deffenbacher, J., McNamara, K., Stark, R., & Sabadell, P. (in press b). A combination of cognitive, relaxation, and behavioral coping skills in the reduction of anger. *Journal of College Student Development.*

Deffenbacher, J., & Michaels, A. C. (1980). Two self-control procedures in the reduction of targeted and nontargeted anxieties — A year later. *Journal of Counseling Psychology, 27,* 9–15.

Deffenbacher, J., & Michaels, A. (1981a). A twelve-month follow-up of homogeneous and heterogeneous anxiety management training. *Journal of Counseling Psychology, 28,* 463–466.

Deffenbacher, J., & Michaels, A. (1981b). Anxiety management training and self-control desensitization - 15 months later. *Journal of Counseling Psychology, 28,* 481–489.

Deffenbacher, J., Michaels, A., Daley, P., & Michaels, T. (1980). A comparison of homogeneous and heterogeneous anxiety management training. *Journal of Counseling Psychology, 27,* 630–634.

Deffenbacher, J., & Shelton, J. (1978). Comparison of anxiety management training and desensitization in reducing test and other anxieties. *Journal of Counseling Psychology, 25,* 277–282.

Deffenbacher, J., & Stark, R. (1990). Relaxation and cognitive-relaxation coping skills in the reduction of general anger. Manuscript submitted for publication.

Deffenbacher, J., Story, D., Brandon, A., Hogg, J., & Hazaleus, S. (1988). Cognitive and cognitive-relaxation treatments of anger. *Cognitive Therapy and Research, 12,* 167-184.

Deffenbacher, J., Story, D., Stark, R., Hogg, J., & Brandon, A. (1987). Cognitive-relaxation and social skills interventions in the treatment of general anger. *Journal of Counseling Psychology, 34,* 171-176.

Deffenbacher, J., & Suinn, R. (1988). Concepts and treatment of the generalized anxiety syndrome. In L. Ascher & L. Michelson (Eds.), *International handbook of assessment and treatment of anxiety disorders.* New York: Guilford Press.

DeLongis, A., Coyne, J. C., Dakoif, G., Folkman, S., & Lazarus, R. S. (1982). Relation of daily hassles, uplifts, and major life events to health status. *Health Psychology, 1,* 119–136.

Dembroski, T., MacDougall, J., Eliot, R., & Buell, J. (1983). Stress, emotions,behavior, and cardiovascular disease. In L. Temoshok, C. Van Dyke, & L. Zegan (Eds.), *Emotions in health and illness.* New York: Grune & Stratton.

Dembroski, T. M., Weiss, S. M., Shields, J. L., Haynes, S. G., & Feinleib, M. (Eds.) (1978). *Coronary-prone behavior.* New York: Springer-Verlag.

Di Nardo, P. A., Barlow, D. H., Cerny, J., Vermilyear, B. B., Vermilyea, J. A., Himadi, W., & Waddell, M. (1985). *Anxiety Disorders Interview Schedule - Revised (ADIS-R).* Albany, New York: Phobia and Anxiety Disorders Clinic, State University of New York at Albany.

Doctor, R. M., & Altman, F. (1969). Worry and emotionality as components of test anxiety: Replication and further data. *Psychological Reports, 24,* 563–568.

Donnerstein, E., & Wilson, D. W. (1976). Effects of noise and perceived control on ongoing and subsequent aggressive behavior. *Journal of Personality and Social Psychology, 34,* 774–781.

Drazen, M., Nevid, J., Pace, N., & O'Brien, R. (1982). Worksite-based behavioral treatment of mild hypertension. *Journal of Occupational Medicine, 24,* 511–514.

D'Zurilla, T. J., & Goldfried, M. R. (1971). Problem solving and behavior modification. *Journal of Abnormal Psychology, 78,* 107–126.

Eastwell, H. D. (1982). Psychological disorders among the Australian Aboriginals. In C. Friedmann & R. Faguet (Eds.), *Extraordinary disorders of human behavior,* pp. 229–258. New York: Plenum Press.

Edelberg, R. (1967). Electrical properties of the skin. In C. C. Brown (Ed.), *Methods in psychophysiology.* Baltimore, MD: Williams & Wilkins.

Edie, C. (1972). *Uses of anxiety management training in treating trait anxiety.* Unpublished doctoral dissertation, Colorado State University, Fort Collins, CO.

Ehlers, A., Margraf, J., Roth, W. T., Taylor, C. B., Maddock, R. J., Sheikh, J., Kobell, M. L., McClenahan, K. L., Gossard, D., Blowers, G. H., Agras, W. S., & Kopell, B. S. (1986). Lactate infusions and panic attacks: Do patients and controls respond differently? *Psychiatry Research, 17,* 295–308.

Eisler, R. M., Miller, P., & Hersen, M. (1973). Components of assertive behavior. *Journal of Clinical Psychology, 29,* 295–299.

Ellis, A. (1962). *A reason and emotion in psychotherapy.* New York: Lyle Stuart.

Endler, N., & Okada, M. (1975). A multidimensional measure of trait anxiety: The S-R inventory of general trait anxieties. *Journal of Consulting and Clinical Psychology, 43,* 319–329.

Engel, B. T. (1972). Response specificity. In N. S. Greenfield & R. A. Sternbach (Eds.), *Handbook of psychophysiology.* New York: Holt, Rinehart & Winston.

Eysenck, H. J., & Eysenck, S. B. G. (1968). *Manual for the Eysenck Personality Inventory.* San Diego, CA: Educational and Industrial Testing Service.

Fairbank, J., Langley, K., Jarvie, G., & Keane, T. (1981). A selected bibliography on post-traumatic stress disorders in Vietnam veterans. *Professional Psychology, 12,* 578–586.

Fairbank, J. A., McCaffrey, R., & Keane, T. M. (1985). Psychometric detection of fabricated symptoms of PTSD. *American Journal of Psychiatry, 142,* 501–503.

Ferster, C., Culbertson, S., & Boren, M. (1975). *Behavior principles,* 2nd ed. Englewood Cliffs, New Jersey: Prentice Hall.

Feuerstein, M., & Gainer, J. (1982). Chronic headache: Etiology and management. In D. Doleys, R. Meredith, & A. Ciminero (Eds.), *Behavioral medicine: Assessment and treatment strategies.* New York: Plenum Press.

Fitts, W. H. (1964). *Tennessee Self-Concept Scale.* Nashville, TN: Counselor Recordings and Tests.

Foa, E., & Kozak, M. (1985). Treatment of anxiety disorders: Implications for psycho-pathology. In A. H. Tuma & J. D. Maser (Eds.), *Anxiety and the anxiety disorders*, pp. 421–461. Hillsdale, New Jersey: Lawrence Erlbaum.

Forman, B. H., Goldstein, P. S., & Genel, M. (1974). Management of juvenile diabetes mellitus: Usefulness of 24-hour fractional quantitative urine glucose. *Pediatrics, 53*, 257–263.

Foy, D. W., Sipprelle, R. C., Rueger, D. B., & Carroll, E. M. (1984). Etiology of posttrauma-tic stress disorder in Vietnam veterans: Analysis of premilitary, military and combat exposure influences. *Journal of Consulting and Clinical Psychology, 52*, 79–87.

Freud, S. (1924). *Collected papers* (Volume I). London: Hogarth Press.

Freud, S. (1936). *The problem of anxiety* (in H. A. Bunker (trans.), *Hemmung, Symptom und Angst*). New York: The Psychoanalytic Quarterly Press & W. W. Norton.

Friedman, M., & Rosenman, R. (1974). *Type A behavior and your heart*. New York: Knopf.

Friedman, M. J., Schneiderman, C. K., West, A. N., & Corson, J. A. (1986). Measurement of combat exposure, posttraumatic stress disorder, and life stress among Vietnam combat veterans. *American Journal of Psychiatry, 143*, 537–539.

Friedman, M., Thoresen, C., & Gill, I. (1981). Type A behavior: Its possible role, detection, and alteration in patients with ischemic heart disease.In J. Hurst (Ed.), *Update V: The heart*. New York: McGraw-Hill.

Frohlich, E. D., Tarazi, R. C., & Duston, H. P. (1969). Hyperdynamic beta-adrenergic circulatory state. *Archives of Internal Medicine, 123*, 1–7.

Fyer, M. R., Uy, J., Martinez, J., Goetz, R., Klein, D. F., Liebowitz, M. R., Fyer, A. J., & Gorman, J. (1986, May). *Carbon dioxide challenge of patients with panic disorder*. Paper presented at the annual convention of the American Psychiatric Association, Wash-ington, D.C.

Gannon, L, Haynes, S., Cuevas, J., & Chavez, R. (1987). Psychophysiological correlates of induced headaches. *Journal of Behavioral Medicine, 10*, 411–423.

Garner, D., Garfinkel, P., Schwartz, D., & Thompson, M. (1980). Cultural expectations of thinness of women. *Psychological Reports, 47*, 483, 491.

Geer, J. (1965). The development of a scale to measure fear. *Behaviour Research and Therapy, 3*, 45–53.

Geller, I., & Seifter, J. (1960). The effects of meprobamate, barbituates, d-amphetamine and promazine on experimentally induced conflict in the rat. *Psychopharmacologia, 1*, 482–492.

Gentry, W., Chesney, A., Gary, H., Hall, R., & Harburg, E. (1982). Habitual anger-coping styles: I. Effect on mean blood pressure and risk for essential hypertension. *Psycho-somatic Medicine, 44*, 195–202.

Gittelman, R., & Klein, D. F. (1985). Childhood separation anxiety and adult agoraphobia. In A. Tuma & J. Maser (Eds.), *Anxiety and the anxiety disorders*. Hillsdale, New Jersey: Erlbaum.

Glass, C. R. & Merluzzi, T. V. (1981). Cognitive assessment of social-evaluative anxiety. In T. Merluzzi, C. Glass, & M. Genest (Eds.), *Cognitive assessment*, pp. 388–438. New York: Guilford Press.

Gleser, G. C., Green, B. L., & Winget, C. N. (1981). *Buffalo Creek revisited: Prolonged psychosocial effects of disaster*. New York: Simon & Schuster.

Goldberg, D., Steele, J., Johnson, A., & Smith, C. (1982). Ability of primary care physicians to make accurate ratings of psychiatric symptoms. *Archives of General Psychiatry, 39*, 829–833.

Goldfried, M. (1979). Anxiety reduction through cognitive-behavioral intervention. In P. Kendall & S. Hollon (Eds.), *Cognitive-behavioral interventions: Theory, research, and pro-cedures*, pp. 117–152. New York: Academic Press.

Goldfried, M. (1988). Application of rational restructuring to anxiety disorders. *The Counseling Psychologist, 16*, 50–68.

Goldfried, M., Decenteceo, E., & Weinberg, L. (1974). Systematic rational restructuring as a self-control technique. *Behavior Therapy, 5*, 247–254.

Goldfried, M., Linehan, M., & Smith, J. (1978). The reduction of test anxiety through cognitive restructuring. *Journal of Consulting and Clinical Psychology, 46*, 32–39.

Goldfried, M., & Trier, C. (1974). Effectiveness of relaxation as an active coping skills. *Journal of Abnormal Psychology, 83*, 348–355.

Goldstein, A., & Chambless, D. (1978). A reanalysis of agoraphobia. *Behavior Therapy, 9*, 47–59.

Good, B., Good, M., & Moradi, R. (1985). The interpretation of Iranian depressive illness and dysphoric affect. In A. Kleinman & B. Good (Eds.), *Culture and depression*, pp. 369–428. Berkeley: University of California Press.

Grant, S. J., & Redmond, D. E., Jr. (1981). The neuroanatomy and pharmacology of the nucleus locus coeruleus. In H. Lal & S. Fielding (Eds.), *The psychopharmacology of clonidine*. New York: Alan R. Liss, Inc.

Gray, J. A. (1985). Issues in the neuropsychology of anxiety. In A. H. Tuma & J. D. Maser (Eds.), *Anxiety and the anxiety disorders*. Hillsdale, New Jersey: Erlbaum.

Haefely, W., Polc, P., Pieri, L., Schaffner, R., & Laurent, J. P. (1983). Neuropharmacology of benzodiazepines: Synaptic mechanisms and neuronal basis of action. In E. Costa (Ed.), *The benzodiazepines: From molecular biology to clinical practice*. New York: Raven Press.

Hamilton, M. (1959). The assessment of anxiety states by rating. *British Journal of Medical Psychology, 32*, 50–55.

Hamilton, M. (1960). A rating scale for depression. *Journal of Neurology, Neurosurgery and Psychiatry, 23*, 56–62.

Hanson, S., & Pichert, J. (1986). Perceived stress and diabetes control in adolescents. *Health Psychology, 5*, 439–452.

Hart, K. (1984). Stress management training for Type A individuals. *Journal of Behavioral Therapy and Experimental Psychiatry, 15*, 133–140.

Hathaway, S. R., & McKinley, J. C. (1967). Minnesota Multiphasic Personality Inventory, Minneapolis, MN: University of Minnesota.

Hazaleus, S., & Deffenbacher, J. (1986). Relaxation and cognitive treatments of anger. *Journal of Consulting and Clinical Psychology, 54*, 222–226.

Hearn, M. D., Murray, D. M., & Luepker, R. V. (1989). Hostility, coronary heart disease, and total mortality: A 33-year follow-up study of university students. *Journal of Behavioral Medicine, 12*, 105–122.

Heide, F. J., & Borkovec, T. D. (1983). Relaxation-induced anxiety: Paradoxical anxiety enhancement due to relaxation training. *Journal of Consulting and Clinical Psychology, 51*, 171–182.

Heide, F., & Borkovec, T. (1984). Relaxation-induced anxiety: Mechanisms and theoretical implications. *Behaviour Research and Therapy, 22*, 1–12.

Helmreich, R., & Stapp, J. (1971). Short forms of the Texas Social Behavior Inventory (TSBI): An objective measure of self-esteem. *Bulletin of the Psychonomic Society, 4*, 473–475.

Helzer, J. E., Robins, L. N., & McEvoy, L. (1987). Post-traumatic stress disorder in the general population: Findings of the Epidemiologic Catchment Area Survey. *New England Journal of Medicine, 317*, 1630.

Hill, E. (1977). A comparison of anxiety management training and interpersonal skills training for socially anxious college students. *Dissertation Abstracts International, 37* (8-A), 4985.

Hillenberg, J., & Collins, F. (1983). The importance of home practice for progressive relaxation training. *Behaviour Research and Therapy, 21*, 633–642.

Hoehn-Saric, R., Merchant, A. Keyser, M., & Smith, V. (1981). Effects of clonidine on anxiety disorder. *Archives of General Psychiatry, 38*, 1278–1282.

Hohnson, E., & Broman, C. (1987). The relationship of anger expression to health problems among Black Americans in a national survey. *Journal of Behavioral Medicine, 10*, 103–116.

Holden, A. E., & Barlow, D. H. (1986). Heart rate and heart rate variability recorded in vivo in agoraphobics and nonphobics. *Behavior Therapy, 17*, 26–42.

Hollingshead, A., & Redlich, F. (1958). *Social class and mental illness.* New York: Wiley.

Hollon, S. D., & Beck, A. T. (1986). Cognitive therapy and cognitive-behavioral interventions. In A. E. Bergin & S. L. Garfield (Eds.), *Handbook of psychotherapy and behavior change* (3rd ed.). New York: Wiley.

Holmberg, G., & Gershon, S. (1961). Autonomic and psychiatric effects of yohimbine hydrochloride. *Psychopharmacologia, 2*, 93–106.

Holmes, T., & Rahe, R. (1967). The social readjustment rating scale. *Journal of Psychosomatic Research, 11*, 213, 218.

Hornsby, J. (1987). *Essentials of neuropsychological assessment.* New York: Springer.

Howard, J., Cunningham, D., & Rechnitzer, P. (1977). Work patterns associated with Type A behavior: A managerial population. *Human Relations, 30*, 825–836.

Hutchings, D., Denney, D., Basgall, J., & Houston, B. (1980). Anxiety management and applied relaxation in reducing general anxiety. *Behaviour Research and Therapy, 18*, 181–190.

Insel, T. R., Ninan, P., Aloi, J., Jimerson, D., Skolnick, P., & Paul, S. M. (1984). A benzodiazepine receptor mediated model of anxiety: Studies in nonhuman primates and clinical implications. *Archives of General Psychiatry, 41*, 741–750.

Jacob, R., & Chesney, M. (1986). Psychological and behavioral methods to reduce cardiovascular reactivity. In K. Matthews, S. Weiss, T. Detre, T. Dembroski, B. Falkner, S. Manuck, & R. Williams Jr. (Eds.), *Handbook of stress, reactivity, and cardiovascular disease*, pp. 417–460. New York: Wiley.

Jannoun, L., Oppenheimer, C., & Gelder, M. (1982). A self-help treatment program for anxiety state patients. *Behavior Therapy, 13*, 103–111.

Jenni, M., & Wollersheim, J. (1979). Cognitive therapy, stress management training and Type A behavior pattern. *Cognitive Therapy and Research, 3*, 61–73.

Jenkins, C. D., Rosenman, R. H., & Zyzanski, S. J. (1972). *The Jenkins activity survey for health prediction, Form B.* Authors, Boston.

Johnson, S. (1980). Psychosocial facets in juvenile diabetes: A review. *Journal of Behavioral Medicine, 13*, 95–116.

Johnstone, E. C., Bourne, R. C., Crow, T. J., Frith, C. D., Gamble, S., Lofthouse,R., Owen, F., Owens, D. G. C., Robinson, J., & Stevens, M. (1981). The relationship between clinical response, psychophysiological variables and plasma levels of amitriptyline and diazepam in neurotic outpatients. *Psychopharmacology, 72*, 233–240.

Jones, I. H., & Horne, D. J. (1973). Psychiatric disorders among the Aborigines of the Australian Western Desert: Further data and discussion. *Social Science and Medicine, 7*, 219–228.

Jonsson, A., & Hansson, L. (1978). Prolonged exposure to a stressful stimulus (noise) as a cause of raised blood pressure in man. *Lancet, 1*, 86–87.

Jorgensen, R., Houston, B., & Zurawaki, R. (1981). Anxiety management training in the treatment of essential hypertension. *Behaviour Research and Therapy, 19*, 467–474.

Joy, V. D., & Lehmann, V. (1975). *The cost of crowding: Responses and adaptations.* Unpublished manuscript, New York State Department of Mental Hygiene.

Kanner, A., Coyne, J., Schaefer, C., & Lazarus, R. (1981). Comparison of two modes of stress measurement: Daily hassles and uplifts versus major life events. *Journal of Behavioral Medicine, 4*, 1–39.

Kanter, N., & Goldfried, M. (1979). Relative effectiveness of rational restructuring and self-control desensitization in the reduction of interpersonal anxiety. *Behavior Therapy, 10*, 472–490.

Katkin, E. S. (1975). Electrodermal lability: A psychophysiological analysis of individual differences in response to stress. In I. G. Sarason & C. D. Spielberger (Eds.), *Stress and anxiety*. Washington, D.C.: Hemisphere Publishing Company.

Kazdin, A. (1974). Self-monitoring and behavior change. In M. Mahoney & C. Thoresen (Eds.), *Self-control: Power to the person*. Monterey, CA: Brooks/Cole.

Kazdin, A. E., & Mascitelli, S. (1982). Covert and overt rehearsal and homework practice in developing assertiveness. *Journal of Consulting and Clinical Psychology, 50*, 250–258.

Keefe, F. J., Kopel, S. A., & Gorden, S. B. (1978). *A practical guide to behavioral assessment*. New York: Springer Publishing Company.

Kelly, D. (1980). *Anxiety and emotions: Physiological basis and treatment*. Springfield, IL: C. C. Thomas.

Kelly, K., & Stone, G. (1987). Effects of three psychological treatments and self-monitoring on the reduction of Type A behavior. *Journal of Counseling Psychology, 34*, 46–54.

Kendall, P., & Braswell, L. (1985). *Cognitive-behavioral therapy for impulsive children*. New York: Guilford.

Kenny, M. (1983). Paradox lost: The latah problem revisited. *Journal of Nervous and Mental Disorders, 171*, 159–167.

Kidson, M. A., & Jones, I. H. (1968). Psychiatric disorders among the Aborigines of the Australian western desert. *Archives of General Psychiatry, 19*, 413–417.

Kilpatrick, D. G., Veronen, L. J., & Resick, P. A. (1979). The aftermath of rape: Recent empirical findings. *American Journal of Orthopsychiatry, 49*, 658–669.

Kleinman, A. (1982). Neurasthenia and depression: A study of somatization and culture in China. *Culture, Medicine, and Psychiatry, 6*, 117–190.

Kleinman, A. (1986). *Social origins of distress and disease*. New Haven, CT: Yale University Press.

Knight, R., Atkins, A., Eagle, C., Evans, N., Finklestein, J. W., Fukushima,D., Katz, J., & Weiner, H. (1979). Psychological stress, ego defenses, and cortisol production in children hospitalized for elective surgery. *Psychosomatic Medicine, 41*, 40–49.

Komaki, J., & Dore-Boyce, K. (1978). Self-recording: Its effects on individuals high and low in motivation. *Behavior Therapy, 9*, 65–72.

Konincyx, P. (1978). Stress hyperprolactinemia in clinical practice. *Lancet, 2*, 273.

Kopel, S. A., & Arkowitz, H. (1974). Role-playing as a source of self-observation and behavior change. *Journal of Personality and Social Psychology, 29*, 677–686.

Krantz, D., Contrada, R., Hill, D., & Friedler, E. (1988). Environmental stress and biobehavioral antecedents of coronary heart disease. *Journal of Consulting and Clinical Psychology, 56*, 333–341.

Krantz, D., & Manuck, S. (1984). Acute psychophysiologic reactivity and risk of cardiovascular disease: A review and methodologic critique. *Psychological Bulletin, 96*, 435–464.

Krug, S., Scheier, I., & Cattell, R. (1976). *Handbook for the IPAT Anxiety Scale*. Champaign, IL: Institute for Personality and Ability Testing.

Kulka, R. A., Schlenger, W. E., Fairbank, J. A., Hough, R. L., Jordan, B. K., Marmar, C. R., & Weiss, D. S. (1988). *National Vietnam veterans readjustment study advance data report: Preliminary findings from the national survey of the Vietnam generation*. Executive Summary. Washington, DC: Veterans Administration.

Lacey, J. I. (1967). Somatic response patterning and stress: Some revisions of activation theory. In M. Appley & R. Trumbell (Eds.), *Psychological stress*. New York: Appleton-Century-Crofts.

Lader, M. H. (1980). Psychophysiological studies in anxiety. In G. D. Burrows & D. Davies (Eds.), *Handbook of studies on anxiety*. Amersterdam: Elsevier/ North-Holland.

Lader, M., Gelder, M., & Marks, I. (1967). Palmar skin-conductance measures as predictors of response to desensitization. *Journal of Psychosomatic Research, 11,* 283–290.

Lader, M. H., & Wing, L. (1964). Habituation of the psycho-galvanic reflex in patients with anxiety states and in normal subjects. *Journal of Neurology, Neurosurgery, and Psychiatry, 27,* 210–218.

Lang, P. J. (1980). Behavioral treatment and bio-behavioral assessment: Computer applications. In J. Sidowski, J. Johnson, & T. Williams (Eds.), *Technology in mental health care delivery systems*. Norwood, NJ: Ablex.

Lang, P. (1985). The cognitive psychophysiology of emotion: Fear and anxiety.In A. Tuma & J. Maser (Eds.), *Anxiety and the anxiety disorders*, pp. 131–170. Hillsdale, New Jersey: Erlbaum.

Lang, P. J., Levin, D. N., Miller, G. A., & Kozak, M. J. (1983). Fear behavior, fear imagery, and the psychophysiology of emotion: The problem of affective response integration. *Journal of Abnormal Psychology, 92,* 276–306.

Lanyon, R. I. (1973). *Psychological Screening Inventory Manual*. New York: Research Psychologsts Press.

Last, C. (1985). Implosion. In A. Bellack & M. Hersen (Eds.), *Dictionary of behavior therapy techniques*. New York: Pergamon.

Lawler, J., Cox, R., Sanders, B., & Mitchell, V. (1988). The borderline hypertensive rat: A model for studying the mechanisms of environmentally induced hypertension. *Health Psychology, 7,* 137–147.

Lazarus, A. A. (1971). *Behavior therapy and beyond*. New York: McGraw-Hill.

Lazarus, R. (1966). *Psychological stress and the coping process*. New York: McGraw-Hill.

Lazarus, R. S., & Averill, J. R. (1972). Emotion and cognition: With special reference to anxiety. In C. D. Spielberger (Ed.), *Anxiety: Current trends in theory and research* (Volume 2), pp. 241–283. New York: Academic Press.

Lazarus, R. S., & Folkman, S. (1984). *Stress, appraisal, and coping*. New York: Springer.

Leary, M. R. (1982). Social anxiety. In L. Wheeler (Ed.), *Review of personality and social psychology* (Volume 3). Beverly Hills, CA: Sage.

Leckman, J. F., Weissman, M. M., Merikangas, K. R., Pauls, D. L., & Prusoff, B. A. (1983). Panic disorder and major depression. *Archives of General Psychiatry, 40,* 1055–1060.

Leelarthaepin, B., Gray, W., & Chesworth, E. (1980). Exersentry: An evaluation of its cardiac frequency monitoring accuracy. *Australian Journal of Sports Science,* 1–11.

Lehrer, P. (1982). How to relax and how not to relax: A re-evaluation of the work of Edmund Jacobson - I. *Behaviour Research and Therapy, 20,* 417–428.

Lent, R., Russell, R., & Zamostny, K. (1981). Comparison of cue-controlled desensitization, rational restructuring, and a credible placebo in the treatment of speech anxiety. *Journal of Consulting and Clinical Psychology, 49,* 608–610.

Levan, I., & Bilu, Y. (1980). A transcultural view of Israeli psychiatry. *Transcultural Psychiatric Research Review, 17,* 7–36.

Levenkron, J., Cohen, J., Mueller, H., & Fisher, E. (1983). Modifying the Type A coronary-prone behavior pattern. *Journal of Consulting and Clinical Psychology, 51,* 192–204.

Liebowitz, M. R., Fyer, A. J., Gorman, J. M., Dillon, D., Appleby, I. L., Levy, G., Anderson, S., Levitt, M., Palij, M., Davies, S. O., & Klein, D. F. (1984). Lactate provocation of panic. *Archives of General Psychiatry, 41,* 764–770.

Liebowitz, M. R., Gorman, J. M., Fyer, A. J., Levitt, M., Dillon, D., Levy, P., Appleby, I. L.,

Anderson, S., Palij, M., Davies, S. O., & Klein, D. F. (1985). Lactate provocation of panic attacks: II. Biochemical and physiological findings. *Archives of General Psychiatry*, *42*, 709–719.

Linehan, M. M., Goldfried, M. R., & Goldfried, A. P. (1979). Assertion therapy: Skill training or cognitive restructuring. *Behavior Therapy*, *10*, 372–388.

Lobitz, W., & Brammell, H. (1981, August). *Anxiety management training versus aerobic conditioning for cardiac stress management*. Paper presented at the annual meeting of the American Psychological Association, Los Angeles, CA.

Long, B. C. (1984). Aerobic conditioning and stress inoculation: A comparison of stress management interventions. *Cognitive Therapy and Research*, *8*, 517–532.

MacDougall, J., Dembroski, T., Dimsdale, J., & Hackett, T. (1985). Components of Type A, hostility, and anger-in: Further relationships to angiographic findings. *Health Psychology*, *4*, 137–152.

Mahl, G. F. (1959). Exploring emotional states by content analysis. In I. D. Pool (Ed.), *Trends in content analysis*. Urbana, IL: University of Illinois Press.

Mahoney, M., & Arnkoff, D. (1978). Cognitive and self-control therapies. In S. Garfield & A. Bergin (Eds.), *Handbook of psychotherapy and behavior change: An empirical analysis* (2nd ed.). New York: Wiley.

Mahoney, M., & Suinn, R. (1986). History and overview of modern sport psychology. *The Clinical Psychologist*, *39*, 64–68.

Malloy, P. F., Fairbank, J. A., & Keane, T. M. (1983). Validation of a multimethod assessment of posttraumatic stress disorder in Vietnam veterans. *Journal of Consulting and Clinical Psychology*, *51*, 488–494.

Maple, S., Bradshaw, C. M., & Szabadi, E. (1981). Pharmacological responsiveness of sweat glands in anxious patients and healthy volunteers. *British Journal of Psychiatry*, *141*, 154–161.

Marcia, J. E., Rubin, B. M., & Efran, J. S. (1969). Systematic desensitization: Expectancy change or counterconditioning. *Journal of Abnormal Psychology*, *74*, 382–387.

Margolin, G. (1987). Marital therapy: A cognitive-behavioral-affective approach. In N. Jacobson (Ed.), *Psychotherapists in clinical practice*. New York: Guilford.

Marks, I. M., & Lader, M. (1973). Anxiety states (anxiety neurosis): A review. *Journal of Nervous and Mental Disease*, *156*, 3–18.

Marks, I., & Mathews, A. (1979). Brief standard self-rating for phobic patients. *Behaviour Research and Therapy*, *17*, 263–267.

Marsella, A. (1980). Depressive experience and disorder across cultures. In H. Triandis & J. Draguns (Eds.), *Handbook of cross-cultural psychology: Psychopathology*, Vol. 6, pp. 237–290. Boston: Allyn and Bacon.

Marsland, D. W., Wood, M., & Mayo F. (1976). Content of family practice: A data bank for patient care, curriculum, and research in family practice—526,196 patient problems. *Journal of Family Practice*, *3*, 25–68.

Martens, R. (1977). *Sport competition anxiety test*. Champaign, IL: Human Kinetics.

Martens, R., Burton, D., Vealey, R. S., Bump, L. A., & Smith, D. E. (1983). *Competitive state anxiety inventory–2*. Unpublished manuscript, University of Illinois at Urbana-Champaign.

Mash, E. J., & Terdal, L. G. (Eds.). (1976). *Behavior therapy assessment*. New York: Springer-Verlag.

Mathis, H. (1978). *Effect of anxiety management training on musical performance anxiety*. Unpublished masters thesis, Colorado State University, Fort Collins, CO.

Matthews, K. (1982). Psychological perspectives on the Type A behavior pattern. *Psychological Bulletin*, *91*, 293–323.

Matthews, K., Helmreich, R., Beane, W., & Lucker, G. (1980). Pattern A achievement striving and scientific merit: Does Pattern A help or hinder? *Journal of Personality and Social Psychology*, *39*, 962–967.

McFall, R. M. (1982). A review and reformulation of the concept of social skills. *Behavioral assessment, 4,* 1–33.

McGrady, A., Woerner, M., Bernal, G., & Higgins, Jr., J. Effect of biofeedback assisted relaxation on blood pressure and cortisol levels in normotensives and hypertensives. *Journal of Behavioral Medicine, 10,* 301–311.

McNair, P. M., Lorr, M., & Droppleman, L. (1971). *Profile of mood states manual.* San Diego, CA: Educational and Industrial Testing Services.

McNally, R. (1987). Preparedness and phobias: A review. *Psychological Bulletin, 101,* 283–303.

Meichenbaum, D. H. (1972). Cognitive modification and test anxious college students. *Journal of Consulting and Clinical Psychology, 39,* 370–380.

Meichenbaum, D. (1985). *Stress inoculation training.* New York: Pergamon Press.

Meichenbaum, D., & Deffenbacher, J. (1988). Stress inoculation training. *The Counseling Psychologist, 16,* 69–90.

Mendonca, J., & Siess, T. (1976). Counseling for indecisiveness: Problem-solving and anxiety-management training. *Journal of Counseling Psychology, 23,* 339–347.

Michelson, L. (1985). Flooding. In A. Bellack & M. Hersen (Eds.), *Dictionary of behavior therapy techniques.* New York: Pergamon.

Miller, I., & Norman, W. (1981). Effects of attributions for success on the alleviation of learned helplessness and depression. *Journal of Abnormal Psychology, 90,* 113–124.

Miller, R. G., Rubin, R. T., Clark, B. R., Poland, R. E., & Arthur, R. J. (1970). The stress of aircraft carrier landings. In: Corticosteriod responses in naval aviators. *Psychosomatic Medicine, 32,* 581–588.

Miskimins, R. W., & Braught, G. N. (1971). *Description of the self.* Fort Collins, CO: Rocky Mountain Behavioral Sciences Institute, Inc.

Morice, R. (1978). Psychiatric diagnosis in a transcultural setting. *British Journal of Psychiatry, 132,* 87.

Mullaney, J. A., & Trippett, C. J. (1979) Alcohol dependence and phobias: Clinical description and relevance. *British Journal of Psychiatry, 137,* 565–573.

Murphy, H. B. M. (1982). *Comparative psychiatry: The international and intercultural distribution of mental illness.* New York: Springer-Verlag.

Mydgal, W. (1978). The acquisition of stress management skills by student teachers: An outcome of stress inoculation and anxiety management. *Dissertation Abstracts, 39,* 5-A, 2839–2840.

Myers, J. K., Weissman, M. M., Tischler, C. E., Holzer, C. E., III, Orvaschel, H., Anthony, J. C., Boyd, J. H., Burke, J. D., Jr., Kramer, M., & Stoltzman, R. (1984). Six-month prevalence of psychiatric disorders in three communities. *Archives of General Psychiatry, 41,* 959–967.

Nally, M. (1975). *AMT: A treatment for delinquents.* Unpublished doctoral dissertation, Colorado State University, Fort Collins, CO.

Neimeyer, R. A., Twentyman, C. T., & Prezant, D. (1985). Cognitive and interpersonal group therapies for depression: A progress report. *The Cognitive Behaviorist, 7,* 21–22.

Nemeroff, C., & Loosen, P. (Eds.)(1987). *Handbook of clinical psychoendocrinology.* New York: Guilford.

Nelson, R., Lipinski, D., & Black, J. (1976). The reactivity of adult retardates' self-monitoring: A comparison among behaviors of different valences and a comparison of token reinforcement. *Psychological Record, 26,* 189–301.

Nezu, A. M. (1987). A problem-solving formulation of depression: A literature review and proposal of a pluralistic model. *Clinical Psychology Review, 7,* 121–144.

Nicoletti, J. (1972). *Anxiety management training.* Unpublished doctoral dissertation, Colorado State University, Fort Collins, CO.

Nicoletti, J., Edie, C., & Spinelli, P. (1971). The public speaking anxiety inventory: Normative data. Unpublished manuscript, Colorado State University.

Nideffer, R. (1986). Concentration and attention control training. In J. Williams (Ed.), *Applied sport psychology: Personal growth to peak experience*, pp. 257–269. Palo Alto, CA: Mayfield.

Ninan, P. T., Insel, T. R., Cohen, R. M., Cook, J. M., Skolnick, P., & Paul, S. M. (1982). Benzodiazepine receptor mediated experimental "anxiety" in primates. *Science, 218*, 1332–1334.

Noel, G. L., Dimond, R. C., Earll, J. M., & Frantz, A. G. (1976). Prolactin, thyrotropin, and growth hormone release during stress associated with parachute jumping. *Aviation, Space and Environmental Medicine, 47*, 543–547.

Novaco, R. W. (1975). *Anger control*. Lexington, MA: Heath.

Novaco, R. (1979). The cognitive regulation of anger and stress. In. P. Kendall & S. Hollon (Eds.), *Cognitive-behavioral interventions: Theory, research, and procedures*. New York: Academic Press.

Orleans, C., George, L., Houpt, J., & Brodie, H. (1985). How primary care physicians treat psychiatric disorders: A national survey of family practitioners. *Archives of General Psychiatry, 142*, 52–57.

Orvashel, H., & Weissman, M. M. (in press). Epidemiology of anxiety disorders in children: A review. In R. Gittelman (Ed.), *Anxiety disorders of childhood*. New York: Guilford.

Ost, L., Jerremalm, A., & Johansson, J. (1981). Individual response patterns and the effects of different behavioural methods in the treatment of social phobia. *Behaviour Research and Therapy, 19*, 1–16.

Paul, G. L. (1966). *Insight vs. desensitization in psychotherapy*. Palo Alto, CA: Stanford University Press.

Paul, S. M., & Skolnick, P. (1978). Rapid changes in brain benzodiazepine receptors after experimental seizures. *Science, 202*, 892–894.

Paul, S. M., & Skolnick, P. (1981). Benzodiazepine receptors and psychopathological states: Towards a neurobiology of anxiety. In D. F. Klein & J. Rabkin (Eds.), *Anxiety: New research and changing concepts*. New York: Raven Press.

Pennebaker, J., Gonder-Frederick, L., Stewart, H., Elfman, L., & Skelton, J. (1982). Physical symptoms associated with blood pressure. *Psychophysiology, 19*, 201–210.

Pensk, W., & Robinowitz, R. (Eds.). (1987). Post-traumatic Stress Syndrome (PTSD) among Vietnam veterans. Special monograph supplement. *Journal of Clinical Psychology, 43*, 1–66.

Perley, M. H., & Guze, S. B. (1962). Hysteria - the stability and usefulness of clinical criteria: A quantitative study based on a follow-up period of 6–8 years in 39 patients. *New England Journal of Medicine, 266*, 421–426.

Peterson, D. R. (1961). Behavior problems of middle childhood. *Journal of Consulting Psychology, 25*, 205–209.

Peterson, D. R. (1968). *The clinical study of social behavior*. New York: Appleton-Century-Crofts.

Phares, E. J. (1968). Test anxiety, expectancies, and expectancy changes. *Psychological Reports, 22*, 259–265, 488–496.

Piasecki, J., & Hollon, S. (1987). Cognitive therapy for depression: Unexplicated schemata and scripts. In N. Jacobson (Ed.), *Psychotherapists in clinical practice* (pp. 121–152). New York: Guilford.

Pipes, R. (1982). Social anxiety and isolation in college students: A comparison of two treatments. *Journal of College Student Personnel, 23*, 502–508.

Pitts, F. N., Jr., & Allen, R. E. (1980). Beta adrenergic blockade in the treatment of anxiety. In R. J. Mathew (Ed.), *The biology of anxiety*. New York: Brunner/Mazel.

Polivy, J., & Herman, C. (1985). Dieting and binging: A causal analysis. *American Psychologist, 40*, 193–201.

Price, D. B., Thaler, M., & Mason, J. W. (1957). Preoperative emotional states and adrenal cortical activity: Studies on cardiac and pulmonary surgery patients. *Archives of Neurology and Psychiatry, 77*, 646–656.

Prince, F. (1987). Tcheng-Larocke culture-bound syndromes and international disease classifications. *Culture, Medicine, and Psychiatry, 11*, 3–19.

Prochaska, J. O. (1971). Symptom and dynamic cues in the implosive treatment of test anxiety. *Journal of Abnormal Psychology, 77*, 133–142.

Prochaska, J. O. (1975). In J. Shoemaker, *Treatments for anxiety neurosis.* Unpublished doctoral dissertation, Colorado State University, Fort Collins, CO.

Quillen, M., & Denney, D. (1982). Self-control of dysmenorrheic symptoms through pain management training. *Journal of Behavioral Therapy and Experimental Psychiatry, 13*, 123–130.

Rachman, S. (1980). Emotional processing. *Behaviour Research and Therapy, 18*, 51–60.

Rapee, R. M., Mattick, R., & Murrell, E. (1986). Cognitive mediation in the affective component of spontaneous panic attacks. *Journal of Behavior Therapy and Experimental Psychiatry, 17*, 245–253.

Rappaport, H., & Katkin, E. S. (1972). Relationships among manifest anxiety, response to stress, and the perception of autonomic activity. *Journal of Consulting and Clinical Psychology, 38*, 219–224.

Rathus, S. A. (1973). A 30-item schedule for assessing assertive behavior. *Behavior Therapy, 4*, 398–406.

Redmond, D. E., Jr. (1979). New and old evidence for the involvement of a brain norepinephrine system in anxiety. In W. E. Fann, I. Karacan, A. D. Pokorny, & R. L. Williams (Eds.), *Phenomenology and treatment of anxiety.* New York: Spectrum.

Resick, P. A., Veronen, L. J., Kilpatrick, D. G., Calhoun, K. S., & Atkinson, B. M. (1986). Assessment of fear reactions in sexual assault victims: A factor analytic study of the Veronen-Kilpatrick modified fear survey. *Behavioral Assessment, 8*, 271–283.

Resick, P., Wendiggensen, P. Ames, S., & Meyer, V. (1978). Systematic slowed speech: A new treatment for stuttering. *Behaviour Research and Therapy, 16*(3), 161–167.

Reynolds, D. (1976). *Morita psychotherapy.* Berkeley, CA: University of California Press.

Richardson, F., & Suinn, R. (1973a). A comparison of traditional systematic desensitization, accelerated massed desensitization, and anxiety management training in the treatment of mathematics anxiety. *Behaviour Therapy, 4*, 212–218.

Richardson, F., & Suinn, R. (1973b). Effects of two short-term desensitization methods in the treatment of test anxiety. *Journal of Counseling Psychology, 21*, 457–458.

Richardson, F., & Tasto, D. (1976). Development and factor analysis of a social anxiety inventory. *Behavior Therapy, 7*, 459–462.

Riskind, J. H., Beck, A. T., Brown, G. B., & Steer, R. A. (1987). Taking the measure of anxiety and depression: Validity of reconstructed Hamilton Scales. *Journal of Nervous and Mental Disease, 175*, 474–479.

Robertson, H. A., Martin, I. L., & Candy, J. M. (1978). Differences in benzodiazepines mediated by a GABA-ergic mechanism in the amygdala. *European Journal of Pharmacology, 82*, 115.

Rose, M., Firestone, P., Heick, H., & Faught, A. (1983). The effects of anxiety management training on the control of juvenile diabetes mellitus. *Journal of Behavioral Medicine, 6*, 381–396.

Rose, R. M., & Hurst, M. W. (1975). Plasma cortisol and growth hormone responses to intravenous catheterization. *Journal of Human Stress, 1*, 22–36.

Rosenman, R., Brand, R., Jenkins, C., Friedman, M., Straus, R., & Wurm, M. (1975).

Coronary heart disease in the Western Collaborative Group Study: Final follow-up experience of 81/2 years. *Journal of the American Medical Association, 233*, 872–877.

Rubin, R. (1982). Koro (Shook Yang): A culture-bound psychogenic syndrome. In C. Friedmann & R. Faguet (Eds.), *Extraordinary disorders of human behavior*, pp. 155–172. New York: Plenum Press.

Rugh, J. D., & Schwitzgebel, R. L. (1977). Instrumentation for behavioral assessment. In A. Ciminero, K. Calhoun, & H. Adams (Eds.), *Handbook of behavioral assessment*, pp. 79–116. New York: Wiley.

Sanderson, W. C., Rapee, R. M., & Barlow, D. H. (1989). The influence of illusion of control on panic attacks induced via inhalation of 5.5% CO^2 enriched air. *Archives of General Psychiatry, 46*, 157–162.

Sarason, I. G. (1985). Cognitive processes, anxiety, and the treatment of anxiety disorders. In A. H. Tuma & J. D. Maser (Eds.), *Anxiety and the anxiety disorders*. Hillsdale, New Jersey: Erlbaum.

Scott, D. (1981). Myofascial pain-dysfunction syndrome: A psychobiological perspective. *Journal of Behavioral Medicine, 4*, 451–465.

Schwartz, G. E. (1978). Psychobiological foundations of psychotherapy and behavior change. In S. L. Garfield & A. E. Bergin (Eds.), *Handbook of psychotherapy and behavior change: An empirical analysis* (2nd ed.). New York: Wiley.

Seligman, M. (1972). Phobias and preparedness. *Behavior Therapy, 2*, 307–320.

Seligman, M. (1983). Learned helplessness. In E. Levitt, B. Lubin, & J. Brooks (Eds.), *Depression: Concepts, controversies, and some new facts* (2nd ed.). Hillsdale, New Jersey: Erlbaum.

Seligman, M. E. P., & Hager, J. (Eds.) (1972). *Biological boundaries of learning*. New York: Appleton-Century-Crofts.

Selye, H. (1956). *The stress of life*. New York: McGraw-Hill.

Serber, M., & Nelson, P. (1971). The ineffectiveness of systematic desensitization and assertive training in hospitalized schizophrenics. *Journal of Behavior Therapy and Experimental Psychiatry, 2*, 107–109.

Shapiro, A., Benson, H., Chobanian, A. Herd, J., Julius, S., Kaplan, N., Lazarus, R. Ostfeld, A., & Syme, L. (1979). The role of stress in hypertension. *Journal of Human Stress, 5*, 7–27.

Shekelle, R., Gale, M., Ostfeld, A., & Paul, O. (1983). Hostility, risk of coronary heart disease and mortality. *Psychosomatic Medicine, 45*, 109–114.

Shoemaker, J. (1976). *Treatment for anxiety neurosis*. Unpublished doctoral dissertation, Colorado State University, Fort Collins, CO.

Shore, J. H., Tatum, E. L., & Vollmer, W. M. (1986). Psychiatric reactions to disaster: The Mount St. Helens experience. *American Journal of Psychiatry, 143* 590–595.

Siever, L. J., & Uhde, T. W. (1984). New studies and perspectives on the nonadrenergic receptor system in depression: Effects of the alpha–2-adrenergic against clonidine. *Biological Psychiatry, 19*, 131.

Sipprelle, C. (1975). Personal communication. In J. Shoemaker, *Treatments for anxiety neurosis*. Unpublished doctoral dissertation, Colorado State University, Fort Collins, CO.

Smail, P., Stockwell, T. Canter, S., & Hodgson, R. (1984). Alcohol dependence and phobic anxiety states: I. A prevalence study. *British Journal of Psychiatry, 144*, 53–57.

Smith, T., Ingram, R. E., & Brehm, S. S. (1983). Social anxiety, anxious self-preoccupation, and recall of self-relevant information. *Journal of Personality and Social Psychology, 44*, 1276–1283.

Snaith, R., Bridge, G., & Hamilton, M. (1976). *The Leeds scales for the self-assessment of anxiety and depression*. Barnstaple: Psychological Test Publications.

Sommer, B. (1978). Stress and menstrual distress. *Journal of Human Stress, 4*, 11–15.

Southern, S., & Smith, R. (1982). *Behavioral self-management counseling for Type A coronary prone university students.* Unpublished manuscript.

Spielberger, C., Barker, L., Russell, S., DeCrane, R., Westberry, L., Knight, J.,& Marks, E. (1979). *Preliminary manual for the state-trait personality inventory (STPI).* Tampa, FL: University of Southern Florida.

Spielberger, C. D., Gorsuch, R. L., & Lushene, R. E. (1970). *Manual for the State-Trait Anxiety Inventory (Self-evaluation questionnaire).* Palo Alto, CA: Consulting Psychologists Press.

Spielberger, C., Jacobs, G., Russell, S., & Crane, R. (1983). Assessment of anger: The State-Trait Anger Scale. In J. Butcher & C. Spielberger (Eds.), *Advances in personality assessment (Volume 3).* Hillsdale, New Jersey: Erlbaum.

Spinelli, P. R. (1972). *The effects of a therapist's presence in systematic desensitization therapy.* Unpublished doctoral disseration, Colorado State University, Fort Collins, CO.

Spiro, M. (1959). Cultural heritage, personal tension, and mental illness in a south sea culture. In M. Opler (Ed.), *Culture and mental health.* New York: Macmillan.

Spitzer, R., & Williams, J. (1987). *Diagnostic and statistical manual of mental disorders,* 3rd ed. rev., DSM-III-R. Washington, DC: American Psychiatric Association.

Stewart, H., & Olbrisch, M. (1986). Symptom correlates of blood pressure: A replication and reanalysis. *Journal of Behavioral Medicine, 9,* 271–290.

Stokes, P. (1985). The neuroendocrinology of anxiety. In A. H. Tuma & J. D. Maser (Eds.), *Anxiety and the anxiety disorders.* Hillsdale, New Jersey: Erlbaum.

Striegel-Moore, R., Silverstein, L., & Rodin, J. (1986). Toward an understanding of risk factors for bulimia. *American Psychologist, 41,* 246–263.

Suinn, R. (1961). Self-acceptance and acceptance of others: A learning theory analysis. *Journal of Abnormal and Social Psychology, 63,* 37.

Suinn, R. (1969). The STABS, A measure of test anxiety for behavior therapy: Normative data. *Behaviour Research and Therapy, 7,* 335.

Suinn, R. (1974). Behavior therapy for cardiac patients. *Behavior Therapy, 5,* 569.

Suinn, R. (1976). The coronary-prone behavior pattern: A behavioral approach to intervention. In T. Dembroski, S. Weiss, J. Shields, S. Haynes, & M. Feinleib (Eds.), *Coronary-prone behavior.* New York: Springer-Verlag.

Suinn, R. (1980). Psychology and sports performance: Principles and applications. In R. Suinn (Ed.), *Psychology in sports: Methods and applications.* Minneapolis, MN: Burgess.

Suinn, R. (1982). Imagery and sports. In A. Sheikh (Ed.), *Imagery, current theory, research and application.* New York: Wiley.

Suinn, R. (1984a). Visual motor behavior rehearsal: The basic technique. *Scandinavian Journal of Behaviour Therapy, 13,* 131–142.

Suinn, R. (1984b). The treatment of generalized anxiety disorder. In S. Turner (Ed.), *Behavioral theories and treatment of anxiety.* New York: Plenum.

Suinn, R. (1986a). Visualization in sports. In A. Sheikh (Ed.), *Imagery in sports.* Amityville, New York: Baywood Publishing.

Suinn, R. (1986b). *The seven steps to peak performance.* Toronto, Canada: Hans Huber Publishers.

Suinn, R. (1988). *Fundamentals of abnormal psychology, updated.* Chicago, IL: Nelson Hall.

Suinn, R., & Bloom, L. (1978). Anxiety management training for Pattern A behavior. *Journal of Behavioral Medicine, 1,* 25–35.

Suinn, R., Brock, L., & Edie, C. (1975). Behavior therapy for Type A patients. *American Journal of Cardiology, 36,* 269.

Suinn, R., & Deffenbacher, J. (1987). Concepts and treatment of the generalized anxiety syndrome. In L. Ascher & L. Michelson (Eds.), *International handbook of assessment and treatment of anxiety disorders,* pp. 332–360. New York: Guilford Press.

Suinn, R., Edie, C., Nicoletti, J., & Spinelli, R. (1972). The MARS, A measure of mathematics anxiety: Psychometric data. *Journal of Clinical Psychology, 28*, 373.

Suinn, R., Edie, C., & Spinelli, P. (1970). Accelerated massed desensitization: Innovation in short-term treatment. *Behavior Therapy, 1*, 303–311.

Suinn, R., Morton, M., & Dickinson, A. (1979). Psychological and mental training to increase efficiency in endurance athletes. *Final Report to U.S. Olympic Women's Athletics Developmental Subcommittee.*

Suinn, R., & Richardson, F. (1971). Anxiety management training: A non-specific behavior therapy program for anxiety control. *Behavior Therapy, 2*, 498.

Suinn, R., & Vattano, F. (1979). *Stress management for tension headache.* Unpublished manuscript, Colorado State University, Fort Collins, CO.

Szpiler, J., & Epstein, S. (1976). Availability of an avoidance response as related to autonomic arousal. *Journal of Abnormal Psychology, 85*, 73–82.

Taylor, J. A. (1953). A personality scale of manifest anxiety. *Journal of Abnormal and Social Psychology, 48*, 285–290.

Terrill, R. (1980). *A biography of Mao.* New York: Harper & Row.

Thompson, J., Griebstein, M., & Kuhlenschmidt, S. (1980). Effects of EMG biofeedback and relaxation training in the prevention of academic underachievement. *Journal of Counseling Psychology, 27*, 97–106.

Uhde, T. W., Boulenger, J. P., Vittone, B., Siever, L., & Post, R. M. (1985). Human anxiety and noradrenergic function: Preliminary studies with caffeine, clonidine and yohimbine. In *Proceedings of the Seventh World Congress of Psychiatry.* New York: Plenum Press.

Uhlenhuth, E. H., Baltzer, M. B., Mellinger, G. E., Cisin, I. H., & Clinthorne, J. (1983). Symptom checklist syndromes in the general population. *Archives of General Psychiatry, 40*, 1167–1173.

U.S. Department of Commerce. (1986). *Statistical abstract of the United States, 1987.* Washington, D.C.: Government Printing House, U.S. Bureau of the Census.

Valentine, C. (1978). The psychology of early childhood. In S. Rachman (Ed.), *Fear and courage.* San Francisco: W. H. Freeman.

van den Hout, M. A., & Griez, E. (1982). Cardiovascular and subjective responses to inhalation of carbon dioxide. *Psychotherapy and Psychosomatics, 37*, 75–82.

Van Hassel, J. (1979). *Anxiety management with schizophrenic outpatients.* Unpublished doctoral dissertation, Colorado State University, Fort Collins, CO.

Van Hassel, J., Bloom, L. J., & Gonzales, A. C. (1982). Anxiety management training with schizophrenic outpatients. *Journal of Clinical Psychology, 38*, 280–285.

Vermilyea, B. B., Barlow, D. H., & O'Brien, G. T. (1984). The importance of assessing treatment integrity: An example in the anxiety disorders. *Journal of Behavioral Assessment, 6*, 1–11.

Waeber, R., Adler, R. H., Schwank, A., & Galeazzi, R. L. (1982). Dyspnea proneness to CO_2 stimulation and personality (neuroticism, extraversion, MMPI factors). *Psychotherapy and Psychosomatics, 37*, 119–123.

Wadeson, R. W., Mason, J. W., Hamburg, D. A., & Handlon, J. H. (1963). Plasma and urinary 17-OH-CS responses to motion pictures. *Archives of General Psychiatry, 9*, 146–156.

Watson, D., & Friend, R. (1969). Measurement of social-evaluative anxiety. *Journal of Consulting and Clinical Psychology, 33*, 448–457.

Watson, D., & Tharp, R. (1981). *Self-directed behavior.* Monterey: Brooks/ Cole.

Wechsler, D. (1955). *Wechsler adult intelligence scale.* New York: The Psychological Corporation.

Wechsler, D. (1974). *Wechsler intelligence scale for children—revised.* New York: The Psychological Corporation.

Weiner, B., Frieze, L., Kukla, A., Reed, L., Rest, S., & Rosenbaum, R. M. (1971). *Perceiving the causes of success and failure.* Morristown, NJ: General Learning Press.

Weissman, M. (1983, September). *The epidemiology of anxiety disorders.* Paper presented at NIMH Conference on Anxiety and the Anxiety Disorders, Sterling Forest, Tuxedo, New York.

Weissman, M. M. (1985). The epidemiology of anxiety disorders: Rates, risks and familial patterns. In A. Tuma & J. Maser (Eds.), *Anxiety and the anxiety disorders.* Hillsdale, New Jersey: Erlbaum.

Weissman, M. M., Myers, J. K., & Harding, P. S. (1978). Psychiatric disorders in a U.S. urban community. *American Journal of Psychiatry, 135,* 459–462.

Williams, D. (1982). The treatment of seizures: Special psychotherapeutic and psychological techniques. In H. Sands (Ed.), *Epilepsy.* New York: Brunner/ Mazel.

Williams, S. L., & Rappoport, J. A. (1983). Cognitive treatment in the natural environment for agoraphobics. *Behavior Therapy, 14,* 299–313.

Williamson, D. (1981). Behavioral treatment of migraine and muscle contraction headache: Outcome and theoretical explanations. In M. Hersen, R. Eisler, & P. Miller (Eds.), *Progress in behavior modification, Volume II.* New York: Academic Press.

Wilson, J. (1988, August). *Anxiety disorders: Current treatments and controversies.* Paper presented at Annual Convention of the American Psychological Assocation, Atlanta, GA.

Wine, J. D. (1971). Test anxiety and direction of attention. *Psychological Bulletin, 76,* 92–104.

Wolpe, J. (1958). *Psychotherapy by reciprocal inhibition.* Stanford, CA: Stanford University Press.

Wolpe, J. (1969). *The practice of behavior therapy.* New York: Pergamon Press.

Wolpe, J. (1973). *The practice of behavior therapy* (2nd ed.). New York: Pergamon Press.

Wolpe, J., & Lang, P. (1964). A fear survey schedule for use in behavior therapy. *Behaviour Research and Therapy, 2,* 27–30.

Wolpe, J., & Lazarus, A. (1966). *Behavior therapy techniques.* Oxford, England: Pergamon.

Woods, S. W., Charney, D. S., Goodman, W. K., & Heninger, G. R. (1987). Carbon dioxide-induced anxiety: Behavioral, physiologic, and biochemical effects of 5% CO_2 in panic disorder patients and 5 and 7.5% CO_2 in healthy subjects. *Archives of General Psychiatry, 43,* 365–375.

Woods, S. W., Charney, D. S., Loke, J., Goodman, W. K., Redmond, D. E., & Heninger, G. R. (1986). Carbon dioxide sensitivity in panic anxiety. *Archives of General Psychiatry, 43,* 900–909.

Woods, S. W., Charney, D. S., McPherson, C. A., Gradman, A. H., & Heninger, G. R. (1987). Situational panic attacks: Behavioral, physiological, and biochemical characterization. *Archives of General Psychiatry, 44,* 365–375.

Wright, R., Contrada, R., & Glass, D. (1985). Psychophysiologic correlates of Type A behavior. In E. Katkin & S. Manuck (Eds.), *Advances in behavioral medicine.* Greenwich, CT: JAI.

Yager, T., Laufer, R., & Gallops, M. (1984). Some problems associated with war experience in memory of the Vietnam generation. *Archives of General Psychiatry, 41,* 327–333.

Ziegler, S., Klinzing, J., & Williamson, K. (1982). The effects of two stress management training programs on cardiorespiratory efficiency. *Journal of Sport Psychology, 4,* 280–289.

Zuckerman, M., & Lubin, B. (1985). *Manual for the multiple affect adjective checklist.* San Diego, CA: Educational and Industrial Testing Service.

Index

Speech anxiety (*cont.*)
    behavioral samplings of, 205
    desensitization for, 40, 41, 44
    SIT for, 130, 131
    SRR for, 135
Speech dysfluencies, 107, 205. *See also*
    specific types
Spielberger Anger Scales, 97, 98, 99
Spielberger State Anxiety Inventory, 50,
    51, 55, 57, 76, 82, 84, 85, 90, 93, 100
Spielberger Trait Anxiety Inventory, 44,
    50, 51, 54, 55, 57, 59, 62, 76, 77, 82,
    84, 85, 91, 93, 97, 98, 100
Sport Competition Anxiety Test, 105
SRE. *See* Schedule of Recent Events
S-R Inventory of Anxiousness, 206–207
SRR. *See* Systematic Rational
    Restructuring
STAI. *See* State-Trait Anxiety Inventory
State anger, 97, 99, 205
State anxiety, 52, 54, 57, 65, 135, 205
    cognitive performance and, 101
    depression and, 93, 94
    in Type A personality, 85
State-Trait Anxiety Inventory (STAI), 205
State-Trait Personality Inventory (STPI),
    205–206
Stomach complaints, 14, 94, 95, 107
    prevalence of, 4
STPI. *See* State-Trait Personality
    Inventory
Stress, 3–31
    contributing factors to, 15–30. *See also*
        specific factors
    multiple sources of, 140, 163–165
    prevalence of, 4–9
    symptoms of, 4
Stress Inoculation Training (SIT), 135,
    136, 137
    for anger management, 98
    applications of, 36
    in performance enhancement, 105
    phases of, 129
    vs. AMT, 128–131
Stress logs, 151, 213–214
    samples of, 327–330
    in session 1, 219, 231
    in session 2, 232, 242
    in session 3, 247
    in session 4, 248, 251, 252

Stress management programs, 4, 100, 101
Structured Interview, 82, 85
Stuttering, 75, 87–88
Subjective Units of Disturbance Scale
    (SUDS), 201–202, 204, 213
Subroutines, 21
Substance abuse, 8, 59
SUDS. *See* Subjective Units of Disturbance
    Scale
Suinn Test Anxiety Behavioral Scale, 39,
    42, 43
Susto, 15
Systematic desensitization (SD), 125, 136
Systematic Rational Restructuring (SRR),
    98, 130, 132–135, 136, 137

Taiwan, 14
Taylor Manifest Anxiety Scale, 46, 50, 51,
    206
Tell-Tale Heart, 38
Temporomandibular joint syndrome, 264,
    297
Tennessee Self-Concept Scale, 60, 61
Termination of AMT, 255–258, 259
Test anxiety, 39, 54, 64, 86, 139
    case illustrations of, 144–147, 220
    compared to performance anxiety, 307–
        308
    desensitization for, 40, 42, 44, 45
    SIT for, 130, 131
    SRR for, 135
Texas Social Behavior Inventory, 88
Theater performance enhancement, 308–
    310
Therapeutic rationale, 117–118, 136
Thought-listing method, 209
Thyroid-stimulating growth hormone, 25
Time monitoring, 116, 251, 259, 308
Topic incident cycle method, 181–182
Trait anger, 99, 205
Trait anxiety, 50, 54, 57, 63, 65, 135, 205,
    206
    anger and, 108
    cognitive performance and, 101
    depression and, 93
    desensitization for, 43, 44
    implosion and flooding for, 128
    in Type A personality, 85, 107
Trait Anxiety Inventory, 50, 52
Tranquilizers, 5, 62